DESIGNED TO
THRIVE

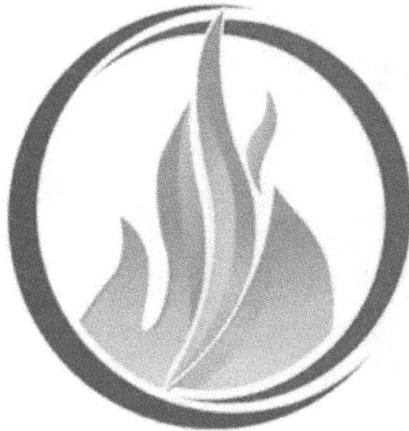

DESIGNED TO
THRIVE

LEARN THE UNTOLD TRUTHS ABOUT HEALTH AND HOW TO MASTER THE KEYS TO LIVING A HEALTHY LIFESTYLE

JASON BERGERHOUSE, D.C.

ISBN (Paperback): 978-1-7347021-0-1
ISBN (Hardcover): 978-1-7347021-2-5
ISBN (eBook): 978-1-7347021-1-8

Library of Congress Control Number: 2020905983

Portions of this book are works of nonfiction.

Printed in the United States of America.

Thrive Spine Center
187 Blue Ravine Rd. Ste. 140
Folsom, CA 95630

https://www.thrivespinecenter.com

Dedication

First and foremost, I dedicate this book to God, for He gave me the inspiration to write it after my beautiful daughter was born. I also want to express my deep sense of gratitude to my parents who raised me to be the man I am today. They instilled in me a strong sense of right vs. wrong. They guided and supported me while I worked on becoming a better version of myself. Thank you, Mom and Dad, I love you very much.

I also want to thank my wife who gave me the space and time every morning that I needed to write this monster. Thank you, Babe, for supporting me and loving me through this painful process of unpacking my thoughts and passions. Thank you for always giving me an encouraging uplift whenever I was down.

A special thanks to Dr. Ken Moger, my mentor. I had the privilege of working with Ken for over three years. During that time, not only did I learn many valuable lessons, but I became a better chiropractor. Thank you, Ken, for giving me the chance to learn from a master!

A special thanks to my Pastor, Francis Anfuso, for showing me a perfect example of what a Christian's heart should look like.

A special thanks to all my "WOKE" friends throughout the world. You continue to inspire me with your bravery and courage

But most importantly, I dedicate this book to you, Rylee, my dear sweet, beautiful daughter. I love you with all my heart. May you become a warrior for truth!

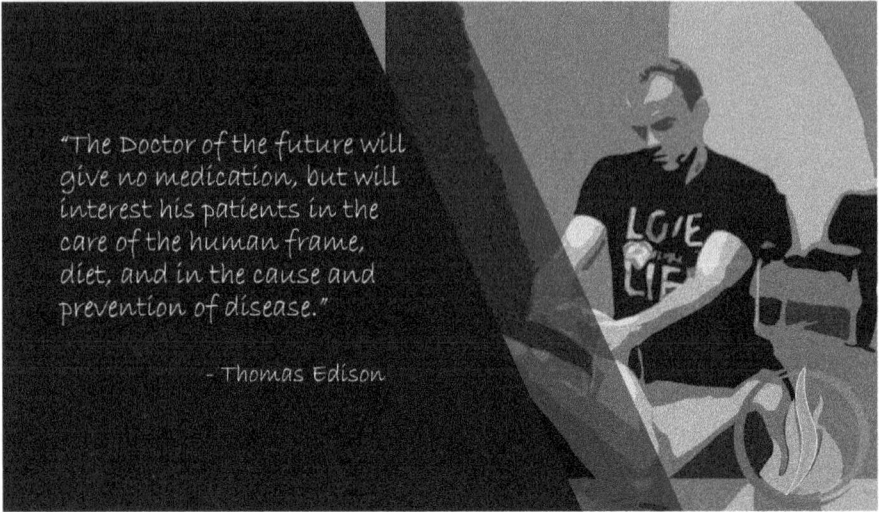

"The Doctor of the future will give no medication, but will interest his patients in the care of the human frame, diet, and in the cause and prevention of disease."

- Thomas Edison

Disclaimer

Designed to Thrive is an immensely powerful book, in that it covers many health-related topics and "alternative," or better yet "holistic" ways of dealing with your mind-body-spirit. In keeping with that, Dr. Jay covers health, fitness, nutritional information, and his opinions, backed up with scientific evidence, regarding medical care. Dr. Jay also covers conspiratorial issues with the hope that the reader will do their OWN due diligence to explore the vast array of topics mentioned. This book is for educational purposes only and is not intended to replace the council of a primary treating physician.

This book details the author's personal experiences and opinions about health. The author is not a medical doctor but has a Doctorate in Chiropractic and has years of experience helping people in this field.

The author and publisher are providing this book and its contents on an "as is" basis and make no representations or warranties of any kind with respect to this book or its contents. The author and publisher disclaim all such representations and warranties, including for example warranties of affiliate products and healthcare for a particular purpose. In addition, the author and publisher do not represent or warrant that the information accessible via this book is accurate, complete, or current. The author has some affiliate links listed throughout the book and when products are purchased using those affiliate links, he will receive compensation.

The statements made about products and services have not been evaluated by the U.S. Food and Drug Administration, the CDC, or any governmental regulating agency. They are not intended to diagnose, treat, cure, or prevent any condition or disease. Please consult your own physician or healthcare specialist regarding the suggestions and recommendations made in this book.

Except as specifically stated in this book, neither the author or publisher, nor any authors, contributors, or other representatives will be liable for damages arising out of or in connection with the use of this book. This is a comprehensive limitation of liability that applies to all damages of any kind, including *(without limitation)* compensatory, direct, indirect, or consequential damages; loss of data, income or profit, loss of or damage to property and claims of third parties.

You understand that this book is not intended as a substitute for consultation with a licensed healthcare practitioner, such as your physician. Before you begin any healthcare program or change your lifestyle in any way, consult your physician or a licensed healthcare practitioner to ensure that you are in good health and that the examples contained in this book will not harm you.

This book provides content related to physical and/or mental health issues. As such, use of this book implies your acceptance of this disclaimer.

Table of Contents

Foreword

I was honored when Dr. Jason Bergerhouse asked me to write a foreword for this book. Countless have been the hours we have waxed philosophical about the health crisis of modern America. Having known him while he attended Life Chiropractic College West, worked side by side with him for a few years after he was licensed, and finally witnessing his focus for making a deeper impact on humanity after getting married and the birth of his first child. I was astounded that he compiled many of our conversations into a book. When it comes to the science of health and the study of the lack there of, I find myself hearing Bilbo Baggins from *The Lord of the Rings* say:

"I don't know half of you half as well as I should like, and I like less than half of you half as well as you deserve."

The complexities and variables in living systems are both beautiful and fascinating while also contradictory and frustrating.

With ever increasing reliance on 'outside in' measures to control the soil, weeds, and pest management of our food supply, it is further complicated by the desire to have infinite shelf life with a perception of freshness.

What past generations once had to "learn to live with," modern technologies promise almost magical solutions. Modern chemistry and genetic manipulations have almost supernaturally provided solutions to food shortages, aches and pains, diseases of all sorts, and even emotional insecurities.

But has the "cure" become the source of the disease?

Donald J. Rumsfeld once said: "Reports that say that something hasn't happened are always interesting to me, because as we know, there are known knowns; there are things we know we know. We also know there are known unknowns; we know there are some things we do not know. But there are also unknown unknowns—the ones we don't know we don't know. And if one looks throughout the history of our country and other free countries, it is the latter categories that tend to be the difficult ones."

While this statement was surrounding military weapons of mass destruction, rising disabilities, and death tolls from medications and treatments originally sold as the "new miracle cure" it also fit the idiom, "unknown unknowns" (unexpected or unforeseeable conditions), which pose a potentially greater risk simply because they cannot be anticipated based on past experience or investigation.

"Known unknowns result from recognized but poorly understood phenomena"- like the potential of a canceled flight. "On the other hand, unknown unknowns are phenomena which cannot be expected, because there has been no prior experience or theoretical basis for expecting the phenomena" – readily fits new and novel treatments later found to be useless, or worse, more dangerous than what they were prescribed for. (Paraphrased from Wikipedia, "Known Unknowns.")

Further muddying the waters is the time factor. The longer a behavior pattern or belief has been held as "safe and effective," the more difficult it is to abandon as new observations are made.

It is quite easy to offhandedly discount things that go against our currently held beliefs. This is especially true if those beliefs are supported by carnal desires such as the love for hollow carbs or comfort foods (my personal nemesis!). Most of us will excuse our choices with the minimizing of bad habits.

Statements such as "all things in moderation" or "you're going to die of something" fill the comment lines on most health-related social media threads.

It is also becoming more prevalent to react to new information that on the surface appears in direct contradiction of truths we accepted in the past as "conspiracy theory non-sense."

On the other hand, as more headlines of corporate fraud and scientific bias that border on corruption appear, doubts begin to arise regarding other commonly held beliefs. What is presented as new information is discovered to actually be old information that was suppressed. We hear about it as gag rules from past settlements expire and the unsealing of former "top secret" government papers occurs.

Ever increasing access to such revelations that point to the old sins of greed and pride can create an attitude for some people to jump on the conspiracy train.

Dr. Jason does a great job of pointing out many of these "half-truths" and "whole-lies" in the chapters that follow. It becomes clear within moments that Dr. Jay sees these revelations from both ends; simple corporate greed and marketing hyperbole, but also something far more nefarious.

His tone is one of passion. Passion for God with a clear awe of that created universe and a deep sense of stewardship of that infinite beauty. Passion for humanity, as one who has dedicated himself to the service of others. Passion for his family, and a deep sense of wanting to protect them from the influences of a chaotic world filled with effects and side-effects of lives lived unnaturally.

As one reads through this book, I suggest one should neither "swallow it whole" nor discount the entirety if one single topic is difficult to accept. Books like this tend to find themselves in the hands of those "believers" (as if preaching to the choir has ever amounted to anything worthwhile), on the shelves, or on the filing cabinet, partially read by those who can't get past a writer's tone or style.

I encourage the reader to be neither. Simply take in the information. Test it against your own beliefs regarding nature/creation. Do you believe that there is in fact a universal intelligence behind the grand orchestration of life and the balance of nature? Do you believe all that exists is only a manifestation of random chemical reactions and material and mechanics flawed by the chaos that is?

Ultimately the discovery about the self is the point, and Dr. Jay is a worthy guide for this part of the journey, and the life hacks within could literally transform your future!

Dr. Kenneth Moger, D.C

Be Inspired Resources

There are resources in the appendix to help inspire you along your journey. They are designed to help you make little changes each day so you can make massive changes later. I once heard Tony Robbins say, "... you should never leave the site of a goal-setting-session without taking some sort of immediate action." These resources are tools to help you do just that. I have included: resources for you to explore, a niacin protocol, my green drink recipe, a glycemic index chart, questions to ask your doctor, and a whole lot more!

References

I also have included a reference section so you can look up the sources referenced in this book. You will also find links to websites, Facebook groups, and books that you can utilize to help guide you further along your path.

Introduction

"You never know how far reaching something you think, say or do today, will affect the lives of millions tomorrow."

B.J. Palmer

I decided to write *Designed to Thrive* because as I looked around at the world we live in, I saw too many people who were sick, tired, and suffering needlessly. Suffice to say, too many people are living well below their full potential. I look at life itself as the greatest gift we could ever be given, and yet so many people squander it because of their ill-health. I see the greatest tragedy in life not as death but dying with your music never expressed. Les Brown said it well:

"The graveyard is the richest place on earth, because it is here that you will find all the hopes and dreams that were never fulfilled, the books that were never written, the songs that were never sung, the inventions that were never shared, the cures that were never discovered, all because someone was too [sick] to take the first step...[1]"

The original quote had the word "afraid" in place of the word sick. In my opinion, I feel too many people in the U.S. aren't living up to their full potential because they aren't in alignment: mentally, physically, and spiritually. Each one of these areas in your life is intimately connected with the other. Therefore, you cannot separate one from the other. In 1st Corinthians, Chapter 6, verses 19-20, it states that our bodies are temples of the Holy Spirit which were a gift from God, thus we must honor God by not defiling our temples. Even if you're not a Christian, I'm sure you

1

could agree on the fact that a healthy body equates to a better version of yourself. I have seen sick people and healthy people in my twelve years as a Chiropractor and I can tell you that there is a very distinct and clear difference between the two. The sick person appears to be in survival mode all the time, as if they are lost at sea and their true sense of self is nowhere to be seen. The healthy person on the other hand, seems to always be striving to be better and do better with a strong sense of who they are. Healthy people rarely ever get sick, rarely ever go to the doctor, and rarely ever take medications, if at all. They are their own health advocates and therefore control their own destinies.

As a Chiropractor I learned three solid principals which govern my decisions regarding my and my family's health care.

1. **The Major Premise:** A universal intelligence is in all matter and continually gives to it all its properties and actions, thus maintaining it in existence.

2. **The Chiropractic Meaning of Life:** The expression of this intelligence through matter is the chiropractic meaning of life.

3. **The Union of Intelligence and Matter:** Life is necessarily the union of intelligence and matter.

Stephenson, R.W. *Chiropractic Textbook*
1927, The Palmer School of Chiropractic

Are you THRIVING or just surviving?

I want you to review your own life and ask yourself this question. Are you lost like so many in a sea of survival, or are you THRIVING? This book is my greatest attempt at inspiring you to connect and realign yourself with your true potential. I believe you were designed *on* purpose *for* an incredible purpose. We are all here for a reason; nothing happens by chance and life is a blessing. We must work to truly THRIVE in life vs. just survive.

"Focus on your *Health* and all else will follow."

Dr. Jay

In hopes of making it easier to read and in making the information more easily understood, I have written this book in three parts. Below you will find a synopsis of each part and what to expect in that part, as well as which chapters are encompassed in the section.

Segment One: Shifting the Paradigm

Chapters I – 3

The first three chapters in this book involve shifting your paradigm about health and why your mindset is so important for you to live your best life ever. In Chapter 1: The Perils of Modern Medicine, I discuss the history of modern medicine and why it is a failing paradigm. In Chapter 2: Remove the Interference, I talk about how the most important thing you need to do in your life is to remove the interference so you can live life without fear! In Chapter 3: The Power of the Mind, I discuss the power of your mindset when it comes to your overall health and well-being. I share some of the phenomenal work done by Dr. Joe Dispenza and Dr. Bruce Lipton on epigenetics and the placebo effect.

Segment Two: Removing the Interference

Chapters 4 - 11

These eight chapters are about removing the interference and allowing your body to naturally heal itself. Within each chapter I discuss getting rid of things that cause interference and adding in things that promote optimal health and function. I speak on a wide range of topics, such as: The Nerve System and chiropractic care, proper diet and nutrition, toxicity and how to cleanse the body, water, reducing your exposure to electromagnetic radiation, healthy sleep, exercise and oxygen, and supplements. There is even an entire chapter on the power of wheatgrass!

Segment Three: Your Divine Sense of Self

Chapters 13 - 14

In the last two chapters I discuss the spiritual dimensions involved in health. These final chapters will explore the concept that we were designed on purpose and therefore MUST have a purpose. This is ultimately the spiritual component that encapsulates who we are as individuals and *why* we are here. I also make the argument that one's health is fundamental to living a life on purpose. Here I discuss action steps, such as the power of meditation, prayer, affirmations, and visualization which can help you create a better life for yourself and your family.

You were designed to THRIVE in life! Don't you think it's time to stop living in the matrix of the system that has caused you to be sick, and to put yourself back in the driver's seat of life? This book is all about gaining your power back and becoming the absolute best version of yourself! It's time to live your best life ever, instead of a somewhat dumbed down version of yourself. Don't you think your family deserves better? What about the world at large? Don't you think you could give more of yourself by expressing the great symphony that sits within you? Why not?! The best time to start is NOW! You are about to embark on a journey that will inspire you to new heights and a much better, more refined version of yourself. My hope is that you will read this book from cover to cover, highlight, take notes, and apply the principles with great fervor and speed! The faster you implement – the better off you're going to be. Remember, *procrastination is the thief of health and the thief of your dreams!*

So, what are you waiting for, dive in, take the journey of all journeys and become renewed! You were indeed,

DESIGNED TO THRIVE!

SHIFTING THE PARADIGM
CHAPTERS 1-3

"Change your paradigm and you change your life."

- Dr. Jay

CHAPTER 1

THE PERILS OF MODERN MEDICINE

Modern medicine is not scientific, it is full of prejudice, illogic, and susceptible to advertising. Doctors are not taught to reason. They are programmed to believe in whatever their medical schools teach them and the leading doctors tell them. Over the past 20 years the drug companies, with their enormous wealth, have taken medicine over and now control its research, what is taught and the information released to the public.

- Abram Hoffer

The United States is one of the "sickest" industrialized countries on the face of the planet. In fact, the U.S. makes up approximately 5% of the ENTIRE world's population, yet, Americans take, on average, 70% of the world's PRESCRIPTION drugs. I put emphasis on those two words because despite the fact that the U.S. makes up a very small percentage of the entire world's population, we take the majority of the world's pharmaceutical drug supply. Yet, when it comes to American overall health and well-being, we are one of the sickest countries! In fact, according to a recent Bloomberg study, the U.S. ranks 35th in the world in overall health. The US ranks 35th, which is five below one of the lowest ranking countries in the world! [2] Americans are diagnosed with more heart disease, cancer, diabetes, and other debilitating diseases than most other countries. This begs the obvious question: If prescription drugs equated to the population being healthier, why are we so sick?!

PILLS WILL MAKE YOU ILL AND SMOKE ALARMS

In 2014, 1.3 million Americans went to the emergency room due to adverse drug reactions (ADR). Out of those 1.3 million Americans, 124,000 of them died according to the CDC and FDA. However, it is thought that this number is grossly underreported, in that it only represents a small percentage of the cases that occur each year. This is in large part due to doctors or pharmacists being fearful of a lawsuit, guilt over responsibility, and a

70% of the entire world's prescription drugs.

lack of interest, or time, or other excuses related to delaying the documentation of ADRs. Despite the under reporting, ADRs are still the 4th leading cause of death in the U.S according to the CDC. This means that the number of deaths caused by ADRs are ahead of pulmonary disease, diabetes, AIDS, pneumonia, accidents, and automobile deaths! [3,5,6,7]

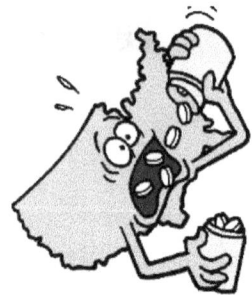

We put more faith in a bottle of pills than in our own body's incredible ability to heal itself, and because of this we have become a nation of "pill-poppers." Half the populous takes two or more pills and this is considered normal! [4] We have become so sick that people think it's weird or abnormal if you don't get sick! Personally, I haven't taken any prescription or over-the-counter medication in over a decade! How is it that being healthy and not taking medication is looked at as the abnormality?!

I'll never forget a patient of mine with a laundry list of medications she was taking. After I quickly counted the number of prescriptions, I realized she was taking a whopping thirty-six medications per day! Rightfully, I thought to myself, "Where is the science to justify this?" In fact, there is no science to show the safety, not to mention the possible adverse events that can occur when taking two or more random medications. It's called polypharmacy. The lady who came into my office was a perfect example of polypharmacy, as well as a walking "science experiment." So, rather than seeking the **CAUSE**, her doctors treated the **EFFECTS** (the symptoms) by merely masking them with medications.

"You cannot poison the body back to health."

Dr. Jay

The main problem with the medical establishment is that their primary goal is to mask symptoms. Symptoms are the red flags - the warning signals your body gives to let you know there is a problem. All medications are designed to mask the symptoms. I can't emphasize this truth enough. I relate masking symptoms to the equivalent of pulling the batteries out of the smoke alarm - so you can go back to bed comfortably - while your house burns down with you in it. I call this the smoke alarm analogy.

On one hand, I get the concept behind mitigating symptoms. If somebody has extremely high blood pressure it is in their best interest to lower it, whether that's with a blood pressure medication, diet, exercise, or other lifestyle change. But, do they need to take the medication for the rest of their life?

Herein lies the problem of masking symptoms with drugs! It never addresses the cause, and all drugs come with side-effects, especially with long-term use.

POTENTIAL LIFE LOST, HUNZA'S, AND MYTHS

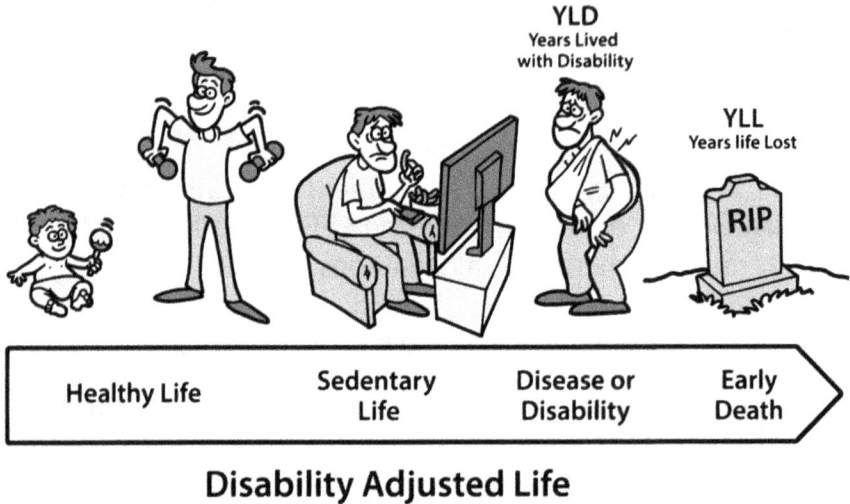

Disability Adjusted Life

But it goes beyond just ADRs! One doesn't have to look very far to see that America has a health crisis. In fact, the U.S. ranks almost dead last when it comes to years of potential life lost *(PLL)*, and that's compared to twenty-nine other industrialized countries! The PLL is a measurement of the average years a person would have lived if they had not died prematurely. [8] This number is calculated by using seventy-five as the reference age. Biblically, we are supposed to live 120 years in good, quality health. And if you think that's shocking, Jeanne Calment of France was born in 1875 and lived until 1997! She lived for 122 years and 164 days on this planet! [9]

The Hunza tribe in northern Pakistan, Jammu, and Kashmir have been extensively studied because they typically live to be over one hundred years old. [9] These centurions survive *and* thrive in their environment. Their main secret seems to be complete isolation from western modern-day-living. They aren't sitting around eating Captain Crunch for breakfast and driving to a nearby Starbucks to get their caffeine hit for the day. They also aren't staring at their cell phones for hours on end, scrolling through Facebook, and getting zapped by all the electromagnetic radiation! Everything they eat is organic and natural; the way God intended things to be. They also move a lot throughout their day, breathing in clean air! And, guess what? They don't suffer from the top disease killers in the U.S., like heart disease, cancer, and diabetes.

THE MYTH THAT KEEPS US SICK

Western medicine's primary goal has always been to treat the sick by chasing the symptoms. In keeping with that, they have always looked at the body from a very mechanistic and linear standpoint. Meaning if someone is having an acute gallbladder attack, they see the problem as the gallbladder, rather than trying to figure out the cause of the inflammation. Doctors are trained to diagnose diseases and conditions and make pharmaceutical recommendations based on the symptomatology. In other words, doctors are trained diagnosticians that hyper-focus on the symptoms, but not the solution. A perfect example of this is cancer. What doctors fail to realize is that cancer is merely a symptom of a greater cause. Cancer isn't the cause; cancer doesn't fall from the sky and it isn't about having bad luck. Inevitably this line of thinking leads to chemotherapy and radiation, two of the most common forms of treatment for cancer. Ironically, both forms of treatment have been proven to cause cancer.

The myth propagated to the American public is that all diseases are due to bad genes and you can't do anything about it, other than mask your symptoms and hope for the best. This level of thinking works great to increase the profits of the pharmaceutical companies. Creating drugs to mask and/ or treat every symptom known to man is what they do best. This mechanistic philosophy is at the core of why Americans are so sick. "The pharmaceutical companies do not create cures; they create customers for life (author unknown)." They aren't interested in teaching mankind what it takes to be healthy. In Chapter III I discuss the "Placebo Effect" and how your environment, both internally and externally, determines what your genes do. In other words, your lifestyle has a more profound effect on your health than your genes do.

Unlike the mechanistic philosophy of healthcare which looks at each part of the body as separate from the whole and takes an outside in approach to health – vitalism sees that everything in the human body is connected. You cannot separate the parts from the whole because everything is interconnected and essential. Every single organ, cell, and tissue is intimately connected. Vitalism sees that true health comes from within the body and not outside the body. Having this philosophy means a person takes a more proactive approach to living their life, rather than a reactive approach. As the saying goes, "An ounce of prevention is greater than a pound of cure." Rather than waiting until you get sick or have a symptom to start taking care of yourself, it would be better to start doing it now.

HOW DID WE GET HERE? BIG PHARMA AND THE ROCKEFELLERS

It might surprise you to find out that you have been indoctrinated to believe what you believe, especially when it comes to health care. As a kid, especially if you are a female, you probably had a "sick baby doll," complete with a fake syringe and "spoonful of medicine" to give as treatment. This is not much different than the fake bubblegum cigarettes created by the tobacco and candy companies used to entice kids into smoking. Also, your parents, like mine, probably gave you Robitussin every time you had a cold or Tylenol for every fever; for pain and inflammation they probably gave you ibuprofen. If these interventions didn't help within a short amount of time, you were probably taken to the doctor for a prescription.

In elementary school we were taught to think that medical advancements, pharmaceutical drugs, and vaccinations are the savior of mankind. Throughout high school and even in college, this indoctrination continued in health-ed classes. On TV, doctors are held up as modern-day heroes, while naturopaths, chiropractors, and other holistic doctors are made to look less-than or unknowledgeable when it comes to health care. It was the American Medical Association that coined the term "quack" for any practitioner who thought outside the box of pharmacopeia and standard medical practice.

Only in America do we get bombarded by direct-to-consumer advertising by Big Pharma. The Pharmaceutical companies OWN the air waves. In fact, they spent over **3.54 BILLION dollars** on drug commercials last year alone. They are one of the largest industries in the TV ad spending category. Because they spend this much money and more every year, one must conclude that they have a strong level of influence and control on the information that people receive about health care. And, if you can control information, especially when it comes to the media, you can control the hearts, minds, and decision making of a populace.

Modern medicine as we know it today began at the turn of the 20th century with John D. Rockefeller. Rockefeller was a monopolist and shrewd venture capitalist. At the time, his oil company, Standard Oil, controlled 90% of all oil refineries in the U.S. At the same time scientists were making new discoveries about how oil could be used to make vitamins, pharmaceutical drugs, and all kinds of petrochemicals. Rockefeller saw this as an opportunity to take hold of not only the oil but the chemical and medical industries at the same time. This meant huge profits for Rockefeller because patents could only be granted for drugs and synthetic vitamins and not for natural/holistic medicines and cures.

The problem that Rockefeller faced was that at least 50% of American doctors and medical schools were practicing holistic medicine! So, with his friend, Andrew Carnegie, he concocted a plan to infiltrate and take over the medical industry. Carnegie had made a fortune on his monopolization of the steel industry. Together they came up with a scheme to send an American educator by the name of Abraham Flexner around the country to report on the status of medical colleges and hospitals. This led to the fancy sounding "Flexner Report." This report was responsible for changing and centralizing medical institutions, which sadly led to more than half of them closing. All holistic medical practices were demonized and severely mocked; doctors were even thrown in jail.

Rockefeller then devised a front group called The General Education Board. The doctors involved were paid to oversee medical institutions to make sure they stayed in line. This gave rise to the current medical system we see today, which resulted in all medical students being taught the same thing – to use petrochemicals in the form of drugs to mask symptoms. What could possibly go wrong?

This is not what healthcare is supposed to be. This should be called "sickcare." Unfortunately, doctors today learn little to nothing about nutrition, holistic practices, and natural medicine. This is one of the main reasons why our nation's health is in crisis. Not only is the healthcare system broken, but the system was poor in the first place because it's all about disease management. Doctors have become the glorified drug dealers for the pharmaceutical companies. [10]

BROKEN SYSTEMS, SCANDELS, AND DOCTOR INCENTIVES

According to a report written by Gary Null, PhD; Dr. Carolyn Dean, MD; Debora Rasio, MD; and Dorothy Smith, PhD; entitled: "Death by Medicine," the number of deaths attributed to medical care is between 783,936 and 999,936, making it the number one killer in the United States, above heart disease and cancer! These numbers are taken from the "total deaths directly attributed to ADRs, medical error, bedsores, infections, malnutrition in hospitals, unnecessary procedures, and those related to surgery."

"The fully referenced report shows the number of people having in-hospital, adverse reactions to prescribed drugs to be 2.2 million per year. The number of unnecessary antibiotics prescribed annually for viral infections is 20 million per year. The number of unnecessary

medical and surgical procedures performed annually is 7.5 million per year. The number of people exposed to unnecessary hospitalization annually is 8.9 million per year." [11]

It seems to me that making your and your family's health a priority and avoiding the "system" would be your best bet!

It is estimated that between 88,000 and 139,000 people in the U.S. had suffered a heart attack and stroke as a result of vioxx.

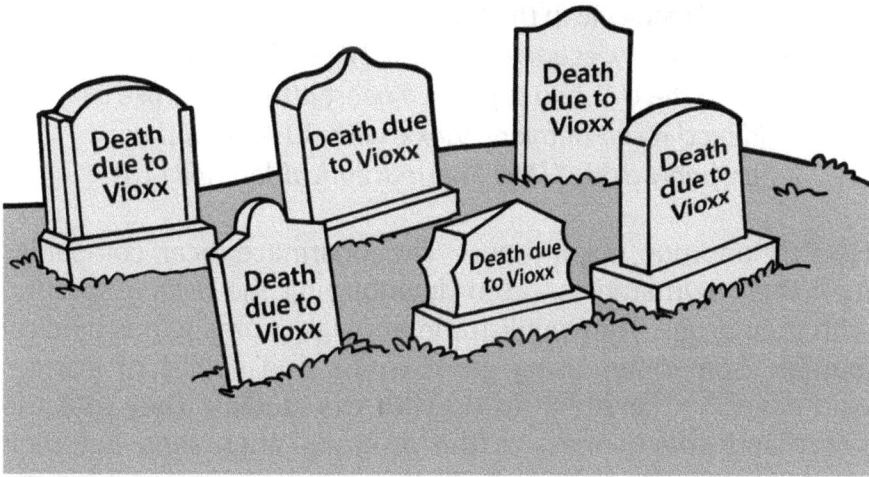

The Vioxx scandal is a perfect example of how broken the medical system is. Vioxx was a painkiller created by the pharmaceutical giant Merck at a time when the drug company really needed a new whiz-bang drug. The patents on several popular Merck drugs were expiring in 2000 and 2001, so Merck was banking on Vioxx to replace the lost revenue. The problem was that Vioxx had been proven to increase cardiovascular problems. A study done in 2000 to compare Vioxx to naproxen in 8,100 Rheumatoid Arthritis patients showed that five times as many patients taking Vioxx had heart attacks compared to those taking naproxen. At the same time, a multitude of doctors and cardiologists came forward to say the drug posed cardiovascular risks. And yet, Merck denied that the increase in heart attacks had anything to do with Vioxx. In 2001, Dr. Eric J. Topol and other cardiologists with the Cleveland Clinic published a study in the Journal of the American Medical Association that concluded both Vioxx and Celebrex (another pain killer) appeared to increase the risk of heart attacks and strokes, but the risk from taking Vioxx appeared to be even greater [12].

Despite all the warnings, the drug remained on the market for four years before finally being taken off in 2004 after wreaking major havoc on U.S. citizens.

> "In a testimony to the US senate committee shortly after Vioxx was withdrawn, David Graham, then associate director for science and medicine in the U.S. Food and Drug Administration's office of drug safety, estimated that between 88,000 and 139,000 people in the U.S. had suffered a heart attack or stroke as a [direct] result of taking Vioxx, with 30-40% of these probably dying." (The Pharmaceutical Journal) [13]

Here is another major issue: The pharmaceutical companies fund their own studies, often downplaying the risks associated with their drugs. They publish the findings in prestigious medical journals, sometimes using ghostwriters and names of doctors who never had anything to do with the studies. They tout the safety and effectiveness of the drug and then send out their good-looking drug reps to "sell" the doctors on prescribing the drug. They offer incentives to the doctors in the form of gifts and "educational" dinners to persuade them into prescribing their premium drugs. In 2012 alone, twenty-four BILLION dollars was spent on marketing drugs to healthcare professionals [14]. So, can we really trust that doctors have our best interest at heart when they have been incentivized to prescribe us certain drugs?

The simple truth is this: the farther we move away from God and nature, the sicker we seem to get. Health is an "inside job" and not an "outside in" job. We seem to forget that God designed our bodies intelligently and we were given all the tools necessary for health and healing. I would argue we should rarely ever try to manage our conditions, symptoms, and ill-health with chemicals. The goal then becomes removing all the things that interfere with our body's natural healing process. Ill health isn't about bad luck or bad genes, it isn't about invisible bugs, parasites, and viruses that you can't see – it's about so much more than that. Shifting your paradigm regarding this is the most important decision you can make in your life.

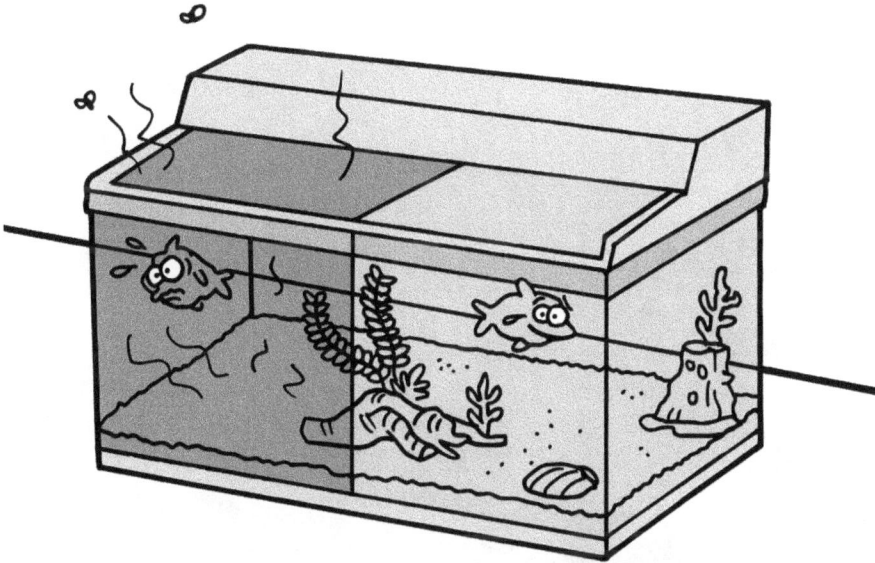

Should you medicate the fish or clean the tank?
Health is an INSIDE job not an outside-in job!

"Much of the scientific literature, perhaps half, may simply be untrue. Afflicted by studies with small sample sizes, tiny effects, invalid exploratory analyses, and flagrant conflicts of interest, together with an obsession for pursuing fashionable trends of dubious importance, science has taken a turn towards darkness."
[15]

Dr. Richard Horton, Editor-in-Chief, The Lancet
(world's most respected medical journal)

"How do you make a dimmed light bright again? Remove the interference. How do you increase health in a diseased person? The same way!"

B.J. Palmer

CHAPTER 2

REMOVE THE INTERFERENCE

*The greatest threat to your health is not disease,
it's interference.*

Dr. Jay

Many people struggle to understand that the body has an incredible ability to heal itself. In fact, your body is a self-healing, self-regulating organism! You were born with all the tools necessary to heal. There is an incredible power within you that has been there since the day you were born. This same power took you from two cells in your mother's womb to 75 trillion cells by the time you were born. This power didn't get up and leave you; it has always been there! If you cut your leg or arm, do you have to look down at the cut and tell it to heal? No, your body automatically heals the wound.

Your blood starts to clot within minutes of a laceration; the blood clots, dries and forms a scab. Amazingly, blood vessels dilate and bring blood, oxygen, and nutrients to the wound for healing. White blood cells are called to the area to help fight infection and repair the wound. All of this happens within two to five days! Over the ensuing weeks, the body repairs broken blood vessels and new tissue grows. Your red blood cells work to create collagen, tough white fibers, and new granulation tissue is formed. The edges of the wound pull together and a scar is eventually formed. [16]

This all happened because of the bodies inborn intelligence called innate intelligence. It is what works to heal the body from the inside-out. If you're healthy, your body will heal itself! The body can heal itself without the use of drugs, lotions, potions, or elixirs. Consider this: people have healed from stage four cancer without chemotherapy or radiation. Even those with diabetes and heart disease have been able to heal through simple lifestyle changes. People all over the world have been able to reverse diseases and ill health without modern medicine. What is the difference that makes the difference?

THE BODY NEEDS NO HELP TO HEAL YOU

How is it possible to have two siblings and one is healthy and the other has cancer, or some other serious condition? If the genes are the same, why does one end up with a debilitating disease and the other one doesn't? What is the overriding difference between the two? There is a fundamental principal you need to understand and learn:

Your body doesn't need any help to heal you, just no interference!

In other words, you don't need to add things to your body to be healthier. For example, if you have a 102° F fever, would it be in your best interest to forcibly lower the fever via Tylenol? Taking drugs to artificially lower your fever could potentially prolong your body's recovery time. Our bodies burn fevers for a reason. A fever supports our immune system's ability to fight off infectious agents like bacteria and viruses. As body temperature increases the white blood cells do their job faster and destroy the invading pathogens.

I'm not saying there isn't a time and place for medical intervention and lifesaving medications. In fact, if a person's fever is extremely high it would be best to err on the side of caution and go to the hospital. We have great lifesaving emergency facilities built to handle people in crisis. However, this notion that we need a "pill for every ill" or that we need a drug for every unpleasant symptom does not work to promote true health and healing within the body, especially in the long run – because again, we are just treating the effects and not the cause.

A wise medical doctor once said, "The person who takes medicine must recover twice. Once from the disease and once from the medicine."

DIS-EASE AND ALIGN 2 THRIVE

All "dis-ease" is created by thoughts, traumas, and toxins that interfere with the body's ability to function normally. First, dis-ease is referring to the lack of ease in the body when a person is unhealthy. In other words, an unhealthy person has a body that is not in harmonious balance with itself. When your body is not in balance and it's not functioning at 100% of its full potential, you will have a harder time adapting to internal and external stressors. This makes you more prone to getting sick, getting an infection, suffering injury, or not performing as well as you could.

Consider diabetes for example. A diabetic is more prone to kidney failure, heart problems, visual loss, and a gangrenous infection than someone who is not diabetic. This is due to diminished blood supply to their extremities. But this doesn't happen overnight. Over months and possibly even years, long before they received the devastating diagnose of Type II Diabetes, their body was already out of balance; they already had blood sugar problems. Referred to as pre-diabetes, this is when the patient's blood sugar levels are only slightly elevated. Despite having felt well, the person was sick. Their body was battling the beginnings of a disease they did not even know they had.

The toxic burden of eating the standard American diet and living a sedentary lifestyle is most likely what led to their diabetes and the dis-ease within their body. If they had removed the interference – the toxic lifestyle behavior- it is likely they would have never been diagnosed with diabetes. And they could have avoided having to take medication or insulin injections for the rest of their "deathspan."

We must redefine our views about what health is; we must re-ground ourselves upon a completely different and opposite view of what it means to be healthy. After years of practicing as a chiropractor, I came up with the slogan, *Align to Thrive*, because I realized that you simply cannot thrive in life unless you're aligned mentally, physically, and spiritually. Think about it, all three of these areas of your life are intimately connected with one another. We know that mental health effects physical health and most definitely the divine sense of self (spiritual as well). We also know that physical health plays a huge role in your mental health. If a person has chronic pain for example, do they tend to be more irritable or less irritable; more stressed or less stressed; more depressed or less depressed? The answer is obvious.

A TRUE WELLNESS MODEL

When we look at a true wellness model of health it should be all encompassing. It should encompass all aspects of health: mental health, physical health, and spiritual health. This means that health is not just about looking good and feeling good. It isn't about being symptomless, in fact, it goes far beyond that. Health isn't about how well you feel, it's about how well your body is functioning. But if we keep waiting until we get sick to finally start taking care of ourselves, we are completely missing the boat on what "being" healthy truly means. In fact, the World Health Organization defines health as: "A state of complete physical, mental, and social well-being, and not merely the absence of disease or infirmity." [17]

Having a strong foundational philosophy of health is paramount to living a healthy life. We must be grounded in our belief and understanding that the body is always striving for our greater good and that the body does have the power to heal itself. We must strive to remove mental, physical, and emotional interference in our lives, making the removal of interference to our bodies our number one priority.

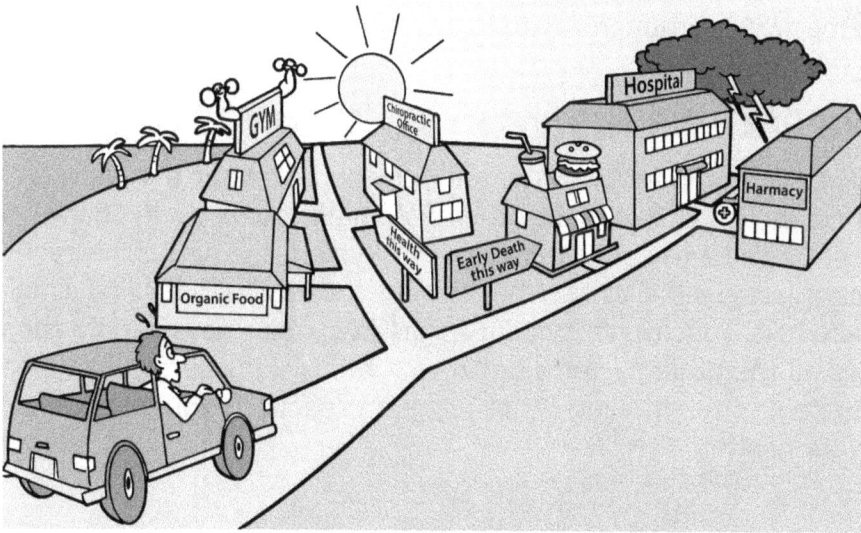

You must put yourself in the driver's seat and take charge of your health. It's about being proactive, not reactive. This means we must go against the grain of everything we once thought to be true about health. And we must understand that our bodies are built to THRIVE!

I see health split into several empowering fundamental tenants. I will now share those tenants with you and why I feel they are so important for a healthy and thriving lifestyle.

THE SIX TENANTS:

#1 *EMPOWERING MINDSET*

This is the most critical component to expressing abundant health and making the absolute best health care decisions for you and your family, but also for living your best life. In the next chapter I will thoroughly explore mindset and why it is crucial to shift your thinking about your health and what you believe is possible. The results you achieve in life have a lot to do with your mindset. The actions you take in life always begin with a thought. Therefore, empowering thoughts lead to an abundant life!

#2 PROPER NERVE SYSTEM FUNCTION

The most important system in your body is your nerve system because it controls all the other systems in your body. In Chapter 4 I will discuss the power of the nerve system and why chiropractic care is essential to stay healthy for the rest of your life. Think about it, your nerve system forms in sixteen days – only then do all the other systems begin to form. Making sure your nerve system is functioning at its highest capacity is foundational to your health!

#3 THRIVING NUTRITION

You cannot thrive in life if you have no energy! You can try and force yourself to push through life, but it's miserable and exhausting. This is why nutrition is SO important! A healthy diet means proper fuel for your body. Proper nutrition will make your body work, run, and function more efficiently – which means more energy! More energy leads to better moods, increased productivity, and ultimately a better quality of life. A healthy diet means you focus more on the nutritional aspects of the foods you are eating and not the calories. *Calories count, but nutrition matters more!* Most companies focused on weight loss, for example, discount this principal and use heavily processed food-like-products which ultimately sabotages health instead of helping it. The problem is most diets put the word "DIE" in diet.

There are a several chapters in the second part of this book that discuss nutrition, superfoods, and diet.

#4 MOTION IS LIFE

Exercise is another important tenant to living a healthy life. Exercise has the incredible ability to instantly change your state. It has the positive benefit of lowering blood pressure and blood sugar as well as decreasing stress and putting us into a state of calm. It also increases our bodies ability to take in and utilize oxygen. Oxygen is arguably the most important nutrient your body needs. Improving your VO2 max ensures that your body is taking in and utilizing more oxygen.

#5 AVOIDING TOXINS

Cleansing the body and avoiding toxins is more important now than ever before. We are exposed to a wide array of toxins on a regular basis that sabotage us. There are toxins in the air we breathe, the plastics in our car that off-gas, mercury fillings, and in our tap and bottled waters. Glyphosate (the active ingredient in Roundup) has been found in everything from vaccines to certain foods we eat. Animal products and meat that are heavily processed contain toxins; they have even found high concentrations of aluminum in random ground samples! The list of toxins is endless, which is why I have an entire chapter in the middle of this book dedicated to detoxing the body and avoiding toxins.

#6 HIGHER PURPOSE

In order to live a life of abundance we must have a purpose that is higher than ourselves. We must use our talents, treasures, and time to serve humanity in a big way. Tony Robbins calls this *growth and contribution*. As we become more and more healthy by living out the healthy tenants listed above, there begins to be a sort of unraveling and discovery of our true sense of self. I call this: discovering your divine sense of self. It is as though you see who you were truly designed to be and what your purpose is when all the interference is removed. You begin to think clearer! Your life becomes a mission; a life lived on purpose. Practically speaking, this could mean being a better parent or a better human being in general!

Living out these empowering tenants is not necessarily an easy road to walk. Often, removing interference causes unpleasant symptoms to manifest – withdrawals can occur, emotional pain can be conjured up, symptoms can become worse. Living a healthier life doesn't come without challenges, discipline, and some degree of suffering, but it's certainly the right way to live life. Principal number six in chiropractic states, *"All healing requires time."* [18] There is NO quick fix if you want to be truly healthy. You can take a pill to feel better, but it isn't going to make you healthier.

Remember, true health is not merely the absence of symptoms. A lifetime coffee drinker who quits drinking caffeine can experience some severe withdrawal affects, such as migraines, extreme exhaustion, irritability, etc. But does this mean that quitting coffee wasn't a good thing for them to do? Absolutely not! I tell all my patients there is a light at the end of the tunnel and that light is them functioning at a much higher level. As you turn up the dimmer switch on your life-light it tends to reveal how "bad" your bad habits are and as a result your body goes through a period of retracing.

I have seen retracing occur as a result of removing neurological interference with chiropractic adjustments. Sometimes patients will experience an increase in pain or have an emotional response to being adjusted. I have had patients laugh, cry, and even become upset because of clearing out neurological interference. This is all part of the retracing affect as "the body tissues themselves have a memory which records the traumas, accidents, and injuries it has experienced." [19] Removing neurological interference, changing one's lifestyle, dealing with negative emotions – these all carry with them the possibility and challenge of retracing. But nothing worth doing is void of a good challenge. Adversity makes it all worth it in the end and is how you grow.

LIVE YOUR LIFE WITHOUT FEAR

Ultimately, your life is better lived when you're grounded upon solid principals of health and healing. Too many Americans stand on a set of weak principals regarding their health. These principals revolve around symptom suppression and disease management. They stand on a faulty premise of health care and believe better living can happen by forcibly altering their biochemistry via drugs. Too many people live their life in fear and make decisions as such.

Having a strong sense of FAITH in your body's ability to heal itself and be healthy allows you to live a life without fear.

Dr. Fred Barge, *A Life Without Fear.*

It isn't about having blind faith either, because when you realize that removing interference in your life decreases your risk of developing any disease, you know that you have more control. Your main goal is to help your body function normally. Diseases are a matter of your body not functioning at 100%. Unlike the medical model, which is entirely based on fear. Because fear sells, this holistic model of health says, the greatest doctor is already within you. It acknowledges that the intelligence that animates the living world is also within us.

We chiropractors recognize there is a universal intelligence in all matter, whether it's living or non-living. Furthermore, this universal intelligence expresses itself within the human body as innate intelligence. Our quality of life has to do with how well this intelligence expresses itself within us. Hence, the reason we need to remove all forms of interference to function at our highest potential! Take some time to consider the principals laid out in this chapter. Begin to remove the interference in your own life so you can live a life of vitality!

"Medicine is the study of disease and what causes man to die. Chiropractic is the study of health and what causes man to live."

- B.J. Palmer

CHAPTER 3

THE POWER OF THE MIND

Your mindset matters. It affects everything - from the business and investment decisions you make, to the way you raise your children, to your stress levels and overall well-being.

- Peter Diamandis

"For as he thinks in His Heart, so is He."

- Proverbs 23:7

Your mind is the most powerful tool when it comes to your health and healing. So, it is essential to have the right beliefs and frame of mind when it comes to your health and the decisions you make regarding health care. As stated throughout the last two chapters, we need to unlearn everything we once thought to be true regarding our health, because, to be frank and in your face – **YOU HAVE BEEN LIED TO!**

We need a complete reformation of our thoughts and ideas surrounding health! And, if you, the reader, are super health savvy, use this information as ammo to go out and preach the "good word" to others. Maybe you're like me and have people you know that think everything the media tells them is the truth and written in stone. Maybe, like me, you have friends and relatives who "worship" at the altar of science. But it's not really science for that matter, is it? It's more of a dogmatic belief system; a religion of sorts that puts more faith in a bottle full of pills and syringes full of God knows what than in our own God given healing power. This form of dogmatic belief has become so common that it has even been given its own name: Scientism. All the more reason to know the TRUTH and spread it!

May THE TRUTH become the infectious agent that spreads throughout the masses!

True science is always evolving and always questioning. It is never settled; it never assumes. The matrix in which we live, the medical complex, has become so corrupted and so full of lies that it is ever more apparent among us who are "WOKE!" Woke is a term coined for those who stand firm in the truth – unwavering. Those who steadfastly speak the truth against any and all forms of opposition, just as the bible tells us to speak light into a world of darkness.

Ephesians (5:11-16) *Have nothing to do with the fruitless deeds of darkness, **but rather expose them**. It is shameful even to mention what the disobedient do in secret. But everything exposed by the light becomes visible and everything that is **illuminated becomes a light**. This is why it is said: "Wake up, sleeper, rise from the dead, and Christ will shine on you." Be incredibly careful, then, how you live – not as unwise but as wise, making the most of every opportunity, because the days are evil.* [20]

Throughout our lives we have been taught that getting sick has to do with bad luck and bad genes. We have been taught that there is no way to prevent disease unless it comes in a vaccine. We have been taught that our genes determine our destiny. We have been told we have faulty genetics and predispositions to certain diseases based on our family history. Even famous movie stars have been duped into this mode of thinking – going so far as to have mastectomies done as a means of preventing breast cancer. This information isn't entirely untrue – but there is way more to the story.

The full story, or what some may call the "real" story, began with DNA and genes. Let me explain. A new science surrounding genetics, called epigenetics, has emerged in the last few decades. This is different from the science we were taught in school. In school we learned that genes determined our health and the quality of life we were going to have (genetics). Any abnormalities, ranging from obesity to cancer and even depression, were thought to be a result of bad genes.

DNA was discovered in 1944. It was one of the biggest discoveries of the 20th century. But even more important was the 1953 discovery by James Watson and Francis Crick which revealed that each strand of DNA contained a gene sequence. Genes are code for something – usually a protein. The length and sequence of a gene determines how large a protein is and what its shape will be. This in turn affects how it will be used in the body. Different proteins combine within the body to make hormones, structural tissue, enzymes, etc. Essentially, "The genes are the blueprints for each of the over 100,000 different kinds of proteins that are the building blocks for making the human body." [21]

With the discovery of human DNA and genes, it was hypothesized that our lives were controlled by our DNA. Since genes code for proteins and protein represents our bodies, we must be controlled by our DNA, right?! Therein lies the problem. This mode of thinking led to the belief that our fates were entirely determined by the genes passed down from our parents; that we are victims with little to no control over our destinies. If you're a pharmaceutical company this mode of thinking is great because if all the genes in the human body were patented, they could be used to make drug products to alter a person's genetic code. Got fat genes, let's give you a skinny gene drug; makes sense, right?!

NEW THOUGHT MODE AND CELL TOWERS

Thanks to the work of Dr. Bruce Lipton, a cellular biologist and author of the book *Biology of Belief*, we now understand that it isn't DNA or our genetics that determines the fate of our cells, thus, the outcome of our lives. It is the environment that surrounds the cell that dictates what the DNA does. Let me explain this further: the nucleus of the cell houses the DNA and has always been considered the brain of the cell, but as it turns out it does not run the show. The controlling structure in cellular biology and gene expression is the cell membrane. This membrane responds and adapts to the chemical makeup that surrounds it (the environment). If the cell is surrounded by a sick environment it leads to dis-ease, interference, and decreased health. Here is the cool thing! If the cell is surrounded by a healthy environment it thrives!

> *The New biology revealed that the brain of the cell is its skin, the membrane, the interface of the interior of the cell and the ever-changing world we live in. It is the functional element that controls life. This is important because understanding its function reveals that we are not victims of our genes. Through the action of the cell membrane we can control our genes, our biology and our life and we have been doing it all along although we have been laboring under the belief that we are victims. I started to realize that the cell was a chip and that the nucleus was a hard disc with programs. The genes were programs. As I was typing this on my computer one day, I realized that my computer was like a cell. It had programs built into it but what was expressed by the computer was not determined by the programs. It was determined by the information that I, as the environment, was typing onto the keyboard. Suddenly all the pieces fell into place: the cell membrane is actually an information-processing computer chip.*
>
> Dr. Bruce Lipton [21]

Consider the fact that you are comprised of trillions of little "cell towers" always responding to the environmental signals surrounding them. According to Lipton each cell has antennae on the membranes that pick up outside signals in the surrounding environment. These signals determine how the cells will respond. However, if the antennae on the outside of the cells are constantly picking up on negative signals from unhealthy thoughts, traumas, and toxins the cells go into survival mode. This is powerful because if we can control the environment through our thoughts, habits, and lifestyle then we can get all the trillions of cells in our bodies to thrive and not just survive. In other words, we program our cells – we are the broadcast that controls our gene expression [21]. A cell that is thriving means that it signals the genes that support life, growth, and abundant health. During this process, your thoughts are most critical and will determine whether you do indeed program your cells.

Do you remember the verse in the Bible that says, "As a man thinketh, so is he?" [22] This statement is more real and truer than you have probably ever considered. Let me begin with a story...

A young man was enrolled in a study for depression. He qualified for the study since he had been experiencing depression and had been unable to find relief on his own. He was taking doctor prescribed pills as part of the study. He felt the anti-depressants were doing their job; his mood was improving, and he was getting better. However, the young man hit an exceptionally low spot after his girlfriend left him. Soon thereafter he decided to down the entire bottle of pills in an effort to kill himself. Realizing he made a mistake he ends up at the hospital. With his blood pressure dangerously low and his breathing severely limited he was on the verge of death. Oddly enough the blood tests found nothing to indicate that any anti-depressants had been taken! It turns out he hadn't been taking anti-depressants. He had been taking sugar pills, aka a placebo. The study he was enrolled in was a blind study meaning some of the participants received the drug and others received a placebo. He had no clue he was taking the placebo which was essentially a simple sugar pill. He thought he was taking the real deal! And don't forget, he got better while taking those sugar pills. When he took the whole bottle of pills, he thought he had overdosed on antidepressants and he began to experience negative effects known as the nocebo effect. His entire physiology changed because of what he believed to be true about the pills he took, even though they were simple, benign sugar pills. [23]

Other studies have shown that when people are convinced they are going to die during surgery, they often do. Or they may have slow recovery times post-surgery. There have even been cases of people being misdiagnosed with cancer, given months to live and then die in that time frame even though they had no trace of cancer! Even "patients given nothing but an IV full of saline, thinking it was chemotherapy actually threw up and lost their hair." [24] Contrast these cases with patients who expected and **BELIEVED** they were going to have great outcomes and did, whether undergoing surgery, taking a sugar pill for pain or depression, or putting on fake Rogaine to grow hair. This is the power of the mind-body-connection!

This is also why a diagnosis and prognosis a patient receives from their doctor can be some of the most detrimental words they ever hear. Once a patient has been given a diagnosis, they take ownership of the disease, therefore giving it power. Add in a devastating prognosis like "you have months to live," "you're going to die unless you do chemo," or "you will have to take this for the rest of your life" and now the patient has a certain mindset about their disease. This mindset, unfortunately, doesn't typically empower people. It takes them out of the driver's seat of their own life, and they end up creating the outcomes that correspond directly to the words they heard from their doctor. The diagnosis and prognosis can be like a voodoo curse over their lives; thus, they manifest a reality that is directly in line with their thoughts and beliefs.

"Your thoughts and beliefs really do become your reality."

Dr. Jay

DD Palmer, the founder of Chiropractic called this autosuggestion. Autosuggestion can be defined as the hypnotic or subconscious adoption of an idea. At the beginning of the 20th century French psychologist and pharmacist Émile Coué developed a whole method of psychotherapy using "optimistic autosuggestion." Coué described autosuggestion as:

An instrument that we possess at birth, and with which we play unconsciously all our life, as a baby plays with its rattle. It is however a dangerous instrument; it can wound or even kill you if you handle it imprudently and unconsciously. It can on the contrary save your life when you know how to employ it consciously. [25]

One of Coué's techniques involved having his patients use the mantra, "Everyday in every way, I'm getting better and better." He would use this mantra in an effort to replace their thoughts about their illness or condition "with a new thought of [a] cure." [25] And lo and behold, his patients got better. He also implemented suggestive techniques in which he would praise the medications he was prescribing. He realized that praising the medications vs. not praising them helped his patients achieve considerably better results. Ultimately, through the power of positive autosuggestion his patients were able to make profound changes in their health. Therefore, patients who perceive the news they hear from their doctor as negative often experience dismal results. It's not necessarily the doctors that make them worse, but their own perception, emotions, and overall mindset about their diagnosis and prognosis. Their negative thoughts play out like a mantra in their mind, thus creating their own self-fulfilled prophecy.

THE CONSCIOUS/SUBCONSCIOUS MIND AND PROGRAMMING

What is the mind and how does it have so much power in our lives? The mind can be split into two categories, the conscious mind, and the subconscious mind. According to Lipton we use our conscious mind about 5% of the time, meaning that 95% of our lives are controlled by our subconscious mind. [26] There is a region of your brain located behind your forehead called the pre-frontal cortex. This is where the conscious part of your mind sits. It is responsible for higher brain functions including creativity, complex decision making, goal setting, expectations based on actions, social control, and personality expression. [27]

Your subconscious mind on the other hand is responsible for storing and retrieving data. [28] Its job is to make sure you respond exactly the way you have been programmed. From a young age we have been programmed with a certain set of beliefs regarding reality. These beliefs have been programmed into us from our parents, television/media, our teachers, authority figures, books we have read, our life experiences, etc. Once those beliefs are instilled in us, they are extremely hard to change. The subconscious mind is extremely powerful!

During the first seven years of life the brain is predominantly in a hypnotic-like-state – a lower brain wave state called Theta. [26] It functions from a more imaginative state of being – a subconscious state vs. a conscious state. In this state, the brain "downloads" behavioral programs and beliefs, etc., from what it observes in the environment. Currently the primary modes of programming during the first seven years of a kiddo's life are the parents (thoughts, beliefs, behaviors), media sources (YouTube, cartoons, other), and the schooling they are immersed in (public/private schooling).

As a child observes their parent's behaviors and learns their beliefs, they download these into their subconscious mind. Whatever media sources they watch, from cartoons to Sesame Street, becomes programming. And with public "schooling" they learn "the rules." They learn what is and what isn't possible, they learn about the "state's" version of reality and, in my opinion, they learn how to become workers rather than creators. This programming plays out throughout our lives and is involved with every decision we make. It's important to note that we *can* break free of our programming and rewire our brains. We *can* create new habits and new thoughts which lead to better decisions and actions.

It's hard to fathom that we have been programmed to think a certain way. Our current lives reflect everything we have ever experienced. Regarding health care, we learn at a young age that we "need" to take medicine when we are sick. We learn that medical doctors are the health authorities and again we learn that genes control our destinies. This programming becomes so hardwired into us that when we do get sick and express symptoms, we have a hard time trusting and having faith in our body's natural healing process. On one hand we may know that taking drugs is harmful to our health, but we conclude that it's a necessary evil. This all goes back to our programming. I have patients who don't want to take drugs, who know without a doubt that the drugs they're taking are harmful but take them anyway because they believe they will die without them. We default back to the programming we grew up with which is reiterated and reinforced repeatedly, over and over again throughout our lives – especially with the "programming" we choose to watch on our television sets.

TEL-LIE-VISION PROGRAMMING

Two movies I watched over the last five years ended with the answer to the zombie apocalypse being a vaccine (*World War Z & I Am Legend*). In another movie I watched Bradley Cooper's character discover a new and mysterious pharmaceutical drug which allows him to utilize all his brain making him somewhat "limitless" (*Limitless*). Suddenly, he could remember everything he learned in his life; he could even learn new things at an astonishing rate of speed. He learns several languages, how to play classical piano, and masters the stock market, all within a matter of months. His character takes a turn for the worse when he realizes he must continue taking the drug every day just to stay alive. If

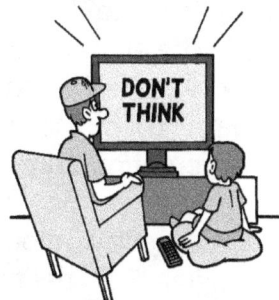

that isn't pharmaceutical propaganda, I don't know what is. The idea that we need a toxic drug to enhance ourselves implies that we as humans are flawed and limited. This is exactly how the pharmaceutical companies want their "customers" to be; automatons who aren't consciously thinking layers deep.

Look at all the cars lined up in the drive through pharmacies, people refilling prescriptions. Or drug commercials telling us to "ask your doctor if such and such is right for you." In both these situations you can see this state of unconsciousness playing out in full effect.

The Emmy award winning show *House* glorified and glamorized western medicine and medical doctors. There is even a TV show, *The Doctors,* which is backed by pharma. The show is merely a panel of doctors that push more of this same agenda. Del Bigtree, a major producer of the Emmy award winning show, quit after he realized how one sided it was. Another example is a cartoon I watched as a child. *David the Gnome* featured a gnome who traveled around the forest on a fox saving animals by using medicine.

I hope you now see just how engrained these beliefs are within you and how heavily they influence the decisions you make or have made in the past.

It's almost comical the level of indoctrination that occurs throughout our lives to make us believe certain things and make certain decisions. I have concluded that we really do live in the Matrix. I even heard Bruce Lipton say one time that, "the Matrix *(the movie)* isn't a fictional tale, it's a documentary." It's like we are living in some dark comedy. It's both funny and sad at the same time. The empowering thing to know is that knowledge is power, but only when acted upon. Hence, we can change our brains by rewiring them. Making different decisions will give us a whole set of different outcomes that will ultimately help us to thrive in life!

In order to rewire our brains, we must first start with our beliefs. Changing our beliefs requires us to completely change our subconscious programming. Beliefs are subconscious and here is how I know that – many people don't even know why they believe what they believe! And when challenged on their beliefs they often become defensive rather than taking a deeper look into why they believe that set of beliefs. It's hard to change beliefs because they are hardwired into us. According to Dr. Joe Dispenza, author of the book *You Are the Placebo*, "A belief is just an extended state of being – essentially, beliefs are thoughts and feelings (attitudes) that you keep thinking and feeling over and over again until you hardwire them in your brain and emotionally condition them into your body." [29] Tony Robbins in his book *Unlimited Power*, describes belief as "nothing but a state, an internal representation that governs behavior." [30]

Remember when you believed in Santa Claus? Year after year, didn't you feel the same excitement around Christmas time because you believed the same fat guy with a white beard was going to bring you gifts? The excitement triggered the same positive emotional chemicals in your body, and you felt energized – a descriptive term for this internal feeling is state of being. Even though the belief was based on a lie – it was true for you because your environment (parents, media, shopping malls) conditioned your belief year after year. And because the belief was so hardwired into your brain, wasn't it devastating when you found out that Santa Claus wasn't real? You probably were in denial, like I was.

Yet, why did we believe in Santa Claus? We believed in Santa Claus because our environment conditioned that belief, even though we really had no solid proof that Santa Claus existed. And, because we believed in Santa Claus for so long it influenced the way we perceived our environment. For example, I never thought it was odd that I saw Santa driving a Lincoln Town Car on Highway 4 one day in December when I was a kid. My perception was that he must be in town for a visit. I also never thought it was odd that Santa's "Ho, Ho, Ho's" in the middle of the night outside my window sounded exactly like my dad. I just perceived that Santa sounded like my dad. Okay, enough about Santa Claus, you get the point.

Dr. Dispenza says, "when you string a set of related beliefs together for long enough, they form your perception about your reality." Your perception about reality is essentially a sustained state of being based on your beliefs. [29] These beliefs are heavily engrained into our subconscious mind. Lastly, our beliefs get reconditioned indirectly and directly through the mechanism of stimulus and response. This means that your perception of your environment (stimulus) will trigger a response which activates your body, thus putting you into a certain state. It then in turn reinforces all that you believe to be true. For example, a person who perceives all their "life's happenings" (environment) as happening for them is going to achieve quite different outcomes than the person who views their life as happening against them. "It is [our] cues from the environment that automatically, autonomically, subconsciously, and physiologically change [our] internal states." [29] Dispenza calls this associative memory and uses the example of Pavlov's dogs. Again, this all happens on an unconscious level and it's recurring.

HOW TO REWIRE YOUR BRAIN

People get trapped into patterns in their life which don't serve them. They end up in the same old relationships, or with the same old health outcomes, or the same old money problems, etc. Whatever the problems are, they are patterns that reflect a person's core beliefs. We end up directly or indirectly creating our reality through thought alone. Thought determines our actions and actions determine our outcomes; our outcomes create our reality. We must breakthrough these subconscious patterns if we are ever going to thrive. In order to change our beliefs and rewire our brains we must bring more consciousness into our lives. We need to become aware of the thoughts, beliefs, and perceptions in our lives that we keep reconditioning on a subconscious level. This means we need to take a proactive approach to our lives by interrupting the negative thought patterns. Tony Robins calls this a pattern interrupt. [30] We need to adopt new and powerful thoughts, beliefs, and perceptions.

REWIRING MY PERCEPTIONS

When I was seventeen, I hit a rock bottom point in my life where I desperately needed to change. As an addict I realized I needed to change my environment if I was ever going to overcome my addiction. My addiction wasn't really alcohol or smoking weed; my addiction was seeking approval from others. Therefore, I engaged in unhealthy behaviors to "blend in" and gain approval from the people I was hanging out with. This was the initial motivator and pattern interrupt I needed to begin to shift my thoughts and perceptions about "my" reality. I immediately stopped hanging out with these people because I realized they weren't really my friends. The second thing I did was to shift my thinking from "man, I'm a loser" to "man, I'm going to change my life and become something!" Because of this shift in thinking I began to work out regularly. I ended up graduating high school on time and I started undergrad shortly thereafter. My new formed thoughts created so much excitement within me that I was creating a new cascade of hormones and chemicals that supported an abundant life. Eventually I was able to abolish those old limiting beliefs. Suffice it to say, if you want to change your life you must change your beliefs about your reality and about yourself; it's a simple concept.

Think about the power of the placebo effect I discussed earlier in this chapter. The belief in their ailment is reinforced and reconditioned by their environment and their thoughts (external and internal stimulus). Once diagnosed, the diagnosis is powerful because it gives them an identity. They begin to identify as their disease. This in turn creates a physiological response that supports and perpetuates the disease. Add in environmental factors that re-condition the negative thought patterns of "I am _____ (depressed, bi-polar, etc.)" or "I have _____ (cancer, high blood pressure, fibromyalgia)" and the body will more than likely not heal. Emotional support from friends and family can work against you in that it reconditions your thoughts instead of interrupting them. However, through the power of the placebo effect a person radically shifts their thoughts and beliefs which changes their physiology from supporting disease and sickness to promoting health and healing. This is exactly what happened with the example of the young man and his depression and me and my addiction. We healed ourselves with the power of our thoughts alone.

ENERGY, FREQUENCY, AND WINNING THE LOTTERY

It all has to do with energy! In fact, everything in the universe is made up of energy vibrating and different frequencies. In other words, all matter is just energy vibrating at various speeds. The faster an object vibrates the higher the frequency and the more energy it has. Even solid objects that don't look like they are in motion – like a couch, for example, are vibrating according to quantum physics. Inanimate objects we can see are typically vibrating at a lower frequency. With humans, our frequency can vary based on what state we're in.

Our states are interdependent on our physical health and mental health. For example, low frequency thoughts lead to a lowering of our state. vs high frequency thoughts that lead to a higher vibrational state. If you believe in the low-vibrational lie that you're not good enough and you continually think to yourself, "I'm not good enough," it will trigger your body to downregulate the chemicals that increase energy in your body. For example, people who are chronically depressed have low levels of serotonin and dopamine. The problem: 90% of the thoughts we think every day are habitual, meaning we primarily think the same thoughts every day. And, every time we think the same thoughts, we are creating stronger neural connections down a single pathway.

This is called a neural pathway and it is how all habits are created. Negative thoughts will always create a low vibrational state, especially when they are repetitive. Since "like attracts like," having a lowered vibrational state will attract things into your environment that will reinforce your state.

Moreover, your energy will attract certain people,
circumstances, and situations into your life that have
the same vibrational frequency.

We radiate a specific "energy signature;" this energy signature is always "broadcasting information as electromagnetic energy." [29] It is as if we are broadcasting our own radio stations. In fact, we are indeed like a radio transmitter and receiver. If you have ever placed your hands on the old-school rabbit ears of a television set and gotten a better picture, it's because your body is working as the antenna and the signal is flowing through you. Your thoughts and beliefs create your electromagnetic energy signature which impacts, influences, and attracts your environment. Want proof of this phenomenon?

Fifty-three-year-old California software account executive, Cynthia Stafford, visualized herself winning 112 million dollars in the lottery and she won exactly that. At the time of her winning Cynthia was raising her late brother's five children in a 1,100 square foot apartment in east Los Angeles. At one point all five children were taken from her by social services. They eventually apologized to Ms. Stafford for their mis-judgement and the children were returned to her care. On the verge of losing her apartment, she found strength in reading the Bible and self-improvement books about positive thinking, visualization, and the law of attraction. One day she decided she was going to win the lottery by manifesting it into her reality. She visualized the exact amount of 112 million dollars, wrote it down daily, slept with the number underneath her pillow at night, meditated on winning it, replaced any doubts with positive thoughts, and got really excited about what she was going to do once she won! She created the thoughts, beliefs, and perceptions that were required to win, and she reconditioned them. She was already a winner before she won. Could it be that her thoughts created an energy frequency that attracted 112 million dollars into her life, or was it merely a coincidence? I would argue that she created her own reality, especially since other people have used similar law of attraction methods to win the lottery or to manifest anything they want in their lives. Whether it's better health, better relationships, or just a better life in general, maybe it's time we start focusing on what we want, rather than what we don't want! [31]

CHANGE YOUR STATE AND INSPIRATION

To get what we want out of life; we must change our state. Reprogramming our minds with new thoughts, beliefs, and perceptions about our reality can take time. If you frivolously try to think positively it isn't going to work. As said before, you must bring more consciousness into your life and condition in new beliefs. In order to condition in new beliefs, you must put yourself into a more energetic state. If there is no shift in your physiology or no shift in your energy when conjuring up new thoughts and new beliefs, then they aren't going to stick. This means changing our thoughts and installing new beliefs needs to be experiential.

A level of physiological change is needed when shifting your thoughts and creating a new reality for yourself. Tony Robbins talks about changing your physiology to dramatically change your state. Have you ever been really pissed off but then you do something, or something happens that instantly changes your state for the better? It could be you were really pissed off and you went to the gym and midway through your workout you noticed that you were feeling better. It could mean someone said something hysterical which instantly interrupted your negative thought pattern of being pissed off because you started laughing uncontrollably. This is because when your physiology changes it changes your psychology. We make better decisions in our life when we are in a more resourceful state. [30] This is also why I think our physical health is so important as well.

In the book *Unlimited Power* by Robbins, he says two things determine our state: our internal representations (how we represent/perceive things to ourselves) and our physiology. For example, a person who is depressed isn't a depressed person, it is just that they are in a "state of depression." They feel depressed as a result of how they interpret their reality (internal representation) and because their physiology reflects that of a depressed person. Usually their shoulders are slouched forward, their breathing is shallow, their back is rather hunched, their gaze is downward, and they move slow or hardly at all (sedentary behavior). In order to get out of a state of depression and program in new beliefs and thought patterns they first have to have a desire to change. And they need to shift their physiology. This means that they would have to change their posture to that of a confident person, regardless of whether they feel that way or not. They need to change their breathing pattern by taking deeper breaths and getting more oxygen into their body. Instead of looking down, they need to look up. Lastly, they need to move!

There is a reason why people who work out rarely suffer from depression. In fact, there was a study that showed exercise worked better than antidepressants for helping with mild to moderate depression! [32] Exercise increases blood flow, increases testosterone and growth hormone that helps you feel more confident, increases endorphins (feel good hormones), helps regulate blood sugar levels, and promotes better sleep. Ultimately, it would be hard to bust out a great workout and maintain your state of depression at the same time. After a bad breakup I would use working-out to dramatically change my state and get over my ex. Working out consistently and conditioning in new internal representations about the breakup helped me eventually get out of my funk. These new internal representations were reinforced by the inspiration I felt while working out.

If I could put a cap on exactly what it is that paves the way for everything in your life to change, it's inspiration. The feeling of being inspired. In my own life I have learned nothing ever changes unless I feel inspired to change. The feeling of being inspired is the ultimate state- change that leads to new beliefs, thoughts, perceptions, and behaviors and therefore outcomes/results.

Instead of waiting on things in our life to change – we need to BE THE CHANGE! We need to first become that person who is to live an extraordinary life before we can manifest an extraordinary life. Inspiration fuels the desire to want to change everything about your life that you feel needs to change. Therefore, we need to do things which "pattern interrupt" our current negative beliefs and thought patterns and create the inspiration for us to change. Below I have listed several examples that can create inspiration in your life.

INSPIRING ACTIVITIES THAT CAUSE A STATE CHANGE

1. Being out in nature and going for a hike can instantly improve your state.

2. Working out is a great way to change your state.

3. Listening to inspiring and instrumental music while practicing meditation is a great way to feel inspired!

4. Talking with a positive person who has manifested a life you're interested in modeling allows you to see what's possible.

5. Reading self-help books.

6. Watching inspirational movies. Watching educational YouTube videos. Listening to motivational podcasts.

7. Go to life transforming seminars (i.e. *Unleash the Power Within*).

8. Church services, community events.

There are many things you can do to feel inspired, change your state, shift your thinking, and create the life you have always wanted to live. Health isn't just about feeling good, it's about knowing that you're creating the life you were destined to live! "Why live an ordinary life when you can live an extraordinary life?" (Robbins) The life you want begins in your head. This is why I chose to write about the power of your mind before I wrote about anything else.

I hope you can now fully appreciate how powerful your thoughts are in creating your life and healing your body. If your mind doesn't change than nothing else in your life ever will.

In the next section of this book you will embark upon several chapters that are designed to inspire you to act regarding your physical health by adding in the good and removing the interference. Remember, in the quest to live an extraordinary life your physical health is key to not only having all that you want, but to be able to fully appreciate and enjoy the life you've created.

"The mind has a powerful way of attracting things that are in harmony with it, good or bad."

Idowu Koyenikan

REMOVING THE INTERFERENCE
Chapters 4 - 11

*"God needs no help to heal
you, just no interference."*

CHAPTER 4

THE POWER OF THE NERVE SYSTEM

*The Nerve System controls and coordinates all of the organs
And structures of the human body.*

- Grays Anatomy

There is an incredible intelligence within each and every one of us that goes beyond any technological advancement ever created. This intelligence is made up of our brain, spinal cord, and nerves which when combined makes up our nerve system. It is because of our nerve system that we can thrive in life and do all that we do!

Did you know that the first organ system to develop within sixteen days after conception is the brain and central nerve system? [33] In other words, nothing in your body develops before your nerve system. Your nerve system controls all the other systems in your body, including all the organs! Your nerve system is really the foundation of everything that is you! That means that everything in your body is 100% dependent on how well your nerve system is working! It is your master control system.

In my opinion, it is the most important system in your body because if it were to cease to function you would be dead. I'll prove it to you; it isn't until a person is pronounced "brain-dead" that they are considered dead by medical standards. [34] In order to keep a person alive at that point machines would need to be used to do the job of the nerve system.

How well your nerve system is functioning should be your number one priority when it comes to your health.

Dr. Jay

A LESSON ON THE NERVE SYSTEM

Think of your brain as the world's best supercomputer. It is estimated that your brain processes a billion-billion calculations per second! [35] That is amazing! Your brain dictates, controls, governs, and regulates what your body does by sending electrical, "life giving" signals down your spinal cord and through your nerves. These messages travel at 300 mph to every single organ, tissue, cell, and muscle of your body. [33]

Your brain is in constant communication with your tissues, organs, and organ systems and all those tissues are in constant communication with your brain. It's this exchange of information between your brain and body that keeps you functioning properly, and it's also responsible for much of the healing that happens.

When your nerve system is working at its optimum it allows you to better adapt to both internal and external stress. It allows you to better adapt to your environment! This means that a person with an optimum functioning nerve system is going to heal faster than somebody who has neurological interference. An optimum functioning nerve system means better balance, better coordination, faster response times, better brain function because of proper CSF flow, decreased stress, and ultimately a better quality of life! When your nerve system is functioning properly it's all systems go, and life becomes better lived! So, read on if you want to better understand how to get your nerve system to function at its highest potential!

THE SPINAL CORD

Your spinal cord is equivalent to a major highway that these life-giving messages are sent through. It is made up of trillions of nerve fibers bundled together (microscopic wires – neurons, axons) and wrapped in a protective sheath called the meninges. [36] As a quite simple and loose analogy, I think of it as a big electrical cord. The outer plastic layer of the cord is like the meninges. If you were to splice the cord open and strip away the outer plastic sheath, you would see hundreds of thin copper wires bundled together to make one big cord.

The nerve fibers in the spinal cord come together to form the nerve roots, which continue out to different parts of your body as peripheral nerves. These nerves transmit and receive all kinds of different messages on sensory information, motor control, and autonomic function. All this information is constantly flowing through the spinal cord for the brain to process and then tell the body what to do; messages are coming in and going out at an extremely fast speed. Hence the reason the spinal cord is considered an "information superhighway!"

THE CSF

Within the meningeal sheath of this superhighway is a fluid that is produced in the brain called cerebrospinal fluid (CSF). This fluid acts as a cushion for the spinal cord and brain, but also provides nutrients and the removal of toxic waste from the system. The proper flow of this clear-water-like fluid is essential for optimum nerve system function.

How well CSF flows through your spinal cord and brain has a lot to do with the proper biomechanics of the spine and how well the spine is functioning (as a whole). [36]

THE SPINE

The brainstem (posterior part of the brain), the spinal cord, and all the precious nerve roots are housed and protected by your spine. Your nerve system is one of the only systems that is 100% encased in bone. Moreover, unlike your lungs, heart, and other organs protected by your ribs, the brain and spinal cord are completely encapsulated in solid bone. The reason for this is clear. Our Creator knew what he was doing when he designed the human body, in that he wanted to fully protect this system. So, he fortified it and surrounded it with a solid protective armor! What better way to protect the nerve system than with a thick round shell, the skull, and the individual moveable vertebral bones that make up the spine.

The spine consists of thirty-three vertebra which are separated into groups. These groups consist of seven cervical vertebra which make up your neck, twelve thoracic vertebra which make up your mid-back, five lumbar vertebra which make up your lower back, the sacrum, and the coccyx bone, which is often called the tailbone. All but one out of the twenty-four upper segments of your spine are separated by fibrous cartilaginous pads called intervertebral-discs, or discs for short. The one bone of the spine that does not have an intervertebral disc is the atlas.

THE ATLAS & OCCIPUT

The atlas is the first cervical vertebra in the neck and is named after the character in Greek mythology who holds the world up in his hands. Like the Greek giant, the atlas supports the entire skull via the occiput. The occiput rests on top of the atlas in

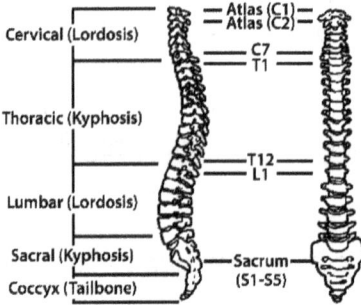

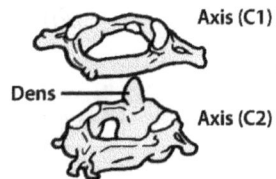

delicate balance. Because of the way these two bones articulate together it allows the skull to rotate and move smoothly in a wide range of motions. Similar to a ball caressing the water it floats on top of, the ball rotates on the water with ease and grace, as the head does on the atlas.

Passing through a hole in the occiput called the foramen magnum (big hole) is the brainstem. Some cultures appropriately refer to this hole as the "Mouth of God" due to its obvious importance. The brainstem, like a plug in an outlet, connects the brain to the spinal cord and is responsible for several vital functions of the body. Some of these functions include respiratory, gastrointestinal, and cardiovascular control. It is a major epicenter of the body because trillions of nerve fibers pass through this area and are responsible for processing an unfathomable amount of information. [37]

The atlas is unique from all the other vertebra of the spine due to its ring-like shape and its housing of the brainstem. It sits on top of the C2 vertebra, aka the axis. The axis has a protruding portion on top called the dens, which the atlas, being a ring, rotates upon. This rotational feature of the atlas accounts for most of our ability to rotate our heads nearly 80°. Thank God for this feature! Can you imagine having to constantly turn your entire body to see over your shoulders?

However, all this range of motion comes with a price. This makes the atlas more prone to misaligning. If the atlas misaligns, even by a few millimeters, it can negatively impact the brainstem and how well it functions. An atlas misalignment can shut down the flow of life between the brain and the rest of the body.

Do you remember Christopher Reeves who played Superman? How did he go from playing one of the most infamous superheroes of all time to being completely crippled in a matter of moments? I'm sure you remember the injury. I remind you of this tragedy to exemplify how important your nerve system is and to further the point that the most important component to your health is a proper nerve supply. Reeves was riding his horse in an equestrian competition when the horse abruptly stopped at one of the obstacles catapulting Reeves into the air. Reeves landed on the top of his head. Even though he was wearing a protective helmet, the force from the impact compressed and fractured the top two bones in his neck thus damaging his spinal cord. In fact, a lot of people think he severed his spinal cord, but he didn't. All he did was bruise his brainstem. In fact, the amount of damage he caused to the area was relatively small. Yet, instantaneously he became a quadriplegic and his body shut down to the point which he had to be put on a respirator because he lost the ability to breathe on his own. Without the advent of modern technology, he would have died within minutes.

What is amazing about Christopher Reeves' story is that he fought hard to live a normal life again. He had dreams of walking again and because of that he broke major scientific grounds on stem cell research. At the time spinal cord injury research was in its infant stages. Reeves did whatever he had to do to make sure his body was functioning at it's very best, despite his injury. He made sure he was receiving the best nutritional therapy available along with daily rehab and physical therapy. Although he made some amazing strides forward in his recovery, he never came close to what he once was because his body lacked the proper neurological communication. While the messages between his brain and his body were blocked, he grew weaker. Sadly, within nine years after his injury he died from complications due to a blood infection caused by a mere bedsore. [39]

SUBLUXATION & CHIROPACTIC

As a practicing chiropractor of thirteen years I know the devastating effects of neurological interference and how it can create ill-health. The reason chiropractors look to the spine is because it houses and protects a major part of your nerve system (brainstem, spinal cord, nerve roots). If you have any interference to your nerve system whatsoever, your body cannot fully function and heal at 100% which leads to dis-ease (lack of ease in the body). This eventually leads to disease, sickness, and an early death. For example, if I cut the nerves that form the cardiac plexus which controls the rate at which your heart beats, guess what would happen? Your heart would miraculously keep beating, but your brain wouldn't be able to communicate with your heart to tell it to slow down or speed up. There would be no heart rate variability, which is critical for survival. Your heart wouldn't be able to function at 100% and your quality of life would diminish greatly.

What if instead of cutting the nerves to the heart, the bones that house and protect the heart's nerve supply shifted out of their normal position causing mechanical stress on the nerves? What

NORMAL   SUBLUXATION

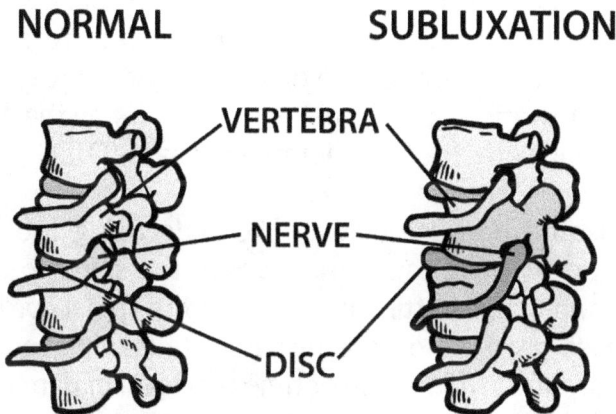

VERTEBRA

NERVE

DISC

Muscle Spasms, Disc Degeneration, Limited Range of Motion, Pain, Inflammation

then? Would the heart still work at 100% of its full potential? No, it would not because the neurological interference caused by the spinal misalignments would inhibit the brains ability to communicate effectively with the heart. It is impossible for the heart, or any other organ, tissue, or muscle, to work at their maximum capacity if the controlling nerve supply is interrupted. In chiropractic practice when a bone or several bones in the spine shift out of their normal position causing neurological interference, we call this vertebral subluxation.

"Vertebral Subluxations cause neurological interference."

Dr. Jay

Vertebral subluxation refers to the loss of normal joint integrity of one or usually several vertebrae of the spine. This loss of normal joint integrity leads to stress on the surrounding soft tissue, spasming of the surrounding musculature, disc degeneration, limited range of motion, pain, and inflammation.

The lack of proper movement combined with the abnormal position of the vertebra(s) leads to neurological interference. And the longer the subluxations remain uncorrected, the worse the problem becomes. An x-ray is one of the best ways to see the pathophysiological changes that occur due to subluxation damage. Long term subluxation damage on an x-ray often shows up as osteoarthritis (oste = bone) or bone spurs on the associated vertebra along with disc degenerative disease (DJD). [40]

The subluxated bones rot away like a decaying tooth. As the bones rot away it can cause the discs of the spine to bulge into the spinal canal thus putting pressure on the spinal cord. This can also increase pressure on the nerve roots leading to decreased nerve supply and function. Over time this level of damage to your spine would eventually lead to symptoms.

As a chiropractor I usually see people when they are at their worst. The problem with this is two-fold. When a subluxation first occurs, there are usually zero noticeable symptoms. This is because only 6% of your nerve system is sensory related. [35] This means you can have neurological interference due to subluxation and not even know it. If there is no pressure on the sensory part of the nerves, you are not going to be able to perceive there is a problem. However, neurological interference can show up as a host of other symptoms. It depends entirely on where the nerves are traveling to and what they control.

Thousands of chiropractors, myself included, have helped their patients with symptoms in addition to back and neck pain by doing specific adjustments to realign the spine and correct spinal subluxations. Below is a list of symptoms I have helped people with in my chiropractic practice.

- Headaches
- Migraines
- Vertigo
- Tinnitus
- Hearing Problems
- Balance Issues

- Sciatica
- Nasal Congestion
- Seizures
- Behavioral Issues (Pediatric)
- Sleep Problems (See Chapter 10)
- Numbness

This does not mean that chiropractic is a panacea – it's not a cure all, end all, be all. Moreover, chiropractors don't diagnose or treat any condition outside of vertebral subluxations. But there is plenty of anecdotal, empirical, and scientific evidence to back up the fact that chiropractic adjustments help people with several issues outside of back and neck pain.

Consider this example as well. Dr. George Bakris, M.D. did a placebo-controlled study on fifty patients to show chiropractic adjustments worked to lower blood pressure as well as two prescription blood pressure medications given in combination! The advantage the adjustments had over the medications was they came without the nasty side-effects! [41]

WHAT CHIROPRACTORS HAVE ALWAYS KNOWN AND X-RAYS

Dr. Henry Windsor, a medical doctor in the 1920's, was intrigued by all the incredible results his patients were getting with chiropractic and osteopathic care. He thought to himself, "How is it possible patients are getting results without drugs or surgery?" He decided to conduct a fascinating study where he dissected both human and animal cadavers to determine if there was a relationship between minor curvatures (misalignments) of the spine and diseased organs. Out of the fifty human cadavers examined forty-nine showed minor curvatures of the spine and one showed a normal lateral curve in the thoracic spine. A whopping 221 diseased organs were observed, "...of these, 212 were observed to belong to the same sympathetic segment [or nerve supply] as the vertebra in curvature." [42] This is what the chiropractic profession has always known since its inception in 1895! Spinal misalignments causing neurological interference can negatively impact the organs and tissues of the body!

In my office we take x-rays because it is the only way to know what your spine looks like. We take a very methodical and scientific approach to correcting the spine through the utilization of digital x-rays. The x-rays help us to pinpoint exactly where the subluxations are and what the overall structure and integrity of the spine looks like. From there we can work on developing a plan of action for correcting the spinal misalignments and helping people live a healthier life. The x-rays also help us to see problems before they become even bigger problems down the road.

When I look at spinal x-rays from the front, I look to see whether the spine is straight or crooked. When the spine is straight it is better equipped to withstand the force of gravity and day to day stress placed on it. Scoliosis is an example of a crooked spine. True scoliosis means that a person has lateral curves in their spine of 10° or more. Any lateral deviation of the spine, regardless of how many degrees it is, means that it is going to be less stable overall. More importantly, a lateral bend in the spine can cause neurological interference.

From the side I want to make sure the spine has all the proper curves. A lordotic curve refers to the normal backwards sloping curve of the spine in both the cervical and lumbar regions. The neck should have a lordotic curve of about 34 to 45° with a person's chin level. The thoracic region of the spine has an opposite frontwards facing curve called a kyphotic curve. All three curves in the spine need to be present for the spine to be stable. Below I will give you an example of this.

Have you ever jammed your finger while playing basketball or something similar? If you are like me this has happened to you more than once. The reason we jam our finger is because the ball impacts our finger while it is completely straight. This compresses the joints in your finger and causes injury. If your finger had even a slight bend in it, you would be less likely to suffer injury. This is because your finger would be able to adapt to the force of the ball impacting it. In the same way the curves of the spine allow us to better adapt to the force of gravity, our body weight, and the impact of our day to day stressors (i.e. sitting, exercise, etc.).

In our office I consider the neck to be the most important part of the spine to work on. The reason for this is your neck houses the very beginning of your spinal cord. So, if it is out of alignment it can negatively affect the rest of your spine and body. In the above paragraph I talked about the neck having a 34 to 45° curve. This curve in your neck is so critical it has been called the "Arc of Life."

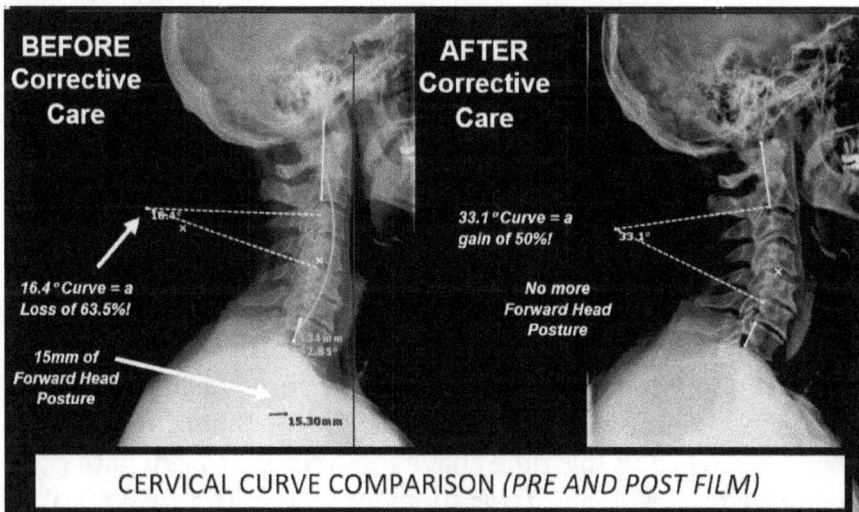

BEFORE Corrective Care

16.4° Curve = a Loss of 63.5%!

15mm of Forward Head Posture

15.30mm

AFTER Corrective Care

33.1° Curve = a gain of 50%!

No more Forward Head Posture

CERVICAL CURVE COMPARISON (PRE AND POST FILM)

A curve in the neck means multiple things:

- The neck has more support for the weight of the head.

- It allows the spinal cord to be more relaxed, thus allowing for better transmission and communication of the information that is sent through it from the brain and body.

- It reduces forward head posture and mechanical pressure on the chest.

- It helps with proper biomechanics of the whole spine.

Most people I see in my office have a complete loss of the normal curve in their neck combined with an average of 30 mm of forward head posture (anterior translation). The loss of curve in the neck leads to a tethering of the spinal cord and neurological interference. Here is what the research shows:

1. Dr. Alf Alfred Breig, neurosurgeon and Nobel Prize recipient, discovered that a loss of the cervical curve can stretch the spinal cord 5 to 7 cm and produce pathological tension, putting the body in a state of disease. [35]

2. Every inch of forward head posture can increase the weight off the head on the spine by an additional ten pounds. [Kapandji, *Physiology of The Joints*, Vol. 3 - 35].

These are just two out of the thousands of studies done and articles written on the cervical spine and its effects on physiology. If the cervical curve is not restored it can lead to severe degeneration, arthritis, and major problems. I demonstrate the importance of the cervical curve in our "Dinner with the Doc Workshop." In the workshop I have people try and take a deep breath in while looking down with their chins jutted forward. You can try this yourself and what you'll find is that it's very challenging to try and take a big deep breath in. Next, I have them take another deep breath in, but this time I have them sit up straight with good posture, chin level, and their shoulders back. The result is they can take an easier and much deeper breath in. Try it now and you'll notice the difference right away.

When forward head posture is present combined with a loss of curve in the neck it puts mechanical stress and tension on the chest. This can decrease your vital lung capacity by up to 30%, which means you would be taking in 30% less air. [35] This inherent shortness of breath puts your body into a state of stress and decreases your overall energy. Just look at how any animal

For every inch of Forward Head Posture, it can increase the weight of the head on the spine by an additional 10 pounds." -Kapandji, Physiology of Joints, Vol. 3

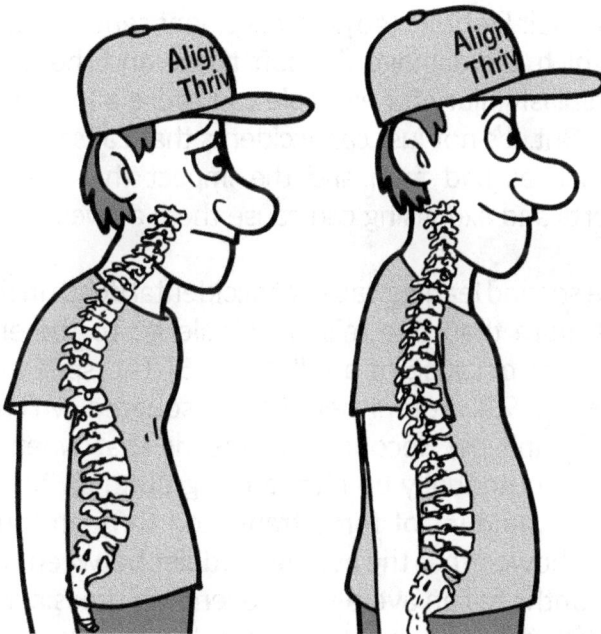

breathes when they are in a state of stress: their breathing is short, shallow, and rapid. Similarly, when your breathing becomes shallow and fast it stimulates the sympathetic part of your nerve system which increases blood pressure and heart rate, increases blood sugar, decreases the function of the frontal neo-cortex part of your brain responsible for higher brain function, and increases muscular tension. [35] If your nerve system is predominantly in a sympathetic state, which argumentatively, most people are, it will run your body into the ground. This is known as sustained sympathetic tone. This is one of the main reasons why correction of spinal subluxation is so important. To correct the spine, I think it's important for you to know what causes it to misalign in the first place.

CAUSES OF SUBLUXATION & SPINAL MISALIGNMENT

The body is a scrap book which means every single injury, insult, and bad postural related stress on your body adds up to exactly what is happening with your spine presently. According to auto insurance experts the average motorist will be in about four car accidents in their lifetime. [43] A car accident sends forces through the back which can damage the soft tissue and the joints of the spine. A whiplash injury for example can cause a loss of the curve in the neck. But, it's not just car accidents that cause subluxations. Traumas, such as bad falls, and the impact that happens from playing sports and exercising can cause them as well.

Falls are the second leading cause of accidental death in the United States and more than one million people go to the emergency room each year because of a fall. [44, 45] The speed of gravity is calculated at 9.8 meters per second squared which equates to about 22 mph per second! This means that when a person falls, they can potentially be hitting the ground at 22 mph! That is a significant amount of force translated through the spine! A 2012 study showed that the average toddler between twelve and nineteen months fell an average of seventeen times per hour and sixty-nine times per hour if they were "new-walkers." [46] This repetition combined with the force of gravity can certainly cause spinal injury and subluxation. When it comes to impact traumas like the ones mentioned above, it makes sense as to how they negatively affect the spine.

One of the very first traumas we experience on our spines happens at birth. This is primarily due to western medicine's complete takeover of the birth process. What they deem "natural" is completely counterintuitive to the way birth should be done. First off, having a woman deliver her baby while flat on her back goes against gravity, rotates her pelvis forward, and narrows the birth canal. This is going to place more stress on the baby, particularly the head and neck, which can cause damage to the spine. The doctor also must pull harder on the head and neck of the child, sometimes rotating the baby's head by 80° or more.

> "Dr. Gottfried Guttman, M.D., former staff member of the Department of Pathology, Boston University School of Medicine, Mallory Institute of Pathology, found that childhood subluxations had received 'far too little attention.' Because of the frequency of problems, especially at birth, he recommended a chiropractic spinal checkup as soon as possible after delivery. Mechanical injury to the upper cervical spinal structures is indicated as a causal mechanism in cases of Sudden Infant Death Syndrome." [35]

It would make sense to utilize gravity when giving birth in a fully upright semi-squat position or to be on all fours. In ancient Greece women did just that and used a birthing stool to deliver their babies in more of a squat position through a hole. [47] But, if going against gravity wasn't traumatic enough on the baby's spine, sometimes doctors use forceps on the baby's head which can cause damage. In fact, the reason why Sylvester Stallone talks the way he does is because he suffered an injury at birth caused by the forceps used. The forceps damaged a nerve on the left side of his face causing paralysis and the slurred speech he is famous for. [48] All and all, the birth process is traumatic on a newborn's spine and it's important to have them checked by a chiropractor that specializes in pediatrics.

Most Americans spend their lives sitting down. Not only do they spend most of their lives sitting down, they also sit with terrible posture. Just look at anybody sitting at their desk or at a coffee shop as they type away on their computers. Usually, they are slouched forward with their arms outstretched, their head is flexed forward about 25° so they can look down at their screens, and their shoulders are rounded forward. They do this on average eight hours per day five days per week for years! And if that isn't enough, they sit with terrible posture in their cars on the way to and from work. All this sitting compresses the vertebra and discs in the lower back and sets off a lot of lower back problems. It can also cause a loss of the normal curve in the neck. Our moms were right when they told us to sit up straight. Not only does a slouched posture look terrible, it is bad for our physiology!

We all know cell phones are bad for our health because of the radiation they expose us to, but cell phones have also caused epidemic proportions of people with terrible necks. This is primarily because as people text and work those thumb muscles their heads are fully flexed forward as they stare down at their phones. It has become so bad that it has been given the nick name "Text-Neck." How pathetic is that? This certainly causes major damage to the cervical spine which can be seen with a lateral x-ray. I have seen twelve-year-olds with a complete loss of the curve in their neck!

D.D. Palmer, the founder of Chiropractic, said that subluxations were caused by thoughts, traumas, and toxins. Furthermore, Palmer believed these three stressors on the body were the soul cause of all dis-ease. In the above section I discussed how traumas could cause subluxation, but what I find fascinating is that emotions and toxicity can also cause your spine to misalign. In short, these non-physical stressors are treated as a threat by your nerve system that in turn causes your muscles to tighten as a way of protecting you. [49] These muscles hold and brace the bones in positions that can cause abhorrent postural changes such as forward head posture and rounded shoulders. Moreover, they can cause regional subluxation patterns and asymmetry of the spine, such as a reversed cervical curve and scoliosis.

It is important to know that no muscle pulls a bone out of its normal position unless the nerve system tells it to do so. As in a pully system, the muscles pull the vertebra out of their normal positions in response to the nerves telling them to fire. These misalignments and changes in spinal curvature only happen because of the internal stress and demand placed on the neurological system due to thoughts, traumas, and toxins. The neurological system must adapt based on the amount of stress placed on it. The more negative thoughts we have, the more physical trauma we suffer, and the more toxins we are exposed to – the greater the demand placed on our nerve systems to adapt. This is also known in chiropractic philosophy as "increased survival demand." [50]

CHIROPRACTIC CARE

Chiropractors work to correct neurological interference by first finding where the subluxations are and then applying a specific chiropractic adjustment. An adjustment is a specific high velocity, low amplitude force done on the spine by hand or with special tools with the intended goal of correcting subluxations. When the spine is in proper alignment it allows for better brain body communication.

We schedule patients for multiple adjustments per week. We don't just do a one "adjustment-wham-bam-and-done." We work to correct the spine so our patients can have lasting changes for the rest of their lives. It takes consistent chiropractic adjustments done for a given amount of time to achieve the desired result of spinal correction. Think about it this way, if you joined a gym and just worked out once, would you expect to increase your muscle mass and improve your cardiovascular stamina? Of course not, it takes time and consistency if you want to create profound physiological changes. So, if someone has twenty-five years of subluxation damage in their spine, it's going to take several visits to correct what is going on. Once the corrections are made, we recommend maintenance/wellness care for life. Similar to working out weekly to maintain your gains, your spine needs consistent maintenance and improvement as well. We make this a normal part of wellness care.

Along with adjustments we also utilize spinal rehabilitation procedures which work to support the adjustments and enhance the effectiveness of care. One of the simplest but most profound things we do is work to restore the cervical curve utilizing an impact-adjustment tool called an arthrostim. The arthrostim works by producing a barrage of messages that are sent to the brain about joint and position. These are known as afferent messages. These afferent messages work to re-educate the brain body connection in what is known as neuromuscular re-education.

We also give all our patients a neck wedge which works by putting the neck in traction. Prolonged traction done on the neck for twenty minutes or more per day over a span of months positively changes the soft tissue that supports the cervical spine, thus, improving the curve. Traction exercise is also great because it helps to relax the upper trap muscles and stimulate the parasympathetic part of the nerve system which puts the body at ease and helps it heal. Several of my patients have reported it's so relaxing they have fallen asleep on the neck wedge.

We do several things in our office to ensure our patients receive the best results, but our main job is to correct misalignments in the spine thus restoring the balance between the brain and the body.

So, how do you find the right chiropractor for you?

FIVE CRITERIA FOR FINDING A GOOD CHIROPRACTOR

1. Make sure they take x-rays. X-rays are an objective measurement of your spine and help a chiropractor to pinpoint exactly where the subluxations are. The x-rays also can help rule out any pathologies that are outside the scope of chiropractic.

2. Make sure they do a thorough consultation. I sit down with my patients and walk through a consultation with them to find out exactly what their chief complaint is, chronicity of symptoms, accident history, what makes it better, what makes it worse, and what their intended goals are. Finding out their goals is my favorite part! A lot of people just want to be able to function at peak performance and lead healthier lives.

3. Make sure they have a good amount of positive reviews online. Most patients who come into our office have looked us up online and read our reviews. A person willing to take the time to write a positive review about an office means they were inspired enough to do so; they were able to achieve their intended goals. This kind of goes without saying, but when an office has several positive reviews you know you are going to be in good hands. Negative reviews are okay as well, especially if the office sees a high number of patients. In my twelve years as a chiropractor I have learned you can't please everyone. But if the overall trend in reviews is good, then you can rest assured you're probably going to be in good hands.

4. Did they answer all your questions? Often a good chiropractic office will have their staff trained to answer common questions such as, "Do you take my insurance?, How much is it going to cost if I have to pay out of pocket?, and Do you work with kids?" The point being, have they answered all your questions and put your concerns at ease? I take pride in the fact that we do this well in our office.

5. Make sure they are close to you in proximity. As mentioned above, I recommend seeing a chiropractor frequently, especially in the beginning phases of care. To correct the spine, it takes time and repetition. I recommend going to a Chiropractor who is nearby for this reason. Preferably one

within a five to ten-mile radius of your home or office. This makes it easier for you to see him or her on a regular basis.

The power of chiropractic can be profound. I have seen the worst of the worst heal. I have witnessed patients get off their nasty pain killers, antipsychotic medications, and a whole host of other drugs. I have watched patients empower themselves and take their health into their own hands. It's quite a phenomenon to watch people go through the process of healing. There is certainly a spiritual connection to the process. I think the medical model severely downplays a person's own power to heal. Instead, this model disempowers people by treating and masking their symptoms via chemicals.

Chiropractic on the other hand has been defined as the study of all things natural. A lot of chiropractors, including me, focus a great deal on preventing spinal misalignment and neurological interference (subluxation) through lifestyle coaching and education. The following chapters in this section deal with the removal of interference by changing the lifestyle factors that cause the interference.

The Truth

WE CHIROPRACTORS work with the subtle substance of the soul. We release the prisoned impulse, the tiny rivulet of force that emanates from the mind and flows over the nerves to the cells and stirs them into life.

We deal with the magic power that transforms common food into living, loving, thinking clay; that robes the earth with beauty and hues and scents the flowers with the glory of the air.

In the dim, dark, distant long ago, when the sun first bowed to the morning star, this power spoke and there was life; it quickened the slime of the sea and the dust of the earth and drove the cell to union with its fellows in countless living forms.

Through eons of time it finned the fish and winged the bird and fanged the beast. Endlessly it worked, evolving its forms until it produced the crowning glory of them all.

With tireless energy it blows the bubble of each individual life and then silently, relentlessly dissolves the form, and absorbs the spirit into itself again.

And yet you ask, "Can chiropractic cure appendicitis or the flu?"

Have you more faith in a knife or a spoonful of medicine than in the innate power that animates the internal living world?

Dr. J G. Gregorson,

Original Title: *Chiropractors Creed*;
Borrowed by BJ Palmer [51]

CHAPTER 5

HYDRATION: THE POWER OF WATER

*Pure water is the World's First
and Foremost Medicine.*

Slovakian Proverb

Why am I writing a chapter on water? Because water along with oxygen is one of the most important nutrients that people are not getting enough of! Most people I see in my clinic are dehydrated and suffer from a variety of symptoms related to dehydration. I tell my patients that water is the oil of the body! Every single organ, joint, and tissue in your body needs water to work properly. And because people simply aren't drinking enough water, nor are they drinking the right kind of water.

The main reason water is necessary for great health is because our bodies are made up of mostly water. In fact, our bodies are made up of an average of 57-60% water. [52] Water helps us absorb nutrients and allows antioxidants to do their job. It is essential for getting rid of harmful toxins from the body. It improves oxygen delivery to the cells, as well as cell to cell communication. It helps to maintain normal electrical properties of cells, thus affecting your energy levels. It even helps with weight loss!

Every single tissue in your body is made up of a collection off cells. Your body is composed of about 75 trillion cells. Collections of cells come together to form different tissues, such as ligaments and organs. Every single cell contains 70% water as it is of critical importance for all the organelles (the cell's organs) within the cell. [53] For a cell to work properly it must have enough water to work with. When dehydration occurs water inside the cell will go to the bloodstream to maintain blood volume. In severe cases of dehydration, it will cause the cell to malfunction and shrivel up. You literally dry up from the inside out. [54]

According to Dr. Zach Bush, MD (triple board-certified physician) cancer seems to happen when the "body is so dry, you're nearly dead. Basically, when you're dehydrated at a cellular level, you get an 'accumulation of oxidative damage,' which negatively impacts the DNA of the cell, which can cause cancer."

Dr. Bush states:

[Cancer], it's simply a lack of water within the cells. You get an accumulation off oxidative damage, which will then do the DNA injury and all of these other things that we think of as being the cancer process... Ideal health, [means that you're fully hydrated]. [Mercola, May 06, 2018, Article on Hydration]

In Bush's study they measure hydration levels using a phase angle. Patients are rated on a scale of 1-10, with ten being "super hydrated" and one being "dead." Bush states that most people in America are between a six and eight if they are considered in good health. This means there is definite room for improvement. Most people, as stated above, are dehydrated on a cellular level.

Just because you are drinking lots of water doesn't necessarily mean you are becoming hydrated.

Dr. Jay

As you can imagine, if your cells aren't able to function at 100% because of dehydration, it will eventually lead to a variety of symptoms such as fatigue, brain fog, tiredness, etc. Some research shows that dehydration can affect things like mood, cognitive abilities, and motor control. There is even research to show that your "brain tissue fluid decreases." [55]

The water we drink is heavily polluted. People load up on coffee, tea, cola, alcohol, etc. all of which contain water, but they don't hydrate the body. All these drinks are also toxic for the body and cause you to urinate more because they act as a diuretic. When you urinate after you drink coffee your body is trying to get rid of the coffee because it treats it as a toxin. Think about it, anytime you drink these types of drinks do you not find yourself needing to go to the bathroom more often? Why is that? When toxic fluids such as coffee or alcohol enter the body, your kidneys must work harder to flush out the toxins. Coffee has a pH of about 4.6 which means it is very acidic. The kidneys act as a buffer and get rid of the excess acid to maintain normal pH levels. [56] Having to work overtime to remove excess toxins from beverages would naturally lead to some level of dehydration.

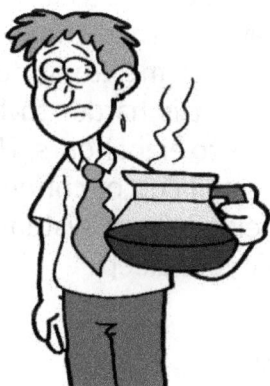

Caffeine is one of the most addictive DRUGS on the planet. Yes, I said it, caffeine is a drug. Caffeine is defined as a drug because it stimulates your central nerve system. It causes temporary alertness because it puts your body into fight or flight mode, but more on this later. According to E-Imports Expresso Business Solutions, as of 2017, "50% of the population, equivalent to 150 million Americans, drink espresso, cappuccino, latte, or iced/cold coffees. [And] Independent coffee shops equal $12 billion in annual sales." [57] There are a lot of Americans addicted to their coffee/caffeine, including me at one time. Since coffee is one of the number one toxins people consume, I offer you five reasons to ditch it.

Top Five Reasons You Should Quit Caffeine:

#1 It overstimulates your adrenal glands

Caffeine causes your adrenal glands to release cortisol, epinephrine, and norepinephrine. This causes your body to be in fight or flight mode. Your body goes into survival mode as blood is drawn away from your digestive system and redirected towards your muscles. This means that your digestion is put on hold while your body utilizes the added energy to process the newly released hormones or to move blood where it needs to be. Cortisol narrows the arteries while epinephrine increases the heart rate. What does this do? It causes the heart to pump blood faster. Imagine drinking coffee every morning, day in and day out, what is this doing to your cardiovascular system long term? [56]

#2 Sleep Problems

Sleep problems are quite common in people who have a caffeine addiction. I was one of them. When I drank caffeine, I had problems sleeping. When your body is in a stressed state melatonin (the sleep hormone) is suppressed and therefore, it is harder to fall asleep. [58] Caffeine has a half-life of about six to eight hours. This means if you have 200 mg of caffeine in a small cup of coffee at 10:00 am, you can still have 100 mg of caffeine in your system at 6:00 pm. This amount of caffeine *can* impair your sleep.

#3 Decreases Insulin Sensitivity

Drinking caffeine consistently can decrease one's insulin sensitivity making it harder to respond to circulating blood glucose. This causes blood sugar levels to spike which leads to sugar imbalances and fluctuations in energy. [60]

#4 Caffeine is Addictive

Most people suffer from caffeine addiction. Caffeine is one of the most unregulated drugs in the US. The caffeine content in tea, coffee, and energy drinks varies widely. But because of its addictive nature companies like to use it in their products. WHY? Because it keeps people coming back for more. The problem with addiction is that being addicted to something makes it much more difficult for the person trying to clean up their diet and lifestyle. Caffeine has some nasty withdrawal affects as well. These include nausea, dizziness, irritability, headaches, and even migraines, among other things. [56] If you can't quit cold turkey then it may be best to try and wean yourself using green tea and/or yerba mate.

#5 Loss of Vital Electrolytes

To reiterate, caffeine is a diuretic meaning it makes you urinate more frequently. Not only does this cause dehydration but it also leeches minerals from your body. Caffeinated beverages like tea and coffee are acidic in nature and cause your body to release minerals to buffer the acid. Minerals are vital for your body to function normally. Perhaps this is one of the reasons people become tired and sluggish with chronic caffeine consumption. [56]

Should you quit caffeine? I would suggest you do. You never needed all that caffeine until you "needed" it, right? People weren't addicted to caffeine until there was a coffee shop on every corner. In my caffeine drinking days I finally got tired of all the stress and anxiety I was feeling. I was tired of the addictive nature of coffee. So, I decided to educate myself and bought the book *Caffeine Blues* by Stephen Cherniske, M.S. I devoured it! It's a great book with about 600 references to research explaining how caffeine isn't so great for us. I feel so much better without caffeine and realize what a dramatic difference it made in my life when I decided to stop. I noticed improved sleep, better energy, and less anxiety. If you too want to kick the habit, I must warn you, the first couple of weeks were very tough for me. I was fatigued and exhausted. I would take up to four naps a day, but I knew my adrenals were healing and there was a light at the end of the tunnel. I fought through all my cravings and my exhaustion and feel so much better now because of it.

Nothing could ever take the place of plain old good water. Water is the best beverage for the body, yet many people think sports drinks are better at hydrating their bodies. The biggest complaint I hear about drinking water is that it's "boring and tasteless." My response is, "Yeah, of course it is because you have become accustomed to drinking other crap." If you are addicted to drinking energy drinks, "mocha crappa latas," or sodas that are loaded with high fructose corn syrup, of course water is going to taste bland!

AMERICANS AND THEIR BEVERAGES

Americans don't drink enough water because we are exposed to all the propaganda that tells us to drink this or that because it's somehow better for us or because it helps with performance. The beverage companies know how to influence the subconscious part of our brain. Therefore, a soda advertisement will usually show young people who appear healthy and vital and are laughing and having fun in some epic setting. Red Bull tells us that their drink will give us "wings." It speaks to the subconscious part of our brain which correlates drinking said beverage to those kinds of positive outcomes. This is called clever marketing and millions of people make decisions every day that destroy their health based on this tactic.

Statistically this marketing works well because according to the beverage marketing corporation the average person in the U.S.

consumes 44.7 gallons of soda and 20.8 gallons of beer every year. [60] This is per person each year. Harvard School of Public Health compiled a list of studies which concluded that men who drank a minimum of one soda per day had a 20% higher risk of having a heart attack or dying of one compared to men who rarely drank soda. They also concluded that women who consumed soda had a higher chance of developing gout than women who rarely consumed soda. [61] Clearly these high caloric and high sugar beverages are contributing to America's health problems.

Diet soda is no better even though it contains no sugar and has less calories. Instead of sugar being used to make diet drinks sweet they contain the chemical aspartame. Aspartame is an artificial sweetener that has been linked to a slew of neurological disorders including multiple sclerosis and Parkinson's disease.

According to an article published in the British Medical Journal, "...although 100% of industry funded (either whole or in part) studies conclude that aspartame is safe, 92% of **independently funded studies** have found that aspartame has the potential for adverse effects." [62] The key word here is independent as opposed to industry. Can we really trust that the industry funded studies are done in the best interest of the consumer? My guess is probably not.

If you Google "aspartame" or "artificial sweetener side effects" thousands of articles will pop up. With so much controversy revolving around one chemical it's probably in your best interest to avoid it all together.

So, let's get back to water, the one pure drink that is good for everyone. We all need to drink more water. How much water should you drink? A good rule of thumb to follow is the eight glasses of water per day rule. This would equate to about 88 ounces of water per day. But this doesn't mean you drink 88 ounces of water all at once. A standard bottle of water is about 17 ounces so if you multiply that by five you get 85 ounces of water. Eighty-eight to one hundred ounces seems like a lot of ounces until you break it up throughout the day. Considering that an average glass of water is about ten to twelve ounces, consider drinking three glasses of water in the morning, three glasses in the afternoon and two glasses in the early evening. Ninety-one ounces (2.7 liters) per day for women and 125 ounces (3.7 liters) per day for men is considered adequate intake of water in the US – from all beverages and foods. [63]

You may not need quite as much water if you're eating fruit throughout the day. Some beverages like almond milk and green drinks are hydrating as well. Your activity level also makes a difference in how much water you will need in a day.

Don't wait until you're thirsty to start drinking water. By the time your brain signals to your body that you're thirsty you are already significantly dehydrated. Remember at the beginning of this chapter when we talked about what happens to your body at a cellular level when you're dehydrated? By the time your cells are drying up, your thirst cravings have kicked in. So be proactive with your water intake rather than reactive.

A good time to start your water consumption is in the morning when you first wake up, a minimum of ten minutes before breakfast. Even though I don't recommend eating early in the morning when you first wake up, I do recommend having a big tall glass of filtered water. You should also drink water ten to thirty minutes before you eat instead of drinking during your meal because it can affect how well your stomach digests and breaks down the food you eat. You don't want to disrupt your digestive system and interfere with the process of digestion.

ENHANCING ABSORPTION

Absorption is not just about drinking a lot of good water. It's also about how much you absorb. If it runs right through you, you are left in the same boat with no water to float in. You want to make sure the water is getting into your cells. As it turns out, much of your ability to absorb water has to do with how healthy your cellular membranes are. In order to pull water into the cell there needs to be a high electrical charge across the cellular membrane. [64] Without this high electrical charge your body will struggle to pull water and nutrients into your cells. This is what happens with dehydration. As you dry up at a cellular level you are speeding up the aging process because your body's cells are less able to bring nutrients in and expel waste products out. A hydrated body is much healthier on multiple levels.

Here are some other things you can do in addition to drinking mineralized water.

- *Increase your Potassium:* Eat leafy green veggies. Spinach, chard, kale, and other greens have a good amount of potassium to help you absorb more water. You can also get lots of potassium from fruits like bananas and avocados. They also contain a lot of fiber which will help the large intestine absorb water. The daily recommended intake of potassium for adults is 4,700 mg. One banana contains about 400 mg of potassium. In Chapter 6: Fuel to Thrive I recommend having a green drink loaded with a good amount of potassium every day.

- *Chia Seeds:* Most of the water we consume is absorbed in the large intestine (colon). Chia seeds contain soluble fiber which soaks up the water. In fact, chia seeds absorb twelve times their weight in water. This water is then carried to your colon where it is slowly absorbed. Sometimes I add chia seeds to my green drink in the morning to boost my plant-based omega-3s.

- *Fulvic Acid:* This humic compound comes from the earth. It is naturally found in soils, rock sediments, and different bodies of water. Back in the day we were exposed to a lot of fulvic acid naturally when playing outdoors in the dirt and soil. As kids we got dirty and it was a good thing. Not so much these days. However, it is recommended by some health professionals and wise medical doctors to supplement with fulvic acid. According to Dr. Zach Bush, MD humic compounds support your cellular membranes, "...allowing for greater cellular hydration." This also means it will help your cells take in more micronutrients. Along with these benefits Dr. Bush points out that it causes your mitochondria to ramp up the reactive oxygen species production in the cells while helping reduce oxidative stress and reduce the aging process. [64,65]

- *Reduce Exposure to EMF Toxicity:* We are constantly being bombarded by high frequency radio waves from all wireless technologies, i.e. cell phones, wireless routers, cell towers, blue tooth, anything wireless! This high frequency radiation interferes with cellular communication and when we are dehydrated the interference is even worse. As Dr. Bush explains, our cells are connected by "10's of thousands of gap junctions, [which] are tubules that resemble fiber optic cables when viewed under electron microscopy. Electrical light energy is sent from one cell to the next across these gap junctions. Healthy cell populations are then one concurrent mass of electrical energy [tuned into their own frequency]." EMF exposure, along with other toxic exposure (chemicals, heavy metals) can damage these junctions between the cells and ultimately screw up cellular communication by reducing this frequency resonance between cells. When cells become toxic due to dehydration and there is less electrical resonance between them – it makes them more prone to "tuning in" and resonating with the high frequency radio waves, otherwise known as the wrong frequency. [64]

ALL WATER IS NOT CREATED EQUAL

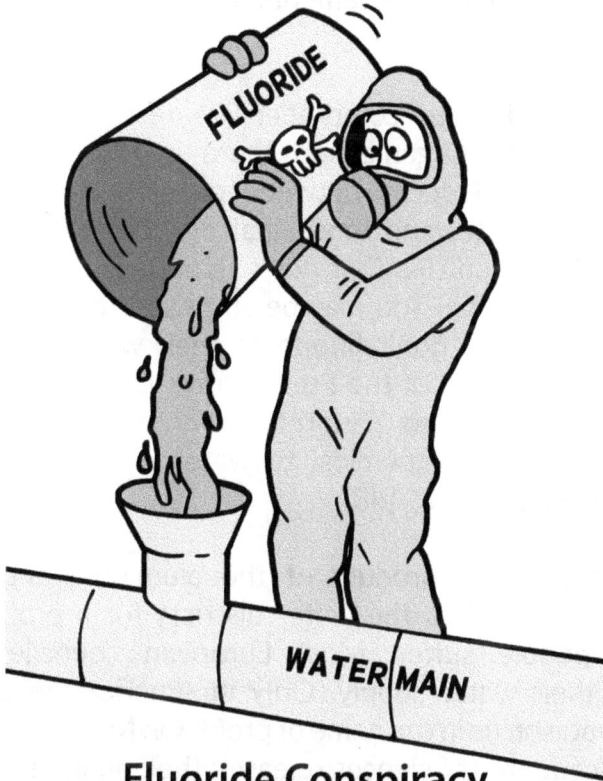

Fluoride Conspiracy

"In point of fact, fluoride causes more human cancer death, and causes it faster than any other chemical."
--Dean Burk -- Congressional Record 21 July 1976

What sounds better to you, "highly filtered water" or "tap water?" Probably the highly filtered water, right? If you have read anything about tap water, you probably know enough not to drink it. Tap water is toxic due to the fluorosilicic acid (form of fluoride) that is added by most water treatment facilities throughout the U.S. This is done due to the FALSE notion that it helps to protect against dental cavities. The CDC has called water fluoridation one of the "top ten public health achievements of the 20th century" because of this false notion. [66]

However, according to comprehensive research compiled by the World Health Organization there is **NO DISCERNABLE** difference in tooth decay between developed countries that fluoridate their water and those that do not. [67] Tooth decay has declined in countries that don't fluoridate their water. This is a significant finding! You may be surprised to learn that most developed countries don't fluoridate their water. According to Hardy Limeback, head of the Preventative Dentistry Program at the University of Toronto, "Fluoridation is no longer [considered] effective. Adding the chemical to water is more harmful [for humans] than beneficial." [68]

Fluoride is a waste product of the aluminum and fertilizer industries. It is sold to the water districts for a profit and the American people suffer. Most European countries do not fluoridate their water supply. Only in America are companies allowed to poison us in the name of profit. On March 22, 2006, the National Academy of Sciences released their analysis of fluoride. The publication stated, "The EPA standard [of just 4mg/L] does not protect against adverse events – [and people drinking water at those levels have an increased risk of bone fractures over their lifetime]." [69]

The history of fluoride reeks of conspiracy which involves companies like Alcoa who produced aluminum for Germany prior to World War II. This gave Germany a distinct military advantage over America. Today Cargill is one of the largest producers of Fluoride and it comes as a by-product of fertilizer production in the form of silicafluoride. To date no studies have been done on the possible health hazards of this toxic compound. [69]

On the side of a tube of Crest toothpaste there is a warning label regarding the active ingredient sodium fluoride. It states, *"Warning keep out of reach of children under 6 yrs. of age. If more than used for brushing is accidentally swallowed, get medical help or contact a poison control center immediately."* The FDA requires this warning label because if a child swallows enough toothpaste containing fluoride, they could suffer acute fluoride poisoning. Some brands of fluoride toothpaste contain enough fluoride to kill a child weighing less than 66 lbs. [70] So if sodium fluoride in toothpaste is this bad, how is it somehow safe in our tap water? There is about 0.7 to 1.2 ppm of "manmade" fluoride in bottled water (0.11 ppm on avg.), which is 14 to 24 times higher than the naturally occurring level in fresh spring water. [71]

Listed below are some of the possible health hazards that can occur after ingesting fluoride.

- Cancer
- Fluorosis
- Neuro behavioral effects
- Pineal gland calcification
- Increased risk of hip fracture
- IQ effects in children

(compiled from *Waking Times*) [68]

NOTE: High amounts of fluoride are found in **cheaply formulated teas**. It's also in some pharmaceutical drugs, especially **antipsychotic medications**. Lastly, it can be found in most **processed beverages** like beer, wine, and fruit juices. [72]

To find out if our tap water was fluoridated, I looked up our municipal water district online and clicked on "Frequently Asked Questions." According to the website fluoride is not added to the water in my city. But just to be sure I also emailed them. As a rule of thumb, I assume all tap water is fluoridated and toxic and therefore choose to only drink filtered water.

WHERE DO DENTISTS STAND ON FLOURIDE?

According to Dr. David Kennedy, D.D.S, "...more damage has been done to animals and crops in the United States from fluoride pollution than any other pollutant." [73] I would expect you to find this just as alarming as I do. Kennedy also stated, "Once you put fluoride in the water it ends up in everything – especially in boxed and packaged foods."

The American Dental Association heavily endorses fluoride as a proactive way to prevent cavities so when a dentist like Dr. Kennedy speaks out against it, I start paying attention. Why would anybody want to risk their reputation and maybe even their license by speaking out against their profession's standard of practice? And he isn't the only dentist speaking out against the dangers of fluoride.

"Once you put fluoride in the water, it ends up in everything – especially in boxed and packaged foods."

- Kennedy

There are a lot of more toxic substances in water than just fluoride. Another harmful toxin in our drinking water is chlorine. Chlorine is the second lightest halogen and it is an extremely reactive element. [74] Chlorine is a particularly good disinfectant, but it reacts with organic compounds in water and forms hundreds of chlorine by-products called DBPs. One such DBP compound is trihalomethanes *(THM)* which are carcinogenic. THM is classified as a Group B carcinogen, meaning it has been shown to cause cancer in laboratory animals. [75]

CHORLINE, HEALTY WATER, AND FILTERS

In a research article published in the journal *Environmental Health Perspectives* and authored by Manolis Kogevinas, MD, PhD, Professor of Epidemiology at the Centre for Research in

Environmental Epidemiology in Barcelona and his research team, they looked at 49 non-smoking healthy individuals after they swam in a chlorinated pool for 40 minutes. The took blood and urine samples and found an increase in "risk markers" related to cancer. This was just from swimming in a pool! [76] So what are the potential biological hazards that could occur from not only swimming in it, but showering in it and drinking it?

The Environmental Protection Agency claims that Americans are getting 300-600 times the amount of chlorine that is considered safe. "According to the U.S. Council of Environmental Quality, the cancer risk to people who drink chlorinated water is 93% higher than among those whose water does not contain chlorine." [77] With all the alarming research which has come out warning us about the dangers of drinking, bathing, and swimming in chlorinated and fluoridated water, it is best to protect yourself and your family.

Now you ask, "How exactly do I protect myself and my family from these toxins?" I assume the tap water in my community is toxic. Having this assumption saves me time and energy. I would suggest you do the same. Most municipal water treatment facilities use chlorine as a disinfectant and according to the CDC in 2012 75% of the U.S. population were served fluoridated water. [78] Their intended goal is to get that percentage to 80% by 2020. Therefore, I think it's safe to assume your tap water is toxic. My recommendation is to not drink tap water. This is the only way to ensure you are not ingesting these chemicals and to protect you and your family from these toxins.

Tests done on tap water across the U.S. have found:

- Chromium-6 (a cancer causing chemical, watch the movie Erin Brockovich)

- Mercury (a heavy metal linked to brain damage and neurological issues)

- Lead (a heavy metal linked to autism and prostate cancer)

- PCBs (a chemical created by Monsanto for industrial purposes)
- Arsenic (a poisonous metalloid element – think rat poison)
- Perchlorate (used in rocket fuel and explosions – attacks thyroid)
- Dioxins (released during combustion – considered carcinogenic)
- DDT (an insecticide in 1940's, banned in 1972 – causes liver and reproduction issues)
- Herbicides/Fertilizers (carcinogenic)
- Pharmaceutical compounds (birth control, antidepressants, etc.) [79]

The only water we drink in our home is highly filtered. The water we drink goes through a thirteen-step filtration process and is slightly alkalized at 8.5 pH with trace minerals then added back in (Ion Thrive System). When it comes to the water you and your family use regularly, you should want nothing but the best!

Cheap filters are good at getting some of the toxins out, like heavy metals and odors, but are not very good at getting the pesticides, fluoride, fertilizers, herbicides, chromium 6, chlorine by-products, bacteria, viruses, pharmaceuticals, and the thousands of other chemicals found in water. I would recommend going beyond the cheap filter in your fridge or water pitcher. Your number one goal should be to make your water as clean and pristine as possible.

I also recommend purchasing carbon filters for your shower heads. Good carbon filters help remove between 80-99% of chlorine, toxic chemicals, and radon from your water. [75] In fact, most of the chlorine you absorb is absorbed through your skin. You can find decent carbon filters for your shower on Amazon for twenty-five to thirty dollars.

Note: I would recommend changing the filters every six months and only taking mild to medium warm showers as filters don't work as well when using hot water.

You may be able to find a health food store in your city or a neighboring city that has a water filtration system. In our town there are three health food stores within a five to ten-mile radius that have their own water filtration systems. We take our five-gallon containers in and fill them every week. It costs about fifty cents a gallon. It's not the most convenient thing to do so we combine these trips with grocery shopping to kill two birds with one stone.

Ideally, we would want to drink fresh spring water containing a few trace minerals and nothing more. But of course, this is not possible. If you're looking for a more home-based filter solution there are whole house filters and filters for underneath your sink. The cost to do this, of course, is initially higher, but you will save money over the long run. I recommend using a reputable system that not only removes toxins but adds minerals back in (re-mineralizes). The last step of any good filtration system would be to re-mineralize your water.

Distilled water is good, but it has no minerals. Reverse osmosis filtered water is good, but it too strips out the minerals that help to hydrate the body.

ALKALIZED WATER

Proponents of drinking alkalized water tout the amazing health benefits, even though there isn't a lot of scientific evidence to support those claims. There is, however, a lot of anecdotal evidence to support the theory that drinking alkalized water is better for you. In addition, there are some scientific studies to support that alkalized water hydrates better than drinking regular water.

One study took thirty-eight healthy young adults with similar activity levels and split them into two groups: Experimental Group & Control Group. Both groups were tested over a four-week time frame. The experimental group was given placebo water (non-mineral water) on the 1st and 4th weeks and high mineral content water (the alkalized water) on the 2nd and 3rd weeks. The control group was given the placebo water all four weeks. The experimental group showed a significant increase in blood and urine pH and less urine output, while the control group had no changes whatsoever. [80] So does this mean we should all be drinking alkalized water? Not necessarily.

The term alkalized water means that it has a higher pH than water that hasn't been alkalized. Alkaline water and food have a pH above 7, which means there are less hydrogen ions and more hydroxide (oxygen and hydrogen bonded together) ions. Acidic water and food have a pH below 7. A standard pH scale is from zero to fourteen. Seven is smack dab in the middle which means it's neutral. [81]

Alkaline water has a pH of 8-10, while regular water is around 7 or lower. There are different pH values in our body depending on the organ and fluids. For example, your stomach is very acidic, it has a pH of 1.2 to 3. The acid in the stomach is needed to breakdown proteins, bacteria, and viruses. Your blood, which is considered an organ, has a pH of 7.365 making it slightly more alkaline in nature. [82] If our bodies were to become too acidic, a condition known as acidosis, or too alkaline, a condition known as alkalosis – we could die. The bottom line is balance is key.

Natural spring water has a pH level anywhere between 6.5 to 9+ and always contains trace minerals. These trace minerals help your cells maintain optimal cellular fluid levels. [83] Before all these fancy "alkalizing" machines were created, what did we drink? We drank from the rivers and streams which consisted of trace minerals. Water picks up minerals naturally as it flows through rock and soil. The minerals alkalize the water which helps the intestines with absorption. Remember, we want to **ABSORB** the water we drink, not just urinate it out of us. According to Dr. Bush if your urine is clear that means you aren't hydrated. Bush says your urine should be a light-yellow color (straw color), which is an indication that your body is getting the water into the cells. [64]

There are two versions of alkalized water worth mentioning. One version uses the chemicals magnesium sulfate, potassium chloride, trace amounts of sodium minerals, and other minerals to artificially raise the pH. Usually these are added to the water after it has gone through a filtration process. For example, Evian bottled water has a pH of 7.4 and contains several minerals (sodium, potassium, calcium, magnesium).

The other version worth mentioning uses electricity to separate water into acid and alkaline components. This process, known as water electrolysis, has been used for over 100 years to make "Electrolyzed Reduced Water." [84] This process involves "disassociating" the water molecules or splitting them up into Hydrogen ions (H+) and Hydroxyl Ions (OH-). As mentioned above, when water has more OH- ions than H+ ions the water becomes more alkaline. This restructuring allows the water to be rapidly absorbed into the cells. And because the hydroxyl ions have a negative charge it makes them particularly good free radical scavengers or antioxidants. Free radicals are a byproduct of cellular metabolism. They are unstable molecules that increase oxidative stress inside the cell.

Oxidative stress "ages" us because of what it does to us at a cellular level. Again, free radicals are unstable molecules making them highly reactive and thereby able to damage the components that make up the cell (i.e. cell membrane, mitochondria, proteins, lipids). Free radicals "increase cell membrane rigidity" and "alter cell permeability" because they react with the lipids (fats) present within the membrane. [85] Because OH- ions have that negative charge they will absorb the unstable free radicals and neutralize them, so they won't cause any damage. A measurement for this is called oxidation reduction potential (ORP). Ionized water has a higher ORP than regular water and chemically alkalized water and can be measured using an ORP Meter.

The key word with drinking water is absorption. The ionization (electrolysis) of water creates a micro-clustering of the water molecules. Normally water molecules are weakly bonded together via hydrogen atoms which form clusters or groups of ten to twenty molecules per cluster. When you zap water with electricity it "weakens these bonds restructuring the molecules into roughly half their original size, or five to eight molecules per cluster." [86] This allows for quicker absorption by the body's cells. The body's cells have small channels called aquaporins which act as the cell's plumbing system. Micro-clustered water can permeate the aquaporin faster than regular water.

I once witnessed a very cool test where the absorption rate of ionized water was compared to the absorption rate of tap water and alkalized bottled water. One tea bag was placed into three separate glasses. Alkalized water was added to the first glass, tap water to the second glass, and ionized water to the third glass. Both the tap and alkalized bottled water only had a hint of color change within ten to fifteen seconds. However, when the ionized water was poured into the glass the color change was instant. The water instantly became the dark color of the green tea. This suggests that the ionized water is absorbed faster by the cells as compared to the two other waters. These micro-clusters can be measured using nuclear magnetic resonance imaging. The evidence was so convincing to me that this is the only kind of water my family and I drink.

Water is essential to life. And yet most people walk around dehydrated. I bet, you, the reader, are dehydrated and you don't even know it. This is because your body cries out for water in subtle ways. I stole the above quote from a phenomenal book titled, *Your Body's Many Cries for Water*, by Dr. F. Batmanghelidj, MD. So, step numero uno is to drink more water. Did you know that many holistic doctors feel most health problems could be resolved if people were to drink more of the "right" kind of water in conjunction with living a healthy lifestyle? Drinking more water should be your first line of focus. Many so-called miracles of people healing everything from allergies to cancer have been proclaimed by people who started drinking better water, and lots of it!

"Thousands Have Lived Without Love, Not One Without Water."

W.H. Auden [87]

At the very least start drinking more purified spring water by finding a local health food store where you can buy filtered water. Pay attention to how you feel. Tiredness and brain fog are common but not so well-known symptoms of dehydration. And when all else fails, try drinking more water because you're probably not drinking enough. When you combine proper water consumption with a healthy diet it will catapult your health into another level!

"Time and health are two precious assets that we don't recognize and appreciate until they have been depleted."

- Dennis Waitley

CHAPTER 6

FUEL TO THRIVE

If it tastes good spit it out!
And if it's made by man don't
eat it.

- Jack Lalanne

In this chapter I intend to give you the fundamental principles that will help guide you to make better decisions regarding your nutrition.

Hippocrates, the father of modern medicine, said, "Let your food be thy medicine and medicine be thy food." Within this timeless statement lies the profound truth that food is the great energy healing fuel source of the body. As Americans we typically live to eat as opposed to eating to live. The foods we choose to eat can either help us to thrive in life or merely survive. I believe one of the main reasons we're so sick in this country is because we don't eat enough "real" foods that will help us thrive. Instead we eat an abundance of synthetic "food like" substances, overly processed foods, and foods that are completely void of any nutritional value.

For example, one is hard pressed to find any food that is completely safe and non-toxic for consumption. There is really no question that anything you find in the supermarket, no matter how "organic" it is still contains trace amounts of heavy metals, pesticides, and other toxins. You simply cannot find something in the supermarket that doesn't in some way, shape, or form poison you at the same time. This is primarily due to the over industrialization, processing, and manufacturing of our food. We will delve more into this later in the chapter.

FOOD VS. POISON

Let's start with two fundamental definitions written in the 1927 book entitled, Chiropractic Textbook, Vol. XIV, written by R.W. Stephenson.

> *"Food is any substance ingested into the body, which when digested and otherwise prepared furnishes wholesome nutrition to the tissue cells."* [88]

> *"Poison is any substance introduced into or manufactured within the living body, which Innate cannot use in metabolism."* [88]

The bottom line on food is this: proper food is going to fuel the body and provide you with energy while "fake food" robs your body of energy and vitality. One form of food gives and the other takes away. Fake food is in fact *poison*.

"Innate" in this context is referring to the invisible intelligence within the body that coordinates every function to maintain homeostasis. Innate keeps the matter within your body in active organization. If your body can't metabolize or utilize a substance you ingest, your body must adapt and neutralize it to maintain homeostasis. This taxes your body and can eventually lead to sickness and disease, especially if you choose to poison yourself daily.

An example of a poisonous substance can be something as benign sounding as a Twinkie or Hostess Cupcake and as volatile sounding as strychnine or arsenic. How poisonous a substance is for the body has a lot to do with its potency and the amount ingested. Water for example can be poisonous if too much of it is ingested at once.

In fact, a twenty-eight-year-old Sac, California woman died due to the excessive amount of water she drank as part of a radio show contest. This is called water intoxication, or water poisoning. Anything can become poison if too much of it is consumed, but poisonous substances will always be toxic to the body, even in trace amounts. Over time a little bit of poison consumed daily becomes a lot of poison consumed over a lifetime. This would gradually lead a person down a road of sickness and ill-health. [89]

My point in all of this is that you should become more aware of the things you are choosing to put down your gullet because they can literally be killing you slowly – this is called a soft-kill.

A general rule of thumb to follow is that the closer a food is to its natural origin, or nature for that matter, the healthier it is going to be for you to consume.

In the 20th century changes were made in the agricultural industry that moved the foods we eat further away from nature. The industrial revolution of agriculture brought about drastic and devastating changes to the American farm. In the early part of the 1900's more than half of Americans were farmers, or they lived in rural communities. Most farmers practiced diversification which meant they had a variety of different crops and animal species on the same farm. Foods were grown in nutrient-rich soils that contained an abundant amount of minerals. The chemical pesticides used today were virtually non-existent. The livestock could roam freely outdoors and get exercise. They were also fed a diet that was more suited to their biology. [90]

The agricultural industrial revolution gave rise to specialization where farmers went from a diversified approach to only managing one to two crops. This was great for the farmer because it made things efficient, but it came with a cost. With this specialized form of farming, farmers planted the same one to two crops in the same place year after year (monoculture). The problem with this is that when you plant the same crop in the same place for years on end the soil ends up nutrient depleted which doesn't provide for healthy plant growth. Therefore, farmers are forced to use chemical fertilizers which are toxic for the environment and toxic for human consumption. Monocultures also lead to more pests. More pests result in toxic pesticides and insecticides used to kill them. The final products are fruits and vegetables that are void of nutrients and loaded with toxins. A similar problem exists with animal farming. [90]

ANIMAL PRODUCTS

Despite the efficiency and increased profits, the industrialization of our primary protein sources in this country has also led to a lot of issues. Whether we are talking about the fish, poultry, eggs, dairy, or meat industry, mass-production (factory farming) is a problem. These concentrated animal farm operations (CAFOs) result in inhumane living conditions and cramped living spaces which makes the animals extremely sick. When there are too many animals confined in a small space and they aren't able to roam freely as they would in the wild, not only does their health suffer but disease flourishes. [90]

Take poultry for example, tens of thousands of chickens that are raised for meat (broiler chickens) are confined to huge metal sheds with no sunlight. The air quality is poor. The air is usually dense with particulate matter from ammonia, feces, feathers, and dust. Sadly, the chickens end up with severe respiratory problems, bacterial infections, and other diseases. Because of this, antibiotics must be used in the animal's feed to combat bacterial infections. This inevitably leads to antibiotic resistant bacteria, otherwise known as "super bugs." To the chicken farmer antibiotics serve a twofold purpose because they also slow down the chicken's metabolism causing them to become fatter faster. In addition to antibiotics, growth hormones and genetic selection have also been used to make chickens grow much larger. In fact, they are much larger than they were seventy years ago which causes heart, lung, and joint problems. Many chickens end up crippled. By the time the chickens are slaughtered they are sick and barely alive. Some studies show by the time your chicken breast hits your plate it may be infected with salmonella and other nasty pathogens. Do you see my point here? [91]

If the animal was sick before it died, you certainly aren't eating something that is healthy for you.

When it comes to animal products, factory farming has really screwed things up. Whether it's beef farming, fish, turkey, pork, or chicken – it's the same theme. Too many animals are:

- confined to cramped living conditions

- fed genetically modified grains (usually corn) which they were never designed to eat

- loaded with antibiotics which fight infection and fatten them up

- given growth hormones

- sick

- slaughtered before they would otherwise die of a wide range of diseases like acidosis.

Again, the farther our food sources are away from "the natural," the sicker we become.

Before the meat hits your plate, it is irradiated. Irradiation is a process where ionizing radiation in the form of x-rays, gamma rays, or high energy electrons are used to kill off microorganisms, bacteria, and molds that spoil food. As it pertains to meat, these pathogens are picked up mainly from the fecal contamination that occurs as a result of the sheer volume of animals that are slaughtered in a slaughter facility. One of the largest meat processing companies, Smithville Foods, for example, can slaughter up to 36,000 pigs per day at their North Carolina location alone! But here's the thing, rather than dealing with the root cause and cleaning up the industry, irradiation deals with the effects. Although irradiation kills most of the pathogens, like e-coli for example, it damages the molecular structure of the meat. This creates free radicals which wreak havoc on the vitamins and enzymes contained therein. Some studies show that irradiation destroys 5 to 80% of vitamins A, K, E, C, and B complex. The free radicals can also create something called unique radiolytic products (URPs) which happens when they combine with other chemicals on the food. Long term studies on the irradiation of our foods have never been done. Therefore, we don't know the long-term consequences of eating foods that have been irradiated. [92]

PROTEINS

You might be surprised to hear that we really don't need all that animal protein in the first place. In fact, you can get all your protein requirements from a full-on plant-based diet. And there are plenty of all-natural plant-based body builders who are healthy. If we really needed all that animal protein to support muscle growth and thrive, how are there vegan bodybuilders who've been able to build lean and muscular physiques without animal products? Some of the largest and strongest animals on the planet are 100% herbivores. Not to compare humans to animals but it's interesting that some of the world's strongest animals (silver-back gorillas, buffalos, giraffes and hippos) aren't even, at the very least, omnivores. I find that amazing! They eat a diet solely consisting of incomplete proteins and yet have an unbelievable amount of muscle and strength.

First, we need to define what protein is. Proteins are made up of strings of amino acids in various sequences which are determined by your body's specific requirements (i.e. tissue repair, muscle growth, enzymatic actions). Different combinations and amounts of the amino acids determine the specific type of protein. There are twenty amino acids split into two groups, nine non-essential (the body makes) and eleven essential amino acids (can only get from diet). A complete protein is comprised of all nine essential amino acids your body needs while an incomplete protein only contains some of the essential amino acids your body requires.

The "protein myth" is propagated on the idea that we need to consume meat because it contains complete protein, fulfilling all our body's essential amino acid requirements. However, when we eat meat the protein is first broken down by our stomach into smaller chains of amino acids which are then broken down further into individual amino acids by our small intestine. The individual amino acids are then absorbed through the microvilli of the small intestine and released into the bloodstream. If protein is broken down within the body into its individual amino acids anyway, couldn't we just eat a variety of plant-based foods to get all of our essential amino acid requirements? The truth is we can. It's also important to note that when you overcook meat it will denature the proteins and can make them harder to digest and breakdown. The denaturing process of meat is what gives it its brown color. Heat sensitive amino acids like lysine get destroyed at high temperatures which would make the protein in meat incomplete. Therefore, it is best to slow cook meat at lower temperatures. [93]

Brown rice with lentils, black beans, or kidney beans will give you your protein requirements for the day. You don't even have to eat these plant-based combinations at the same time. You can eat a variety of different plant-based foods throughout the day. Your body will combine the different proteins you eat from different plant-based sources to form complete proteins as needed. The key word here is VARIETY. Therefore, when choosing a vegetarian diet, you need to make sure you are eating a variety of plant-based foods.

Here is the rub, I am not advocating that you give up all animal-based foods if you don't want to. All I'm saying is that you can get your protein from plants. Besides, I realize there are some health benefits to eating healthy organic animal foods. However, I specifically advocate not to eat animals or animal products that are factory farmed.

If you are going to eat animal – you might as well get the best of the best which means grass-fed and ORGANIC.

Over the last five years I have stuck to mainly a plant-based-diet and have noticed several improvements in my overall health. First, I was able to maintain muscle mass; I didn't deflate. In fact, I have been working out every week since I was eighteen years old, and I didn't stop once I went plant based. Within the last five years I have gained muscle weight going from 185 lbs. to 200 lbs., entirely fueled by plants. I have noticed a difference and improvement in my cognitive abilities and energy patterns. I even opened my own chiropractic office and have had the energy and the stamina to build it successfully. I'm not alone in this either. There's plenty of anecdotal evidence to support the health benefits of switching to a plant-based diet. There are a lot of people who heal themselves of all sorts of diseases and ailments on a 100% plant-based diet, which goes against the grain of traditional thought. The well-known but controversial all-natural Gerson Therapy Method for detoxing the body and helping people to heal from all sorts of chronic diseases, including *some* cancers, utilizes only a strict plant-based diet. [94]

DAIRY IS SCARY

The dairy industry is another industry of controversy. The clever advertising slogan that "milk does a body good" is a myth. Yet in this country we love our milk. I have heard the question posed, "Why are we the only species in the animal kingdom that drinks another animal's milk secretions and think it's actually good for us?" Hmm, maybe it's because the USDA tells us to consume three servings of dairy per day as part of a healthy diet! As it turns out the USDA Dietary Guidelines Committee has members directly connected with the dairy industry! This is called "Politics 101" - they have a vested interest in making sure Americans regularly consume dairy. Can you say, "Conflict of interest?" Once you take a deep dive into the industry itself it is likely you will never consume dairy again. [95]

**How healthy the animals are during their lifespan plays a
direct role in the quality of the animal-food product
and how healthy it is for you.**

Starting at about fifteen months of age the dairy cow is brutally impregnated using artificial insemination because just like humans, she must give birth to produce milk. Once she gives birth to her calf the calf is removed within thirty-six hours. This distresses her to the point where she will bellow for days and sometimes weeks calling for her calf. If the calf is male it will be slaughtered or sold for veal which is a nasty industry in and of itself. If the calf is a female, she will live out the same meager existence as her mother. [96]

The cows are usually milked three to four times per day while standing on concrete. The amount of work the cows go through just standing in one position for hours leads to a crippling lameness. Milking for hours every day also leads to mastitis, a potentially fatal infection of the mammary tissue. As a result, a certain number of white blood cells called somato cells end up in the milk. The USDA allows for up to 750,000 somato cells per milliliter of milk. Therefore, farmers must give their cows antibiotics to keep the infections at bay. These antibiotics end up in the dairy products you consume. "Got pus?" would be a more honest advertising slogan for the dairy industry. [97]

Pasteurization is the process in which a liquid is heated to 165° F or higher to kill off bad bacteria. The problem with this is the heat is not selective and it also destroys the beneficial bacteria which is needed to help build a healthy gut and strong immune system. It also destroys other beneficial nutrients in milk like the enzyme phosphatase which helps you to absorb the calcium in milk. If you can't absorb the calcium in milk how can it be good for your bones? Pasteurization also destroys an enzyme called lipase which is needed by your body to help complete the breakdown of fats. Pasteurization even destroys or severely decreases vitamins B12, C and D. In fact, food manufacturers will replace the vitamin D destroyed in the pasteurization process with synthetic vitamin

D which is never as good as the real thing! Is it any wonder why the countries with the highest levels of dairy consumption have the HIGHEST numbers of osteoporosis, the U.S. being one of them? The absolute opposite is true for countries with the lowest milk consumption. Hmmm, that should make you think. [98]

Milk also contains high amounts of estrogen because dairy cows are impregnated by artificial insemination while still secreting milk from their previous pregnancy. Milk from pregnant cows contains far higher hormone levels than milk from nonpregnant ones – five times the estrogen during the first two months of pregnancy according to one study and a whopping thirty-three times as much estrogen as the cow gets closer to term. [99] A study was done using seven men, six prepubertal children, and five women. All the subjects were given dairy milk to drink. This was the shocking outcome.

"After the intake of cow milk serum estrone (E1) and progesterone concentrations significantly increased and serum luteinizing hormone, follicle-stimulating hormone, and testosterone significantly decreased in men. Urine concentrations of E1, estradiol, estriol, and pregnanediol significantly increased in all adults and children. In four out of five women, ovulation occurred during the milk intake and the timing of ovulation was similar among the three menstrual cycles." [100]

Why does this matter? Increased estrogen has been linked to the development of many cancers including prostate, uterine, ovarian, and breast cancer. Dairy has even been linked to young girls starting their periods before hitting their teenage years and early breast development. For men, having lowered testosterone levels can affect a variety of issues including loss of bone mass, decreased muscle mass, mood changes, decreased sperm count, difficulty sleeping, and a decreased sex drive among other things. [101]

Some dairy cows, especially conventional "non-organic" cows, are injected with Monsanto's recombinant (genetically engineered) bovine growth hormone (rBGH). Cows treated with this genetically engineered hormone produce 10 to 25% more milk which is great for the dairy farmer. So, what's the problem? The milk from cows injected with this hormone has been shown to contain increased levels of insulin-like-growth-factor (IGF-1) which promotes tumor growth. There is also a higher incidence of mastitis in rBGH-injected cows which equates to more antibiotic usage. [102]

The bottom line is we never needed the dairy in the first place. We just fell for the clever marketing schemes of the dairy industry. We once thought the dairy industry was just like the beautiful pictures on their packaging. The truth of the matter is dairy cows live out a horrible existence and that directly affects the quality of the end-product. Whether it's cheese, cottage cheese, creamer, whole fat, or non-fat milk, it's simply not good for you. There are better non-dairy options out there like nut milks (almond, cashew, hazelnut, etc.). If dairy is a must for you, the absolute best option would be organic grass-fed raw milk and cheese. Raw dairy is always more expensive and tends to be harder to find. This is mainly because raw dairy farmers aren't subsidized. I have enjoyed raw dairy products myself, but I primarily consume unsweetened organic nut milks.

SUGAR

Another powerfully addictive food culprit that has plagued America's health is sugar. American's love sugar and food manufacturers know this. Manufacturers add sugar to everything to make their products taste better. In fact, there are about sixty-one different sugar additives that manufacturers utilize in varying combinations to make their products taste better. [103] For example, if you were to read the ingredient label on many kinds of packaged products in the grocery store you might see the words high fructose corn syrup, maltose, sucrose, dextrose, dextrin, and rice syrup among others. And they don't just put it in packaged junk food either. They put it in **EVERYTHING**. I'm not sure if I can emphasize that point enough. Sugar is added to everything from almond milk, to tomato paste, to cereals, to almond butter. It is in everything! You get it?!

This is how the average American unknowingly consumes seventy-two grams of sugar per day which equals seventeen whopping teaspoons! If we were to add all this sugar up the average person is eating fifty-eight pounds of sugar per year! Obviously if a person consumes high amounts of sugar like this year after year, it's going to be disastrous to their health. And with obesity rates sky rocketing, Americans should be genuinely concerned with the amount of sugar they are consuming. [104]

Physiologically we know excess sugar leads to increased weight gain and the reason for this is clear. Because sugar is toxic the body works hard to protect us from large amounts of sugar circulating in our blood stream by storing it as fat. If our bodies weren't intelligent enough to do this, we wouldn't live long. In fact, some researchers think the reason why the body stores excess sugar as fat around our waists and hips is to keep it away from our organs. Excessive amounts of fat around your organs and within them, like in the case of fatty liver disease, severely disrupts their function. A healthy body has less than a teaspoon of sugar (glucose) in the blood stream at any given time or about 80-100 mg/dl. According to the American Diabetes Association a person is a diabetic when their fasting blood sugar levels are over 126 mg/dl. This means that the difference between a healthy person and a sick person is merely a quarter of a teaspoon of sugar! To get there, however, takes years. [104]

To receive a diagnosis of Type II diabetes you must EARN it. It's often a seven to ten-year process in the making. Consistently eating excess sugar, and foods that convert to sugar fast (breads, rice, pastas, etc.), in combination with a sedentary lifestyle eventually leads to prediabetes and then diabetes if steps aren't taken to drastically reverse it. The good news is that diabetes (type II) can be reversed, but it's important to understand the mechanism behind it in order to reverse it.

First, sugar is not all bad. In fact, both glucose and oxygen are used by the mitochondria in the cells as energy sources. Glucose is also so essential to the function of your brain that your body has several strategies to maintain normal blood sugar levels using protein and fat. This is what happens when a person is on a zero-carb diet. The foods that are broken down into glucose for energy are called carbohydrates. Carbohydrates are comprised of fiber, starch, and sugar and can be broken down into three categories: Simple, Complex, and Refined. Simple and refined carbohydrates will cause your blood sugar levels to rise much faster than complex carbs because the fiber has been stripped, leaving just the sugar and starch. Refined foods are going to be your sodas, juice concentrates, syrups, packaged sweets (candy and cookies), white breads, and cereals. Foods that are considered complex carbohydrates are your whole grain breads, unprocessed grains (quinoa, barley, buckwheat), fruits, veggies, beans, and tubers (root veggies). The more fiber a complex carbohydrate contains, the slower it is converted to glucose in the body. Examples of these kinds of foods consist of vegetables grown above the ground, such as legumes, lentils, and fruits with high fiber skins (apples, blueberries, etc.). [105]

The glycemic index is a scale used to assess how quickly carbohydrate foods convert to sugar and raise your blood sugar levels. The index rates foods on a scale of 1-100. According to the American Diabetic Association foods given a number of seventy and higher are considered high glycemic foods. Foods rated from fifty-six to sixty-nine are considered medium glycemic foods and anything below fifty-six is considered low. Pumpkin has a high glycemic index vs. sweet potatoes which are rated low. Quick oats have a medium rating. What the glycemic index doesn't account for is portion size (glycemic load) and how the food is prepared. Obviously, the more carrots you eat for example, the higher your blood sugar levels are going to go up. And if you juice the carrots which strips away all the fiber, your blood sugar levels will skyrocket. [106] (For a thorough GI list, see the appendix).

It's also important to note that if you combine your carbohydrates with healthy fats (coconut oil, olive oil, sesame oil, avocados, nuts, and seeds) and fiber (leafy greens) it will slow down the digestion process and how fast your body breaks down a food into glucose. Foods like flax, pumpkin, and chia seeds are a great combination of both fat and fiber. We want to slow down how fast our bodies convert a food into glucose and we want a gradual rise in our blood sugar levels as opposed to a radical rise. [107]

When our blood sugar levels rise, insulin, a hormone produced by the pancreas is released into the blood stream which tells the liver, muscle, and fat cells to "open up" and accept glucose. Once the liver and muscles have stored up all the glucose they need as glycogen any excess glucose is converted to fat. Eating a consistent diet that is high in carbohydrates, especially simple carbs, and sugary food like substances, puts our pancreas into overdrive. As more and more insulin is pumped out (hyperinsulinemia) the liver and muscles become insensitive to insulin which leads to a condition called insulin resistance which then leads to hyperglycemia. It's a vicious cycle. This also leads to increased triglycerides and fats in the bloodstream which are stored in the adipose tissue. Hence, this is why obesity rates are through the roof. This is also why insulin is known as the fat storage hormone. [108]

One major sign of a healthy person on a cellular level is their sensitivity to insulin. A healthy body that is sensitive to insulin has a much easier time regulating blood sugar levels and maintaining balance as opposed to somebody who has insulin resistance. A person who suffers from insulin resistance will usually have huge spikes in their blood sugar levels after a meal, followed by a huge dip in blood sugar levels hours later. They're on a blood sugar roller coaster ride as they go from hyperglycemia to hypoglycemia. This negatively impacts their energy levels as well as their ability to think. Brain fog, for example, is a common symptom of low blood sugar levels. The good news is that a healthy diet, intermittent fasting, sleep, increased water intake, and exercise can improve your sensitivity to insulin which will undoubtedly increase your energy levels – more on this later.

> *"The Higher Levels of Healthy Energy you have in Life*
> *Equate to a Higher Quality of Life Lived."*

Dr. Jay

Does sugar "feed" cancer? Better yet, can it cause it? What's interesting about cancer is that it has a high rate of glucose metabolism. Cancer is extremely metabolically active which is what makes it so dangerous and it uses glucose as its primary fuel source. A PET scan is an imaging test used to diagnose cancer. Doctors inject the person with a radiotracer which is radioactive glucose because the cancer cells eat up glucose faster than healthy cells. A doctor can easily detect cancer, see if it has spread, and determine whether or not treatment is working from reviewing results of the scan. If sugar is what cancer thrives on, shouldn't we be more mindful of how much sugar we consume daily? Absolutely we should. [109]

In 1968 a study (Project 259) was funded by the Sugar Research Foundation to see how sucrose (table sugar) affected the bacterial organisms in the GI tract of rats vs. those fed starch. The author of the study noted that the rats who were fed a basic diet of starch contained an inhibitor of the *enzyme beta-glucuronidase* in their urine vs. the rats fed sucrose. At the time of the study research had already been done showing the link between increased beta-glucuronidase and bladder cancer. As soon as this link was made by the author of the study the Sugar Research Foundation stopped funding the study. Coincidence? Probably not. [110]

There's a lot more research pointing to the correlation between sugar and cancer than I want to go into in this book, but I do need to discuss artificial sweeteners!

ARE ARTIFICIAL SWEETENERS BETTER?

First, any artificial food like substance consumed is toxic to the body regardless of the amount consumed. One of the arguments I hear a lot of times is, "But everything in moderation Dr. Jay." My response is always, "What is a moderate amount of poison to be putting into your body?" Artificial sweeteners are no exception to this rule as they are completely toxic for human consumption. In fact, the history of artificial sweeteners is loaded with conspiracy, conflicts of interests, controversary, and tens of thousands of health claims. These alone are enough to say, "Don't consume them, take caution!"

THE BIG FAKE FOUR

The artificial sweetener Cyclamate which used to fill the tiny pink packets of Sweet N Low was banned in the late 1960's after it was proven to cause bladder cancer in rats, only to immediately be replaced by saccharin.

Saccharin is a derivative of coal tar that was discovered in the early 1900's which may be carcinogenic. It also has been linked to diabetes and weight gain. The FDA even required a warning label to be placed on all products containing saccharin up until the year 2000. [111]

In 1981 another controversial player called aspartame came to market. Otherwise known as NutraSweet or Equal. Aspartame has been used to sweeten everything from bubblegum, to diet soda (Diet Coke), to a ton of products that say sugar free on the packaging. This sweetener is about 200 times sweeter than real sugar and it is extremely addictive. It's chemical composition of 50% phenylalanine, 40% aspartic acid, and 10% methanol makes it a potent neurotoxin.

In fact, the world-renowned neurosurgeon, Russel Blaylock, M.D., described aspartame in his book *Excitotoxins* as a potent excitotoxin, meaning it "excites" nerve cells in the brain to death.

This is one of the main reasons why aspartame has been linked to several neurological disorders including multiple sclerosis and Alzheimer's Disease. Other research shows a possible link between aspartame and a wide range of health issues including cancer, seizures, dizziness, headaches, depression, and ADHD, to name a few. According to Dr. Betty Martini, the Founder of Mission Possible International, aspartame brings more complaints to the FDA than any other food additive. [112]

How aspartame was approved for consumption in the US is one big conspiracy involving G.D. Searle, Donald Rumsfeld, Monsanto, and Dr. Arthur Hull Hayes which goes to show when you mix money with politics you get *BAD* politics.

It's a shame that people still consume aspartame. Needless to say, natural is always going to be better than artificial. It would be best to avoid artificial sweeteners all together as they cause major interference.

The last artificial sweetener I want to touch upon is Splenda because in my opinion there is nothing splendid about it. Splenda, aka sucralose, came about in 1976 because scientists figured out a way to bond sucrose with chlorine. If it sounds like weird science that's because it is. The FDA approved sucralose for use without ever proving it was safe for human consumption – more shady politics. One of the most astonishing things I found about Splenda during my research was a 2008 study which found a small dosage of sucralose (1-11mg/kg) significantly decreased the gut microbiome in rats after twelve weeks of administration. The significance of this has to do with the connection between your gut and immune system. Scientists are only now unraveling the mystery of how trillions of good bacteria in your gut play an intricate role in your immune system. Roughly 70% of your immune system is in your gut. When your gut is negatively affected, mainly due to diet, toxins, and stress, it can cause your body's immune system to attack its own cells. This is all the more reason to eliminate toxins from your diet, including Splenda. [113]

ARE THERE HEALTHIER OPTIONS?

The best option is always going to be to extremely limit the amount of sugar you consume daily, especially refined and processed sugar. This also means extremely limiting your consumption of carbohydrate containing foods (breads, rice, pastas, refined foods, potatoes, high glycemic fruits – melons, pineapple), especially if you have been diagnosed with a disease. Popular diets like the Paleo Diet and most recently the Keto Diet, are both very restrictive on carbohydrate consumption. Healthy protein and fat intake are at the core of both these diets, with the principal goal being to get your body to utilize fat and protein for energy instead of sugar. This not only helps for weight loss, but it also radically reduces inflammation which is the number one culprit for all diseases. In a sense a person becomes a "fat burner" instead of a "sugar burner" on these diets. But know that if you must go sweet there *are* healthier sweetener options.

By now I'm sure you have heard all the wonderful things regarding stevia and how it's a great "all natural" sweetener. Stevia is an herb that has been used as a medicinal tea for centuries as it has a vast array of health benefits. However, when discussing the health benefits of Stevia, we are mostly talking about the whole leaf which of course *isn't* approved by the FDA. The stevia you find at your local grocery store is the highly processed version and therein lies the problem.

Whenever you take a plant and use commercial processing techniques to extract the isolates it can have a negative effect on your biochemistry. The store-bought versions are usually loaded with a bunch of fillers, and shockingly even sweeteners! For example, the popular brand "Stevia in the Raw" lists dextrose as its number one ingredient and stevia leaf extract second! Here is the rule, if you're going to use stevia, get the least unadulterated version, which means avoiding the fillers and added sugars. Adding sugar to a no calorie sweetener sort of defeats the purpose of using it in the first place, don't you think? [114]

Xylitol is a sugar-alcohol used in many products as a substitute for sugar because it doesn't raise blood sugar levels. It occurs naturally in some plants, however, the kind used to sweeten bubblegum and packaged foods is highly refined. The more refined a substance is the less likely it's going to be good for you. In fact, too much xylitol can lead to digestive issues like gas, bloating, diarrhea, and some people even report that it causes them headaches. Xylitol has no nutritional value and is considered an empty calorie. When used in moderation it can be a great alternative to sugar and artificial sweeteners when you need to add a bit of sweet into your life. Make sure to buy non-GMO, organic, and the least refined versions of the product. This of course means study up on the products you buy for your household. [115]

WARNING: Although xylitol is generally considered safe for humans it is not safe for your pets, especially dogs.

THE LOWDOWN ON FATS

There is more controversary and misinformation surrounding dietary fat than any other food group. Scores of non-sense dietary books have been written encouraging people to go low-fat. Along with that the "Tel-LIE-vision" via the media has done a great job of propagating the myth that fat is bad for you and makes you fat! So called "nutritional experts" in the "Mercedes 80's" and early 90's also took the available mis-information and vomited it out through every major media channel. I can remember my mom buying low-fat dairy products and snack foods for our home thinking low fat somehow meant healthy. To this day food manufacturers still advertise on their packaging the words "low fat" and people keep buying into the myth. Fat has become enemy number one and yet the BRAIN is the FATTEST organ in your body. Yes, your brain is made up of nearly 60% fat! But "by all means America," continue to starve your brain of this extremely valuable macronutrient. [116]

Two things you need to know: Good fat is good for you and bad fat is bad for you. Seems a bit self-explanatory, right? But let's dive deeper into it.

"Bad Fats" are a modern-day invention. Highly processed and refined polyunsaturated vegetable oils like corn, safflower, sunflower, and canola (rapeseed) are made up of an overabundance of omega-6, omega-9, and trans-fats. An overabundance of these fats in the diet increases inflammation and has been proven to cause cancer. There are even studies that link these nasty fats to insulin resistance. These bad fats are also a major cause of heart disease. You cannot find any of these highly processed fats in nature, thus a major reason why they cause so much interference with our body's ability to normally function. These refined oils can be found in over 4,000 packaged products at your local grocery store. [117] Most salad dressings, for example, contain canola oil as a top ingredient. Potato chips contain one or more of these refined oils as well.

The war on fat started in the 1950's due to the ever-increasing rise in cardiovascular disease. It was determined that saturated fats caused LDL levels to rise. LDLs are considered the "bad cholesterol" because they clog your arteries and cause cardiovascular disease. The problem with this level of thinking is that LDLs can't necessarily be a bad thing if your body naturally produces them. This level of thinking was based on the research of Ancel Keys who linked an association between the amount of saturated fat communities ate and their incidence of cardiovascular disease. However, Keys failed to look at the entire picture such as the amount of sugar and processed foods people were eating on top of everything else. Keys only found an association between saturated fat and heart disease and never proved unequivocally that this was indeed the cause. Keys used his false information and influencing powers to join the nutritional committee for the American Heart Association (AHA). And what I find interesting is that in the 60's the AHA took a huge donation in the sum of 1.7 million dollars from Proctor and Gamble, the makers of Crisco! [118]

Traditionally Americans have eaten animal products containing a considerable amount of saturated fat. This would be your red meats, bacon, egg yolks, and of course, butter. After skewed research started coming out linking these saturated fats to heart disease the USDA went to war on the traditional American diet coming out with new dietary guidelines. This would eventually lead to our current standard American diet or SAD for short. The main staple of the USDA dietary guidelines at the time, and even to this day, recommends that Americans consume a lot of whole grain-based foods and low-fat dairy and animal meats. We know that a high carbohydrate diet consisting of grains leads to higher blood glucose levels, but what you may not have known is that low-fat products contain a lot of refined SUGAR!

So, food manufacturers took heed of this incredible opportunity and launched the era of highly processed unsaturated fat (low-fat) food like substances. They replaced the vilified healthy saturated fats with highly refined vegetable oils (Trans Fat) and refined sugars. In fact, they are so heavily refined and processed that they NEVER go bad! And if a so-called food never rots, common sense says – DON'T EAT IT. Hence, therefore Jack Lalanne said, "If it's made by man, don't eat it." [119]

The problem with these man-made trans-fats is that they clog you up at a cellular level. Every single cell in your body is surrounded by a cellular membrane. This membrane is composed of a phospholipid bilayer, cholesterol, and protein. The membrane is responsible for letting nutrients into your cells and expelling waste. It also plays a crucial role in cellular communication which is how one cell communicates with its environment and other cells. Unfortunately, your cells can't determine the difference between a healthy fat or a bad one. When it comes to trans-fats they are absorbed into the cellular membrane where healthy fats should be. This screws up cellular transport, making it harder for the cell to take in nutrients and expel waste. It also negatively impacts cellular communication leading to a wide range of problems. Once inside the cell membrane, your body can't get rid of these fats very readily which means they will accumulate over the long run. Thus, the symptoms show up years to decades later. Hundreds of studies have shown that trans-fats cause a variety of deleterious effects. [120]

Some examples of Trans-Fat Problems [116, 121]

- Increased coronary heart disease
- Increased LDL and decreased HDL
- Increased risk of heart attack and stroke
- Increased CRP levels (measure of inflammation)
- Makes arterial walls soft and weak, but also stiff leading to abrasions, injury, and plaque buildup
- Trans-fats pass from the placenta to the developing baby negatively impacting the baby's metabolism
- Diets high in trans-fats seem to correlate with a higher rate of Type II Diabetes
- Infertility
- Weakened bones
- Prostate cancer
- Liver dysfunction

I'm not surprised to see that trans-fats, like fully hydrogenated and partially hydrogenated fats and oils are still used in many products today. The reason why food manufacturers love using hydrogenated oils in their products is because it gives them a longer shelf life – sometimes years. To make hydrogenated oils the food manufacturers breakdown healthy seeds and beans (soy, corn, sunflower, safflower, rapeseed, cottonseed) using chemical solvents. Then as a final step hydrogen gas is added under intense pressure and heat. This saturates the polyunsaturated fat with hydrogen atoms which is what makes it stay solid at room temperature. [122] So rather than getting a healthy fat, what you end up with is a "Fraken-Fat." This Fraken-fat is added to everything from twinkies, to cake mixes, to fast food French fries (it's in the oil used in the fryer). It can be labeled in the ingredients as partially or fully hydrogenated vegetable, cottonseed, safflower, sunflower, and coconut oil or sometimes it's more covertly labeled as shortening or margarine. Margarine is still touted as a great alternative to butter, but it's loaded with trans-fat!

Instead of banning ALL foods containing trans-fats like other countries have already done (Denmark), the FDA allowed manufacturers to label only whether their products contained trans-fat or not. The problem with this is multifaceted. First, the FDA is heavily influenced by industry and lacks the proper concern for the American public – time and time again this has proven to be the case. Second, as long as the food contains 0.5 grams of trans-fat PER SERVING or less the FDA has permitted the manufacturers to label their products as having, get this... ZERO grams of trans-fat! [117] So all manufacturers must do is make their servings smaller and "wallah" you get zero grams of trans-fat! This little loophole has led to millions of Americans consuming bad and unhealthy products because they say the words Healthy, trans fat Free, or zero grams of trans-fat, when all along they contain this silent killer! It's INSANE! Arguably this is one of the main reasons why heart disease is still a top killer.

Let's do some math...

If a person eats four servings of a product containing 0.5 grams of trans fat, then they have unknowingly consumed two grams of trans-fat. Let's say conservatively that they consume roughly two grams of trans-fat per day for seven days. That equates to fourteen grams of trans fat. Multiply this by fifty-two weeks and you get 728 grams of trans-fat! Remember, this is a conservative estimate. We'd being doing well if this was all the average American consumed. Sadly however, it's not even close!

A study published in a 2007 issue of the journal "Topics in Clinical Nutrition," reported that the average American is consuming 5.6 grams per day! Multiply this by 365 days and you get 2,044 grams of trans-fat consumed per year! [123] This doesn't surprise me!

HEALTHY FAT?

In order to be healthy, we must eat an abundance of good, healthy fat! Whether it's saturated, monosaturated, or polyunsaturated, as long as it's healthy it's good for you to consume it. We should also be using fat as our primary fuel source vs. carbohydrates. When your body becomes a fat burner vs. a sugar burner you not only lose weight, but you also improve the quality of your life. In fact, Dr. Joseph Mercola states,

> *When your body is able to burn fat for fuel, your liver creates ketones that burn more efficiently than carbs, thus creating far less reactive oxygen species and secondary free radicals that can damage your cell membranes, proteins, and DNA. [120]*

This notion that the preferred fuel of the body is glucose and that saturated fat is bad for you is a pervasive myth that has led to many of the health problems we see today. There are so many great foods that contain an abundance of healthy fat we need to be consuming. In this chapter I have listed several amazing, healthy fat containing foods that you should eat more of.

BENEFITS OF HEALTHY FAT

Any healthy fats are going to be good for your body, including saturated fat and cholesterol. The main thing is that they must be as close to their natural form as possible. Coconut oil for example, is made up of a ton of saturated fat and has some amazing health benefits. In fact, coconut oil is about 50% lauric acid which is a medium chain fatty acid. It is broken down into monolaurin which has great anti-microbial properties (viral, bacteria, parasite). Medium chain saturated fats work as an immediate source of energy for the body because they skip the gallbladder during digestion and easily enter your bloodstream. [124] Long chain saturated fats help with the structure and integrity of cellular membranes. They also help your brain, are used in protein metabolism, and help to fuel the muscles and the heart. [125]

FAT BREAKDOWN

Saturated Fat

Saturated fats are thus named because they have no double bonds in their structure and are "saturated" with hydrogen atoms. This allows them to remain solid at room temperature. As mentioned above, food manufacturers love taking a polyunsaturated oil and saturating it with hydrogen atoms via the hydrogenation process because it gives their products a longer shelf life. The problem with doing this is that it creates a ton of trans-fats. It's also important to note that saturated fats like raw butter and virgin coconut oil are going to be your best fats to cook with because they are highly resistant to oxidation at high heat levels. A good rule of thumb to follow is that if the oil starts to smoke in the pan it has gone bad.

EXAMPLES OF GOOD SATURATED FATS:

- Virgin coconut oil

- Raw butter

- Raw dairy products (cheese)

- Beef from grass-fed cows (proper balance of omega-6 to omega-3 fat ratio)

- MCT oil (medium chain triglycerides)

EXAMPLES OF BAD SATURATED FATS:

- All refined oils

- Canola oil (GMO rapeseed oil)

- Meat from grain fed animals (including fish, poultry, pork, and beef)

Monosaturated Fat

Monosaturated fat has only one double bond in its structure therefore making it easier for the body to digest. This makes it a great source of energy. Monosaturated fats help with insulin sensitivity and have been shown to reduce LDLs and increase HDLs which support cardiovascular health. [125]

EXAMPLES OF GOOD MONOSATURATED FATS:

- Avocados (my favorite). Interesting fact: Avocados contain more potassium than bananas!

- Olive oil (unrefined/virgin).

- Almonds, walnuts, pistachios, cashews, brazil nuts, hazelnuts, macadamia nuts, and pecans.

- Nut butters (almond, cashew). Make sure they are raw butters instead of roasted.

BAD MONOSATURATED FATS:

- Heavily refined oils (avocado, olive oil)

- Canola oil (usually highly refined and made from genetically modified rapeseeds)

- Peanut oil (peanuts are high in molds which produces aflatoxin known to cause cancer as well as inflammation)

Polyunsaturated

Poly means many or much, therefore polyunsaturated means that two or more double bonds are in its structure. Polyunsaturated fats remain liquid at room temperature and are very prone to becoming rancid when exposed to heat. This makes them terrible fats to cook with. However, polyunsaturated fats like omega-3 and omega-6 are essential for overall health and wellbeing. In fact, they are called essential fatty acids because our bodies don't make them. [125]

Omega-3s reduce inflammation, support healthy cell membranes, and healthy hormones, may help to prevent cancer, are good for the skin, and can even help with sleep. [125, 126]

Omega-6s support healthy brain and muscle function. The problem, however, is because of the Standard American Diet (SAD) Americans eat way too many omega-6 fatty acids which causes increased inflammation. [125, 126]

GOOD POLYUNSATURATED FATS:

- Wild caught salmon (contains a healthy amount of omega-3 fatty acids (EPA & DHA) and is loaded with protein and potassium.

- Flax seeds. Supplement that can be used ground, milled, or as cold-pressed oil. You can also purchase raw flax seeds and grind them yourself. Contains high amounts of alpha-linolenic acid (ALA), an omega-3 fatty acid found in plant-based sources. You can add flax seed to smoothies or put them on different foods you eat as a nutritional bonus.

- Pecans. Loaded with healthy levels of Omega-3 fatty acids. Also contain more than nineteen vitamins and minerals).

- Cod liver oil (A supplement rich in Omega-3s found in capsule or liquid form. It is extracted from the livers of cod fish. Also loaded with Vitamin A and D. Only buy the least refined version, i.e. extra virgin).

- Walnuts (Great to add to smoothies and loaded with fiber)

- Chia Seed (Rich in calcium and high in protein. Chia seeds are a great source of soluble fiber as well).

- Seaweed (Great source of plant based DHA & EPA omega-3 fatty acids.)

- Chlorella (A plant alga super food that is packed with nutritional properties. It contains more beta carotene than carrots and is loaded with protein. Chlorella also contains a ton of other nutrients including vitamins B, C, D, E, K, and minerals (calcium, phosphorous magnesium, zinc, iron). It's also a potent detoxifier in that it binds to heavy metals and helps safely remove them from the body).

- Spirulina (Like chlorella, spirulina is an alga that is packed with nutrients and protein. In fact, one teaspoon of spirulina contains four grams of protein and more protein per ounce than a steak.)

- Grass- fed beef (The ratio of omega-6 to omega-3 in grass-fed beef is optimal. Animals fed a good, clean, organic diet that is true to their biological make up ALWAYS have a better ratio of omega-6 to omega-3. Grass- fed beef contains two to five times more omega-3s than grain fed which balances out this vital ratio. Grass- fed beef also contains conjugated linoleic acid (CLA), another type of polyunsaturated fat which research shows is a potent antioxidant and can help reduce the risk of all three types of disease killers. Along with all these wonderful benefits, grass- fed also contains a lot more antioxidants, vitamins, and minerals than grain fed).

- Olive oil (cold pressed and best used as a salad dressing)

A WORD ABOUT CHOLESTEROL

Cholesterol is vital for the body. In fact, your body uses cholesterol in the production of many hormones such as testosterone, estrogen, progesterone, and cortisol. Cholesterol is so important for your health that your liver and intestines make most of it while approximately 20% comes from the foods you eat. When it comes to your brain, cholesterol is found in the white matter and is critical for normal function. Then what's wrong with this fat? It does a lot of good things and is needed by our body, yet we are told to avoid it at all costs. We have been plagued by the LIE that cholesterol is the bad guy because it causes plaque to buildup in the arteries leading to heart attack or stroke. But when you look at the body, our physiology tells us a different story. Our bodies NEED cholesterol, in fact, 90% of the cholesterol we consume is reabsorbed in the gut. When we starve ourselves of this vital nutrient the liver overcompensates by overproducing cholesterol from the carbohydrates we consume.

Ironically, we are told not to consume dietary cholesterol, therefore the liver goes into hyperdrive producing more cholesterol than we need. This of course raises total cholesterol numbers which is what prompts your doctor to put you on a cholesterol lowering medication (Statin). Statins work by poisoning your liver so it will stop producing cholesterol but at a detrimental cost. The danger of taking a statin medication is that it substantially depletes your body's own natural reserves of CoQ10. [116] CoQ10 is a coenzyme that helps to generate energy in your cells. Low levels of CoQ10 have been associated with several health conditions including brain disorders and heart disease, the very disease doctors prescribe statins to prevent. In fact, "CoQ10 may be the single most important nutrient for the functioning of the heart." [116] What is probably the most peculiar thing about statins is they have never been proven to reduce one's risk of having a heart attack which of course begs the question – "What is the point of taking them?"

Cholesterol is only a problem in the presence of systemic inflammation. Therefore, the standard eating habits of the average American (high-carbohydrate, high-sugar, and highly processed foods) are a problem. The standard American diet leads to widespread inflammation throughout the body. The inflammation causes the cholesterol to oxidize which leads to plaque buildup in the arteries. Another point to make here is that your HDL/LDL numbers are a snapshot of what is going on inside your body and serve mainly as an indication that you need to change your lifestyle. [116]

HDL and LDL are protein transport mechanisms for cholesterol – THEY AREN'T CHOLESTEROL. In fact, LDL isn't BAD! Again, if your body naturally produces it, how could it be bad? LDL takes cholesterol from the liver to the extremities and organs so your body can make things like vitamin D and important hormones. HDL grabs this used up cholesterol and returns it to the liver so it can be recycled. If cholesterol was so bad for you, why does your liver repeatedly recycle it?

Lastly, cholesterol is also used by the body to patch up areas of arterial damage created by systemic inflammation. Thus, LDL levels rise as a result of your body trying to *survive* in its current environment. Without this mechanism it is likely we would keel over a lot sooner. Taking a statin to artificially lower cholesterol and stop your body's natural response to systemic inflammation isn't the answer. Medicine has it all wrong! I like what Nora T. Gedgaudas, CNS, CNT states in her book, *Primal Body, Primal Mind*.

Going in with statin drugs to stamp out cholesterol is the equivalent of preventing the firemen who arrive to put out a fire from doing their job - and blaming them for the fire. Elevated glucose or insulin levels, for instance, damage arterial walls and lead to an increased need for cholesterol to repair them.

[116, Pg.]

Bottom line is you need healthy fat in your life. You must disparage the myths, the lies, and the misinformation you thought were right regarding this vital macro-food. Remember that fat doesn't make you fat, nor does it make you unhealthy. The only fat you want to avoid is bad fat. The other food or "food-like substances" you need to worry about are refined and simple carbohydrates, especially if they are consumed in excess! The refined carbs you find in a box or a package aren't "real" food anyway.

CALORIC RESTRICTION

One of the best things you can do for your health is restrict the number of calories you consume in a day and limit the number of hours you spend eating food. Caloric restriction is the one habit proven time and again to improve your health. In fact, in the animal kingdom whenever an animal is sick, they will abstain from eating to allow their body to fully heal and recover.

Digestion requires a tremendous amount of energy. So, giving your body a rest from the digestive process allows your body to utilize all the extra energy to cleanse, heal, and repair itself at a cellular level. In fact, fasting upregulates a cellular process called autophagy.

Autophagy is a process where your cells clean out old cellular components, mainly organelles, proteins, and cell membranes. This process allows your body to run more efficiently. This would be like replacing the old spark plugs or changing the oil in your car so your car will run better. Fasting causes an increase in the peptide hormone glucagon. Glucagon is released by your pancreas and causes your liver to convert glycogen into glucose. This process allows your body to maintain normal blood sugar levels during periods of starvation. The rise in glucagon is also what stimulates cellular autophagy. [127] In contrast, eating stimulates the release of insulin by the pancreas which downregulates this process. Therefore, leading nutritional experts are telling us to make fasting a daily practice.

BENEFITS OF FASTING

- Decreases inflammation
- Increases insulin sensitivity and glucose regulation
- Helps with weight management
- Helps to convert your body from a Sugar Burner to a Fat Burner.
- Decreases cortisol and increases melatonin (sleep hormone)
- Increases growth hormone (intermittent fasting)

When people hear the word "fasting" it can conjure up feelings of anxiety. The practice of caloric restriction is not a habit Americans are accustomed to. I'm here to tell you that it isn't all that bad, it just takes discipline. There are several different ways to fast. Technically fasting means to abstain from all or some types of food and/or drink for a period of time. This period can range from hours, days, weeks, and even for life. For example, a strict "vegan for life" person has chosen to give up animal products for the rest of their lives. Others may choose to give up simple carbs. For our purposes I am going to focus on short term (intermittent) and long term fasting from all food and caloric beverages.

The first book I ever read about fasting was written by Paul Bragg. The title was "Miracle of Fasting." In the book Bragg talked about fasting for one whole day out of every week and ten whole days every quarter. In his book he talked about being able to outpace and outlast ten young college athletes on an empty stomach while on a thirty-mile Death Valley hike. In fact, he was the only one who was able to finish the hike and he never got ill under the sweltering 130° F! The only thing Bragg put into his body that day was distilled water. [128]

Another beautiful example of fasting can be found in the Bible. Before Jesus was tempted by the devil he went into the woods and fasted for forty days and forty nights. One would think that having done a prolonged fast Jesus would be at his weakest, yet he was mentally strong enough to quote scripture to the devil and not fall into temptation (NIV, Mathew 4:1-11). If you think what Jesus did was a myth or absolutely impossible, know that others have done it as well.

Natural health guru and certified detoxification specialist Dan A. McDonald recently did a complete forty-day water fast – meaning he drank nothing but water for forty days. In forty days, he lost a total of forty-nine pounds. Once he completed the fast, he was able to healthfully return to 182 pounds on a raw vegan diet! He stated on his Facebook page:

"Don't listen to people who object to fasting. They don't truly understand health and healing. Diet and exercise are only half the equation. Periodic fasting and detoxification is just as important."

As mentioned above, fasting isn't really all that difficult to do, but discipline is key. The current popular way to fast is intermittent fasting. Intermittent fasting is done by giving yourself a very narrow window of time in which to eat, therefore spending most of the day not eating. Dr. Mercola recommends fasting for sixteen to eighteen hours per day. Although this sounds a bit daunting, it can easily be done if you refuse to eat anything past six or seven at night. If you stopped eating at 7:00 pm and had a late breakfast around 11:00 am, you could accomplish a sixteen hour fast. Mercola recommends only giving yourself a six-hour window to eat. He recommends this window be from 12:00 pm to 6:00 pm. [129] You could also start out by doing a ten to fourteen hours intermittent fast. The point is to figure out exactly what is right for you, but also give yourself some time.

The first three to seven days of an intermittent fast can be discouraging because you may feel like absolute crud. You can get headaches, feel lethargic, and you may even feel yourself becoming "sick." As said in previous chapters, feeling "sick" is your body expressing health. The symptoms are a result of your body going through a healing process. However, it's the unpleasant symptoms that cause people to discontinue their fasting program, but as Arnold Schwarzenegger appropriately said, "No pain, No gain." This is relatively true for your body as well.

The symptoms you may experience during a fast are due to several reasons. Here are some examples of symptoms you may feel when fasting.

Withdrawal

Eating multiple meals everyday as well as snacks in between has become the standard American way. We have become addicted to eating a robust amount of food multiple times daily. As a result, our bodies are physically addicted to eating. When you fast, a withdrawal affect occurs because your body must get used to the fact that you aren't eating an abundance of calories anymore. There is a transition that takes place as your body goes from burning sugar to burning fat.

Detox

Your body will also start getting rid of toxins that have plagued it. A lot of toxins are stored in your fat cells. Some of these toxins are persistent organic pollutants (POPs). POPs are comprised of industrial chemicals, pesticides, pharmaceuticals, and other chemicals. POPs do not break down very readily in the environment and end up bioaccumulating in the adipose tissue of all living organisms, mainly through diet. This means that the higher up the food chain you go the more POPs you are going to ingest and be exposed to. Things like DDT and Glyphosate (Roundup) will bioaccumulate in your fat cells, therefore, when your body starts burning fat for fuel the toxins are released into the bloodstream where they are processed through your liver and eventually eliminated out of your body through the excretory system. As toxins are released into your bloodstream it can create a "detox" effect that can set off a vast array of symptoms. Be aware that you might get worse before you get better. [130]

Hormone Imbalance

Your hormones, like insulin, ghrelin, and leptin go through a period of balancing themselves out during a fast. The standard diet tends to burn out the receptors on your cells which causes your body to adapt and release more of a particular hormone so your cells will respond, as with insulin resistance. There will be another transition period as your cells grow new receptors and your hormones balance themselves. This can cause problems with energy levels. In fact, in the beginning you may feel like you need to sleep more. I suggest taking more periodic *powernaps*, especially if you have a full-time job. This can easily be done in ten-minute increments in your car, on your couch, or outside on the grass!

A healthy pattern of eating should become your way of life. Unfortunately, the word diet has become synonymous with healthy eating. The problem is most diets tend to be short lived and are so far removed from anything healthy for us that they should just take the "T" right out of the word so you're left with only the word "Die." A positive change in the way you eat should become the normal.

So, here is a "Top Ten List of Rules" I have comprised for eating healthier.

Rule Number 1: *EAT LESS and FAST MORE*
To reiterate, eating less and practicing caloric restriction allows your body to work more efficiently. Give yourself a small window in which to eat your food and don't eat anything past 6 or 7 pm.

Rule 2: *EAT MORE GREENS & FRUITS*
In Genesis 1:29, God said to Adam and Eve, "*I give you every seed-bearing plant on the face of the whole earth and every tree that has fruit with seed in it. They will be yours for food (NIV).*" In this context it is clear that God designed us to be vegetarians. Even animals were originally designed to eat "every green plant for food." It was only after the fall of man that we started eating the flesh of animals. "A 2017 study published in JAMA showed that consuming just 3% less animal protein and replacing it with plant protein was associated with up to a 19% lower risk of death from **ANY** cause." [131]

One of the wonderful things about eating more greens and fruits is that they are loaded with phytochemicals that protect us from toxins. Plants are densely packed with vitamins, minerals, and antioxidants which we desperately need to live an abundant life. In the chapter I wrote on wheatgrass, I cover a lot about chlorophyll. Chlorophyll is what gives a plant its green color, and studies show it can help increase the red blood cell (RBCs) count in your body. Increased RBCs means that your body will be better at delivering oxygen to the tissues. Therefore, the greener the food the more chlorophyll it contains. Plant algae like spirulina and chlorella are rich sources of chlorophyll. My breakfast in the morning is always a healthy green drink loaded with protein which is ALL plant based. See the Appendix for my green drink recipe titled, "Dr. Jay's Green Drink Recipe."

Rule 3: *SHOP THE PERIMETER*
Shopping the outside of a grocery store and avoiding the middle sections are going to make it easier for you to find healthier food options. The center aisles usually contain nothing but highly processed and refined foods. Although there are some healthy options found in the middle of the store, as a rule of thumb avoiding the middle will serve you well. In the middle sections you literally need to become an expert food-label reader because most of the "food" items are found in a box or a package. Work on improving your ability to know what is in the foods you eat.

Rule 4: *BUY ORGANIC & NON-GMO*
It's important that you invest in foods that contain less toxins and are healthier for you. Organic foods tend to mean better nutrition and less toxins. We already know organic grass-fed beef contains more CLA and a better ratio of omega-3 to omega-6 fatty acids than factory farmed meat. And, organic produce means slightly better nutrition and ultimately less toxins. About 150 years ago we never needed the term organic because most foods were "ALL natural." Today the term is used in labeling food that hasn't been heavily sprayed with pesticides and herbicides or grown using synthetic fertilizer. For animal products, the term means that the animals weren't given growth hormones, antibiotics, and other toxic chemicals as part of their upbringing. It also means the animals weren't genetically engineered, they were raised outdoors and ate natural organic non-GMO grass and feed.

I must warn you, however, because there's a dark side to the organic industry and you can't just trust a product because it says "organic" on the packaging. You must do your due diligence and study up on the products you buy to ensure that you are buying the healthiest products available. Organic produce and fruits contain a five-digit bar code that starts with a nine (Organic Bananas = 94011), while conventional produce has a four-digit bar code that starts with a four (Conventional Bananas = 4011). For meat, eggs, and dairy products you must read the packaging to determine whether it is grown organically or conventionally. Also, you can get to know your local farmers by going to your local farmer's market and finding out their farming practices. There are also plenty of online sources that will deliver high quality organic food right to your front door at a good price!

Rule 5: *CUT BACK ON ANIMAL PRODUCTS*
Even though I have been a vegetarian for the last five years, I still think there is some benefit to eating healthy animal products. but my feeling is that we need to eat way less. In fact, you don't have to eat the flesh or excretions (Milk) from animals every day. Too much animal protein leads to fatigue and a buildup of uric acid in the body. If uric acid isn't detoxed from the body fast enough, it ends up in bodily tissues forming "crystals." This leads to inflammatory arthritic conditions like gout. It can also cause bladder stones and kidney stones. Though it's interesting that some people with rheumatoid arthritis have reported that their symptoms improved drastically when they switched to an all plant-based diet and/or choose to cut out red meat.

Too much animal protein has been shown to increase the workload on the kidneys because it increases the blood flow within the kidneys. Over time this could cause damage to the kidneys, although no conclusive studies have shown this to be fact. However, studies do show that people with kidney damage have a worsening of symptoms when they eat a high protein diet. My recommendation is to always buy the healthiest forms of meat, fish, and animal products. Make sure to always buy organic – non-GMO! Stay away from factory farmed meats and fish. And remember that you don't have to eat animal protein every day to be healthy.

Rule 6: *JUST SAY NO TO "NUKING" YOUR FOOD*
Isn't it funny that microwaving your food is considered "nuking" your food? Have you ever considered why there is a slang term used to describe microwaving your food? I haven't used a microwave in years, but I remember when I was a kid that if I microwaved food in a Tupperware container for too long the plastic would melt! Odds are, you know what I'm talking about. I also remember that the food would come out piping hot and sometimes there would be a rubber-like texture to it.

Anytime your food is piping hot you can rest assured that you just destroyed all the nutrients in it. Microwaves work by heating the water molecules in the food. This is because the water molecules resonate with the high microwave frequency which essentially cooks the food from the inside out. A study published in the Journal of Agricultural and Food Chemistry showed that vitamin B12 was changed from the active to the inactive form and there was a 40% loss of the vitamins in foods that were microwaved. [132]

I found an article in The Journal of Pediatrics which showed breastmilk heated in a microwave for thirty seconds on both high and low settings resulted in the destruction of powerful bacteria-fighting agents. [133] Still other studies showed microwaves can create carcinogens, change the components in your blood, and even change your heart rate. [134] There is no need to use a microwave; they are merely a convenience and not a necessity. Cooking food fast for the sake of convenience is always going to negatively impact the quality of the food you eat.

Rule 7: *DRINK MORE WATER*
In the chapter I wrote on water I discussed the need for people to drink an adequate amount of highly filtered water. Most people barely drink enough water and with all the diuretics people drink regularly (coffee, tea, soda, and alcohol) it's imperative that

people make sure they are staying fully hydrated. Our bodies are comprised of roughly 70% water! And our cells need water to be able to absorb the nutrients from the foods we eat and to flush out toxins.

Unfortunately, by the time you feel thirsty you are already well into a state of dehydration. So, pay attention to what your body is saying to you. Once your urine is a light-yellow color you know that your cells are absorbing the water. The first thing you should do in the morning is drink a full glass of clean, pristine water. For more specifics on what kind of water to use, refer to Chapter 5 as a reference.

Rule 8: *EAT DINNER WITH THE FAMILY*

As Americans, we need to get back to our foundational core fundamentals and values that built this great nation – which is to say we need more quality family time. I remember several years of my youth sitting down at the dinner table and eating with my family. It was a time for us to spend good, quality time together and slow down. When it comes to eating food, it's good to slow down, chew more, and take your time.

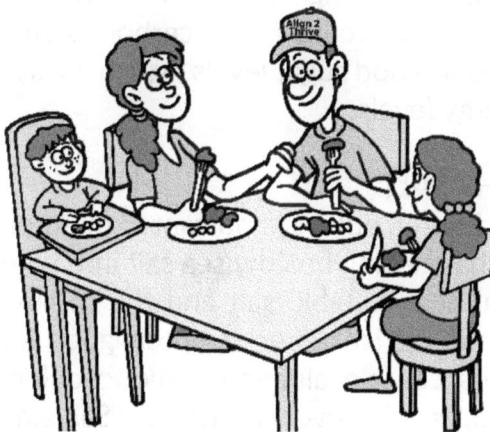

Having dinner together as a family serves two purposes. You receive insight into your kids and spouses lives *and* you are less likely to wolf down your food. Science shows that slowing down to eat is good for your health too! Slowing down to eat gives appetite suppressant hormones which control hunger, enough time to signal to the brain that you're full and to stop eating. What's even more amazing is that studies show obese people tend to eat faster than those who maintain a normal weight. [135]

The easy way to eat less is to slow down and have a conversation with your loved ones while you eat.

Rule 9: EAT MORE HEALTHY FAT, NOT LESS
We talked a great deal about eating healthy fat in this chapter. Hopefully, you are now convinced that eating more good fat is a necessity for living a healthy life. Coconut oil is one healthy fat that you should be consuming on a regular basis. It is loaded with great medium chain FAs and as we discussed previously, is one of the best oils to cook with. Healthy omega-3 FAs found in wild caught fish are essential as well. You can also get omega-3s from healthy vegetarian options like organic nuts and seeds. I always add a healthy fat option to my green smoothies. Usually raw almond butter or a full avocado.

Remember that healthy fats also help your body to absorb fat soluble vitamins and slow down the digestive process. Simply slowing down how fast your body breaks down carbohydrates into sugar will help stabilize your blood sugar levels, which always lead to more sustainable energy levels.

Rule 10: EAT MORE HEALTHY SALT
I didn't talk about salt in this chapter, but it's important to mention here. Current research says that getting healthy sea salt into your body is essential for optimal health. Table salt and the sodium used in a ton of packaged products isn't even remotely good for you. In fact, many table salts contain aluminum, monosodium glutamate, and processed sugar. However, Celtic Sea Salt and Himalayan salt contain essential minerals along with sodium and potassium to help your body function. The key thing to know is that healthy forms of salt are vital to the body because they help you to stay hydrated. To stay hydrated your body needs to have a good balance of sodium and potassium, making natural salts the best option vs. table salt. Sodium is also critical for your nerve system because it helps to balance water flow and is required for sending and receiving signals (electrical conduction). [136]

The biggest thing you can do regarding eating healthier is to use your gut instinct – no pun intended! You must use your commonsense radar to find what works for you and your body. Everybody is different, but there are universal laws that apply to everyone. For example, highly processed and refined foods are bad for everybody, refined sugar is bad for everybody, artificial sweeteners and hydrogenated oils are bad for everybody. Don't think you can have your cake and eat it too and not face any consequences. Ultimately, as far as the exact right diet regimen, research seems to suggest that intermittent fasting and eating less throughout the day is the healthiest way to go. Caloric restriction is still the most uncomplicated and best thing you can do for yourself overall. I have used my own body as a guinea pig and have been able to figure out what works and what doesn't work for me. But I'm also constantly refining my diet according to my lifestyle.

I hope you use the information in this chapter as a guide to help you discover the right eating habits for you and your family. Nutrition is a vast subject and trying to tackle it in one chapter was a challenge to say the least, hence, why it is my longest chapter. As always, I would encourage you to do your own research, but don't get lost in a sea of analyses.

In a world plagued by self-induced interference, diet is probably one of the biggest factors. We need our nutrients; however, we seem to struggle with getting our nutrients from diet alone.

"Take care of your body, it's the only place you have to live."

- Jim Rohn

CHAPTER 7

THE POWER OF WHEATGRASS

Drinking grass just might
save your ass.

- Dr. Jay

For many people the idea of eating grass grosses them out. They think eating or juicing grass is for hippies. But if they understood the powerful healing benefits in a blade of grass, maybe they would adjust their thinking. In this chapter I will talk about the amazing benefits of wheatgrass and why it is considered a superfood, especially by many of us health nuts. My hope is that after reading this chapter you will change your thinking and be inspired to get more of this powerful substance down your gullet and into your system. I also hope you will add the power of wheatgrass to an otherwise healthy diet!

I always knew that wheatgrass was amazing, but whenever I tried it, I would get nauseous and couldn't get over the "grassy" taste of it. I eventually was able to get over my nausea and negative conditioned response. I knew it was too good not to consume and so I figured out a little trick to help me out, but more on that later.

There is no doubt that one of the biggest reasons Americans are so sick is because we consume an incredibly SAD diet. As discussed previously, SAD stands for *Standard American Diet*. Unfortunately, the SAD diet is void of the necessary micronutrients that create abundant health. This modern day pattern of eating consists of: A high amount of red meat, processed meats and foods, packaged foods, fried foods, dairy products, eggs, white breads, sugar, and flower, heavily refined grains, genetically modified foods, high amounts of corn, products that contain ingredients comprised from corn, potatoes, and refined sugars. Moreover, Americans drink copious amounts of alcohol, soda, and coffee. This is a recipe for disaster! [137]

Is it any wonder why we are, quite literally, one of the sickest industrialized countries on the planet? I believe this "disaster diet" to be one of the chief culprits as to why we are so plagued with disease in this country. I also believe it to be one of the chief reasons we take more medications than all other industrialized countries. We are so far removed from nature and what we need to do to thrive, it has turned us into survivors. Hence, the question, "Are you thriving or just surviving?" To thrive in life, we must get back to nature.

You're not going to find the nutrients you need to truly thrive in all those processed foods or synthetic food-like substances. You find the nutrients in the plants. The largest mammals (remember the silverback gorilla in Chapter 6?) eat a diet that consists mainly of leafy greens! WHY?! Because that's where most of the vitamins, minerals, and antioxidants are found! The greener the food the more nutrient dense the food is. The problem is Americans don't like greens, so we don't eat enough of them, or we just avoid them completely.

We also discussed chlorophyll in Chapter 6. It's what makes many green foods so powerful, remember? Wheatgrass is green due to chlorophyll. This pigment is responsible for making plants green and it is also considered the blood of the plant. This powerful molecule converts sunlight into energy within the plant. Wheatgrass is approximately 70% chlorophyll, a remarkably high amount. The fascinating thing about chlorophyll is that its structure is almost identical to human blood. In fact, Ann

Wigmore, founder of the Hippocrates Health Institute, points out in her book, *The Wheatgrass Book*, that a study done in 1930 showed that injecting chlorophyll into healthy animals increased their red blood cell count! Since then, numerous studies have been done showing the positive benefits of chlorophyll for the blood and the body. [138]

When I drink wheatgrass juice, I feel energized! Perhaps this is because it helps my body create more hemoglobin as some studies have pointed out. Increased hemoglobin means your blood will carry more oxygen. Oxygen rich blood to your brain, as well as other organs and tissues, means that they will function better. It also has a powerful detoxing effect and can help rid your body of carbon monoxide, other pollutants, and even some heavy metals.

When we eat a diet rich in greens, we are ingesting not only the energy of the sun, but vital nutrients as well. That's why I call wheatgrass a nutrient rich food! In fact, the nutrient density in about one ounce of freshly squeezed wheatgrass is equivalent to 2.2 lbs of leafy green veggies. Wheatgrass is heavily loaded with iron, copper, calcium, and vitamins C, B-12, K, A, folic acid, and pyridoxine. There is more vitamin C in wheatgrass than oranges and it has twice the amount of vitamin A compared to carrots! Did I mention that wheatgrass is up to 30% protein and contains ALL essential amino acids?! Along with chlorophyll, these nutrients are also essential blood building components. [139]

WHEATGRASS IS A SUPERHERO

Below are some evidence-based conditions and symptoms that wheatgrass has been proven to help and/or alleviate: [140, 141]

- Inflammation
- Reduction of cholesterol
- Cancer
- Blood sugar regulation
- Gastrointestinal issues
- Diabetes
- Detoxification
- Skin issues (*eczema*)

- Weight loss
- Infections

- Arthritis
- High blood pressure

Let's explore the detox capabilities of wheatgrass a little more since that is one of the main things it's known for. The chlorophyll in wheatgrass helps to purify the liver. And, as I like to say, "You need your liver to live." Your liver is one of the largest organs in your body and is responsible for many vital functions in your body including, energy, metabolism due to the breakdown of fats, storing excess sugar in the blood as glycogen, metabolizing protein, and production of proteins used for blood clotting. One of its main jobs, however, is to cleanse the blood coming in from the digestive track by neutralizing toxins before they pass into the rest of the body. This is how your body can detox from substances like alcohol and get rid of the toxins created from the breakdown of medications. Without your liver, you simply could not live. [142]

The liver is an incredible organ, but over time it can become fatigued from a poor diet that is high in bad fats, sugar and processed carbohydrates, long term medication usage, and alcohol consumption. In these cases, the person ends up with fatty deposits in their liver cells. This is called non-alcoholic fatty liver disease (NAFLD). Although scientists generally consider NAFLD to be a benign condition, fat in the liver is not normal. NAFLD can lead to another more serious condition of the liver called non-alcoholic steatohepatitis (NASH). This is when fat in the liver causes inflammation of the liver cells and scarring. This inevitably can lead to cirrhosis. Cirrhosis of the liver happens when most of the liver is scarred and it is not able to work properly. Although NASH is rare and only 3-12% of the populous suffers with it, NAFLD is more common with numbers ranging between 30-40% in the U.S. [143, 144]

According to research, most people who have NAFLD have no symptoms. However, the question begs, can a person really function at 100% if they have all this fat accumulation in their liver? This is one of the main reasons why I think wheatgrass is so essential for your overall health. Wheatgrass works as a powerful detoxifier for the liver since the chlorophyll it's loaded with helps to cleanse the blood before it enters the liver. Some of the research shows that it can stimulate the regeneration of damaged liver cells. In a 2014 study published in the Journal of Membrane Biology it was concluded that "...wheatgrass effectively protects the liver against alcohol and fatty induced changes and preserves cell membrane integrity." [145] This is how powerful wheatgrass is!

We are exposed to an unprecedented level of toxins in our environment from the air we breathe, food we eat, medications we ingest, vaccines we inject, mercury in amalgam fillings, aluminum in our deodorant, and the toxic chemicals we spray inside our home, to name a few. Our toxic exposure is extremely high! All these toxins, which many people are unaware of, are carcinogenic, mutagenic (can alter DNA and genes to affect generations to come), neurotoxic (negatively impact the nerve system), hormone disrupters, and they negatively impact the thyroid and the glandular system. Basically, these toxins negatively affect every system in your body and are extremely detrimental to your health. If your body isn't efficient at detoxing from this toxic onslaught you are not going to live a very long life, nor will you add quality to those years. Fortunately, plants can bridge the gap between our toxic exposure and our body's ability to detox from them.

GRASS CAN SAVE YOUR ASS

Plants have an amazing ability to purify and neutralize the air of pollutants and other toxins. This is one of the reasons why I recommend you have lots of plants inside your home. Grass on the other hand, is unlike other plants in that it has an even more powerful air purifying capability because of the enzymes that are found within. It stands to reason that ingesting a grass capable of such detoxifying powers can help us to do the same, and that's just what the research shows.

For example, in her book, Ann Wigmore writes about Japanese scientists showing that the enzymes and amino acids in young grass have the power to deactivate the carcinogenic and mutagenic potential of 3,4 Benzpyrene, a substance created by charcoal-broiled meats. Wheatgrass has also been shown to neutralize the carcinogenic effects of automobile exhaust. And, along with its nutrient rich content it contains an abundance of super oxide dismutase (SOD) a highly potent antioxidant enzyme that protects you from free radical damage! I also mention SOD and its relationship with melatonin in the chapter on sleep. [138]

Growing wheatgrass isn't really that hard to do and the great thing is you can grow it inside your own kitchen, or in your back yard. The most important thing is to have fun with it! Get your children involved with the process! I wish my parents had grown wheatgrass inside our home when I was a kid! One thing is for sure though, you are teaching your child something phenomenal that they can utilize the rest of their life! And, you're also building great memories as a family!

In order to grow wheatgrass, you need indirect sunlight and an area with temperatures of about 65-75° F when you start your tray(s). You will also need multiple trays because one tray will only yield about eight ounces of wheatgrass juice. Once you decide on your location you will need several things. With the power of the internet you can purchase an entire kit for growing wheatgrass which comes complete with trays, soil, wheatgrass seeds, and fertilizer. I purchased my first kit from Amazon. But, if you want to go "old-school" and you don't want to wait a few days for delivery, you can usually find all you need at your local home and garden store. As an FYI, seeds are sometimes called wheat seeds or wheat berry seeds. I have listed directions below, in full detail, about how to grow your own wheatgrass at home!

INSTRUCTIONS FOR GROWING WHEAT GRASS

1. Make sure the seeds are organic and that they haven't been treated with pesticides! (especially important) Avoid over-sprouting or sprouts may not root in the soil for growing wheat grass.

2. Prep the seeds by washing them using filtered/clean room temperature water in strainer. Measure out about one cup for a 10x10 tray.

3. Soak the seeds. Once the seeds are thoroughly washed, soak them in a bowl of cold, filtered/clean water. If you are soaking one cup of seeds you will need about three cups of water. Make sure to cover the bowl with a lid and soak for about ten hours. Drain the water and repeat the process. Repeat three times or until the seeds sprout roots. Once the seeds sprout roots you are ready to begin the next step.

4. Make sure the soil you use in your trays is organic and free of pesticides and other chemicals. You can find good topsoil at your local home and garden store. You can also purchase a coconut coir block; they work great for growing wheatgrass.

5. Prep your tray(s) by lining it with a non-toxic liner. Organic paper towels work well and will prevent the roots from shooting out the bottom. Be sure to get trays that are thick and durable, close to 2 mm in thickness.

6. Add an even layer of organic all-natural fertilizer to the bottom of your tray(s).

7. Add an evenly distributed one-inch layer of topsoil to your tray(s). Make sure to moisten your soil using filtered/clean water. Do not soak the soil, only moisten it.

8. Sprinkle sprouted seeds evenly across soil, breaking up clumps as needed. Add a light layer of topsoil over the seeds. Make sure to keep the topsoil damp using a spray bottle.

9. Place tray in an area with indirect light, at 60-80° F and cover with moistened organic all-natural paper towels. Or you can buy a humidity dome which will improve seed germination. Be sure to keep the trays wet by removing the covering and spraying them at least once every morning. Remove the covering after 3-4 days. The humidity dome traps the moisture and keeps the temperature levels even which speeds up seed germination.

10. Keep your trays in partial sunlight to make sure they don't get too much sun. Watch it grow!

After about ten days your wheatgrass will be ready for harvest. Now it's time to party! Once your grass has reached five to eight inches tall it will be ready to be cut. You will positively know it's ready when another blade of grass begins growing out of the first shoot. This means your grass has reached its full nutritional peak! If you cut it too early you miss out on getting 100% of the potential nutrients contained within! So be patient.

When you're ready to put some wheatgrass juice in your system, cut your wheatgrass just above the root using scissors or a very sharp blade. Collect your grass on a napkin or in a bowl and prepare to juice it. You also have the option of refrigerating your wheatgrass after you harvest it, but you will lose valuable nutrients each day after harvest. Personally, I juice my wheatgrass right away. Once you have completed your harvest, water the remaining roots to obtain a second harvest.

Now for the fun part! After you cut your wheatgrass place it in a bowl. Make sure it doesn't smell putrid or have any mold on it. It's important to note that if you find any mold on your wheatgrass you should toss out the whole batch. Mold will make you incredibly sick, so it's best not to take the risk. Once you've determined there is no mold on your wheatgrass, rinse it off using filtered/clean water. Once the wheatgrass is clean it is ready to be juiced.

To juice wheatgrass, you need a slow masticating/churning juicer. You will not get enough juice to have enough of a therapeutic effect using a high-speed centrifugal juicer. Centrifugal juicers are more for your high fibrous fruits and veggies that contain a ton of water, like carrots, apples, celery, beets, etc. Electric wheatgrass juicers are one of your best options, but they tend to be a little pricy. But, if price is of no concern, get an electric wheatgrass juicer. Your other option is a mechanical hand crank wheatgrass juicer. These can be kind of fun, but they require a ton of hand cranking and a bit more of your time to get the same amount of juice you could have gotten with virtually zero effort using the electric version. The advantage is the cost is only about 10% of what an electric juicer will cost.

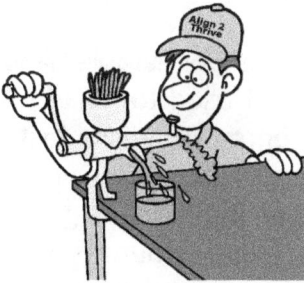

To juice you will need several handfuls of wheatgrass. Roll good size chunks into a wad and put it into the mouth/top of the juicer; juice it and drink it within twelve hours. I would recommend slamming a nice two to four ounce shot within seconds of acquiring the juice. Why? Wheatgrass is very volatile meaning it starts degrading soon after it has been cut and you don't want to lose out on those vital nutrients. [146] Make sure to drink the wheatgrass juice at least thirty minutes before a meal, always on an empty stomach. You can store freshly cut wheatgrass in the refrigerator for up to seven days, but even then, you will lose some of the nutrients. It's always best to juice it right away! After you have juiced it, always clean and rinse your juicer using non-detergent soap and hot water. I have a stainless still hand crank juicer which takes me about two minutes to clean after each use. Start by drinking one to two ounces at a time.

ALLERGIES TO WHEATGRASS

Although allergies to wheatgrass are extremely rare, some people might have a reaction once consumed. If you are allergic to wheat or grass, be cautious. Wheatgrass is different from wheat because it's considered a vegetable and not a grain. But if your allergy is to a wheat protein (Gluten Sensitivity) you might have a reaction to wheatgrass because the same protein could be present in the grass. If you have celiac disease or gluten sensitivity look for certified gluten-free wheatgrass products. If you are concerned about an allergic reaction, it is recommended you consult with your doctor, although odds are, he may not be fully up to date on the healing benefits of wheatgrass. I recommend always consulting with professionals who are well versed on the subject. Your local naturopath or chiropractor likely knows more than your general practitioner does about using wheatgrass and what the precautions are. Lastly, if your doctor isn't healthy, it is always best to look for health advice somewhere else.

MIDIGATE THE GRASSY TASTE

For some people, the taste of juiced grass is unbearable. And, like I said at the beginning of this chapter, it used to make me nauseous because of its strong and concentrated grassy taste. Now that I'm used to it, I love the taste of grass juice. But if you're a beginner, there are a few ways that you can mitigate the grassy taste. I recommend a beginner start with one to two ounces a day for a week and then bump it up to two to four ounces after that. My goal is to get wheatgrass into my body everyday as part of a daily health regimen. Because of its potency and detox potential however, one to two ounces per day is what you should start with.

So, here is how you mitigate the grassiness. Use an orange wedge immediately after taking a shot, similar to what people do with a shot of tequila and a lime - only wheatgrass doesn't destroy your liver! This was something that really helped me in the beginning. The other thing you can do is add apple juice, carrots, celery, and other water rich fruits and veggies to it. As a rule of thumb, keep the ingredients few and simple. Meaning, don't overdo it on how many things you add into the mix. Below I have listed a good and tasty go-to recipe.

DR. JAY'S GO TO RECIPE FOR WHEATGRASS

- 4 ounces of wheatgrass
- 1.5 small Granny Smith apples *(low glycemic)*
- 1 stick of celery

This remarkably simple recipe is a powerful way to start every morning. I believe the absolute best time of day to get wheatgrass into your body is in the morning on an empty stomach.

Think about it, you have been fasting all night and the greatest thing you can do for yourself is feed your body some nutrient dense juice as soon as you awake.

When it comes to adding things to your life to help you thrive, wheatgrass is something you're going to want to include! With all the benefits I have gone over in this chapter, you need not wait any longer. Get on it! Don't procrastinate! For about $120.00 you can get a hand crank juicer and an entire organic wheatgrass growing kit. Within ten days of planting the seeds in the soil you will reap a bountiful harvest and you'll be ready to "juice up!" It's time to thrive in this lifetime and wheatgrass is one of the top things I have added to my life in order to thrive. I hope you do the same!

Now... on to the next life enhancing chapter!

"The first wealth, is health."

-Ralph Waldo Emerson

CHAPTER 8

MOTION IS LIFE

The human body is an amazingly complex system of bones, joints, muscles, and nerves, designed to work together to accomplish one thing: Motion. Remember that motion is life and [life is motion].

- Discover Wellness

I always tell people that their number one asset is their health and that if they don't know what actions they need to take in life, focusing on health is always a good place to start. And, when it comes to the fundamentals of health, motion is everything! Most people simply do not move enough! The title of this chapter says it all: "Motion is LIFE!" And nothing is BIGGER than LIFE! In this chapter you will discover how exercise can help balance out your pH and other benefits. You will also learn about the phenomenal power of oxygen and how to improve your ability to take it in and utilize it (VO2 MAX) using a specific workout method called burst training. Lastly, I also want to touch upon the benefits of using hyperbaric O2 chambers and exercising with oxygen to maximize your potential! Let us begin!

I have always liked the expression, "motion is life" because if you're not moving you might as well be rotting away. Most people spend their lives sitting down. They sit in their car on their way to work, they sit at a desk to type away at a computer all day, they sit in their car on the way back to their house once they get off work, and when they get home exhausted from a grueling day, they sit on the couch to watch TV. They sit, and then they sit some more. According to a survey done by Ergotron, a global manufacturer of digital display furniture, mounting and mobility products, including sit-stand desks, the average American sits for roughly thirteen hours per day! Let's say the average person sits for thirteen hours per day five days per week – that's sixty-five hours per week. Multiply that by fifty-two weeks and you have 3,380 hours. Divide 3,380 hours by twenty-four and you get 141 (rounded up). That's 141 days per year that a person sits on their arse! That is a whole lot of not moving very much! If you spend most of your life not moving, how is that going to negatively impact your health? Our bodies are designed to move. The same study also reported that only 31% of Americans go to the gym, even though the vast majority know that exercise is important! [147]

In fact, many people have sought out medical treatment for pain related to excessive sitting. Sitting has become the new smoking. In a study done by the American Journal of Preventative Medicine researchers found that sitting more than three hours in a day will greatly increase your risk of an early death. In fact, sitting for three plus hours per day is responsible for 3.8% of all-causes of deaths across fifty-four countries. This accounts for over 430,000 deaths every year, just from sitting! How exactly is this possible? One, you burn fewer calories than you would if you were standing. Secondly, sitting can lead to sedentary lifestyle behaviors that contribute to disease. [148]

MOVE MORE, SIT LESS

So, what is the answer? The answer is to move more and sit less! Because sitting more and moving less has become the cultural norm, we need to interrupt that pattern of behavior with daily movement and exercise. For example, I recommend to all my patients that they take a break from sitting every forty-five minutes to an hour. This means that when that forty-five minutes or one-hour mark hits, they must get up, walk around, and do some stretches. I have included one of my stretches for "office athletes" in the appendix section. When we get up and move around, we are re-energizing ourselves, getting the blood flowing, and reducing tension and stress. People who take more breaks at work and move around are more productive. One study in the Journal Cognition showed that even brief diversions from a work task can lead to a dramatic increase in focus and productivity on a task for prolonged periods. [149] It's important for business owners to know that letting their employees take quick breaks from their tasks can increase their overall production for the business.

Moreover, sitting for prolonged periods of time can negatively impact one's psychological health. A study out of the University of Tasmania showed that employees who sat for longer than six hours at a time had a remarkable increase in anxiety and depression compared to those who sat for less than three hours per day. The study also concluded that women seemed to be more impacted by sitting than men did. [150]

The other thing I recommend is walking at a brisk pace for a minimum of twenty minutes per day. A Cambridge University study of 334,000 people revealed that increasing your level of physical activity prolongs your life. The study concluded that walking briskly for a minimum of twenty minutes a day, "...burning between 90 to 110 calories" can cut the risk of premature death by up to 1/3 in people considered the least fit. Obese people can expect a 16% reduced risk of dying early, while those of a healthy weight could expect a 30% reduced risk. This study suggests that even a little activity among those least active has substantial benefits. [151] There is also an obvious conclusion to make from this study. If a person of any BMI were to do longer bouts of exercise while upping the intensity levels, they would benefit even more.

I was fortunate growing up because I had parents that exercised regularly. Growing up in the 80's, Gold Gyms, step aerobics, leotards, and bodybuilding were immensely popular. My parents were into all of it. I can still remember to this day my mom taking me to the local "Club" as they called it. Delta Athletic Club was a big two-story building with weightlifting equipment, racket-ball courts, and a basketball court, and that was just the downstairs. The upstairs consisted of cardio equipment along with a nice size group fitness room. Even though I was stuck in the Kids Care Center, my mom taking me to the gym played a huge role in my workout habits today. My mom was planting a seed and she didn't even know it.

My dad also played a role in me now working out regularly. In his hay-day my dad weighed a good 240 lbs. and at 6'2" he was a giant! He would take me to the police department gym to workout with him. He taught me how to do things like preacher curls and bench press. At the time I could barely bench press the bar and I probably weighed 130 lbs. sopping wet! When I turned seventeen, I really got into working out and lifting weights every week. And even though my workouts have changed, the habit of working out multiple days every week hasn't. If you have kids, your kid's habits are a direct reflection of your habits. Your actions will play a role in the decisions they make for the rest of their lives. This is especially true when it comes to diet and exercise.

A study of 554 Southampton, U.K. moms, along with their four-year-old children, showed a "...direct correlation in physical activity levels among mothers and their children!" This is a no brainer! If moms make exercise a priority, their kids will engage in more physical activity! The reverse is also true, sadly, if mom leads a sedentary lifestyle the child is more likely to follow suit. As taken from a CBS report:

"But this study is also one of many that demonstrate how mothers often serve as ambassadors for the health and wellness of their family, especially their youngest children. The authors of the paper suggest a family's health can be improved by implementing

programs that encourage mothers and their children to engage in exercise together." [152]

If you make working out and eating healthy a regular thing in your household, it just becomes the norm, period. Often, I have heard parents say that they just can't get their kids to eat healthy. But, after digging deeper, I found out that the parents weren't eating healthy either. Suffice to say, to get your kids to lead healthy lives you must be the leader and set the tone. Kids follow their leaders. It's time more parents consider themselves to be leaders in their family and follow it up with congruent action!

> **"Exercise is King, and Nutrition is Queen:**
> **Together you have a Kingdom."**

-Jack Lalanne

EXERCISE IMPORTANCE

The definition of exercise is: *"activity requiring physical effort, carried out, especially to sustain or improve health and fitness."* I like

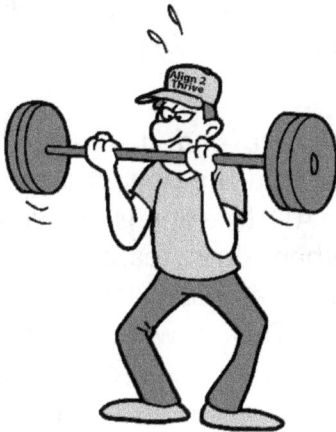

this definition; it's simple and to the point. Exercise increases one's overall health and fitness levels. The science behind exercising consistently is sound. With all the different ways to workout, the question becomes what can you do efficiently and easily to get the biggest benefit for your effort? Are there more efficient ways to exercise? Certainly! I am going to give you one of the best ways to work out that has been proven to increase testosterone, balance blood sugar, and burn fat fast.

The form of working out I'm talking about is interval training. This form of working out is also called burst training, surge training, HIITT (high intensity interval training). These are all just variations on a theme. Interval training consists of low to high intensity exercises with periods of rest between sets or timed intervals. The major advantage to this form of exercise is that the benefits are gained in less time than a traditional workout. All it takes is about 12-15 minutes per day five days per week. And, who doesn't have an extra fifteen minutes per day to work out? Well, dead people don't. Described below are the five major health benefits of burst training.

BENEFITS OF BURST TRAINING

1. *Improved Aerobic Capacity, aka Vo2 Max: Vo2 Max means maximal oxygen consumption.* This measurement indicates how well the body can take in oxygen, distribute it, and utilize it for energy production. This is huge! Research shows that as little as five minutes of HITT training a few days per week can increase the size of the left chamber of the heart (left ventricle) and therefore strengthen cardiac contractility! [153] In 2011 the American College of Sports Medicine reported that two weeks of HIIT improves aerobic capacity as much as six to eight weeks of endurance training. [154]

2. *Increased mitochondria in both size and number:* The mitochondria in a cell are considered the powerhouse of the cell. The mitochondria utilize ATP (the energy molecule of the cell) to produce energy. When you increase numbers of dense mitochondria this increases muscular strength and muscular endurance! [155] This is what makes a sprinter different from a marathon runner. A sprinter has more muscle mass so he can sprint at maximal capacity. In contrast, the marathon runner usually looks weak and tired.

3. ***Increased Fat Burning:*** A study showed that six weeks of interval training significantly increased fat and carbohydrate metabolism within muscle tissue. In this study, "untrained recreationally active" individuals were tested doing high intensity interval training for one hour three days per week. The intervals were split into ten four-minute intervals at "90% of maximal oxygen consumption (VO2 Max)," followed by two minutes of rest. Here is the conclusion of the study.

"This study demonstrated that 18 hrs. of repeated high-intensity exercise sessions over 6 weeks is a powerful method to increase whole-body and skeletal muscle capacities to oxidize fat [breakdown] and carbohydrate in previously untrained individuals." [156]

According to the American College of Sports Medicine (ACSM) you can burn more calories doing a HIIT style workout than longer, lower intensity workouts like running. Also, ACSM explains that the reason why HIIT workouts work so well is because it challenges your heart by taking you in and out of an anerobic (without oxygen) state. Your heart is pushed to 80% of its "maximum heart rate" (MHR) which doesn't happen as often with lower intensity workouts. [157]

4. ***Increased Testosterone:*** High intensity interval training may help to increase both testosterone and human growth hormone. [158] These are the primary hormones involved in weight loss and increased energy levels. Testosterone helps to support lean body mass and increased muscle size. A study published in the open access journal, *Endocrine Connections*, showed that six weeks of HIIT training for endurance athletes made considerable improvements in strength and testosterone. The kicker was that these endurance athletes were sixty *(+/- 5 years)* and yet, were still able to increase their "Peak Power Output" (Sprinting)

as well as their free testosterone, despite their age. As a bonus, cortisol levels also decreased! [159]

5. *Normalizes Blood Sugar:* When you burst train, you are tapping into stored muscle glycogen (stored sugar for your muscles) in a big way. This stored glycogen is broken down into glucose and is used by the muscles for energy when they contract. The muscles can store up to 500 grams or approximately 2,000 calories worth of glycogen. Therefore, the body will utilize glucose in the blood to replenish the glycogen used up during the workout. This helps to balance blood sugar levels. "In fact, a single bout of exercise [can] increase insulin sensitivity for up to 48 hours into recovery as well as improve glycemic control in individuals with Type 2 Diabetes!" [160]

These are just a few of the benefits of burst training. The cool thing is most people can do this type of workout. It just comes down to a matter of doing it. I always loved the Nike commercials that tell us to, "Just do it." That's a very simple but profound statement.

THE ANATOMY & PHYSIOLOGY OF BREATHING

One of the health benefits of working out and moving more is we breathe more. I would argue that most people don't really think about how important breathing is and how it changes when we challenge our bodies. The anatomy of breathing goes something like this.

When we take a breath the diaphragm contracts and moves downward which opens-up space in the chest cavity. The lungs expand into this open space and as they do this air is sucked in through the mouth and nose. The air travels down the trachea (windpipe), through the bronchi (passages), and finally through the bronchioles (like branches or roots of a tree) into these little air sacs called alveoli. The alveoli are tons of tiny bubbles with thin walls surrounded by blood vessels called capillaries (pulmonary capillaries). This is a point of gas exchange, mainly oxygen and carbon dioxide. The alveoli are so important there are about **300 million** in each lung to assist in transporting oxygen into the blood. [161, 162, 163]

When we breathe the alveoli fill with air and oxygen diffuses into the blood while carbon dioxide passes from the blood into the alveoli. When we exhale, we are primarily exhaling carbon dioxide. Oxygen rich blood is carried through a network of capillaries to the pulmonary vein which delivers it to the left side of the heart. The left side of the heart pumps this blood to the rest of the body. [162, 163]

Breathing is both a conscious and unconscious endeavor, but it is mainly something we do without thought. At the base of our brain lies the brainstem which contains a respiratory center (medulla and pons portion of brainstem). This respiratory center sends continuous messages down the spinal cord, through the nerves, and into the muscles (Diaphragm, Neck mm, Intercostal mm, abdominal mm) that control breathing. [163] What's cool is that you have various chemoreceptors located in your brain, blood vessels (carotid artery, aortic arteries), lungs, and muscles that "sense" changes in carbon dioxide and pH. These changes in CO2 levels cause you to increase or decrease your respiratory rate accordingly. There are both central and peripheral chemoreceptors.

The central chemoreceptors located in the brain detect changes in the pH of the cerebrospinal fluid and are responsible for slow changes in breathing. This is where you get the more rhythmic and even flow of breathing. Peripheral chemoreceptors located in the carotid and aortic arteries monitor immediate changes in CO2, O2, and pH and automatically adjust your breathing short term. This means when you have higher concentrations of CO2 than O2, your respiration rate automatically increases to expel excess CO_2 until the chemical concentrations in your blood become balanced. Once the chemical concentrations in your blood become balanced, your breath rate becomes slower and even. What's miraculous is that this happens without thought – it's automatic and happens hundreds if not thousands of times every day. [163] Consider this, **the average person takes 17,280 to 23,040 breaths a day!** [164]

This equates to 8,409,600 breaths per year, which means that the average eighty-year-old will have taken about **673 MILLION** breaths in their lifetime! [164]

When we exercise our breathing becomes heavier because our bodies produce more carbon dioxide. The faster respiratory rate combined with deeper inhalation during exercise leads to an equal amount of CO_2 production and CO_2 removal. Therefore, CO_2 levels never get out of hand. [165] It's important to note that our bodies are producing more CO_2 during exercise because we are consuming more oxygen. The benefits of taking in more oxygen are vast, which is one reason why exercise is so important.

With any type of exercise that challenges your breathing – mainly aerobic (cardio, burst training), your body adapts and becomes more efficient at taking oxygen in and utilizing it. Aerobic means using or with oxygen. Aerobic exercise consists of running, biking, cardio fit classes, walking briskly, etc. When you do cardio and your breathing becomes challenged your heart gets stronger and more efficient at pumping blood throughout your body. Your lungs become more efficient at getting oxygen into your blood while removing carbon dioxide. Lastly, all your muscles involved in breathing get stronger, especially your diaphragm. [166]

All these things help to improve your Vo2 max, which is an important measurement for everybody, regardless of whether a person is an athlete or a desk jockey. Exercise, according to Dr. Buteyko (creator of the "Buteyko method of breathing"), is the "most efficient method to increase cellular oxygen levels." [167]

After exercise, breathing slows down and body oxygen levels are higher and can remain that way for up to two hours. [166]

Many doctors and health professionals believe that we aren't getting enough oxygen because of the way we breathe. Most people breathe too shallow and too rapid which negatively affects the whole body. On top of this, they also breathe through their mouths. Shallow and rapid breathing through the mouth sets off the sympathetic nerve system which is responsible for the fight or flight mode. This inevitably raises blood pressure and heart rate while simultaneously shutting off blood flow to the digestive system. Also known as over-breathing, it constricts the airways and reduces the body's ability to oxygenate itself. Blood vessels also become constricted with over breathing and most of the oxygen is directed to the limbs and not the organs. Not surprisingly, long term shallow breathing can lead to major health problems. [168, 169]

BREATHING AND THE BOHR EFFECT

According to conventional medicine thought, a healthy person will take about ten to twelve breaths every minute and consume about five to six liters of air. However, a sedentary person over-breathes taking in double or even triple the number of breaths in a minute! Healthy breathing has a lot to do with what is called the Bohr Effect. The Bohr Effect tells us that oxygen is released by hemoglobin in the presence of appropriate amounts of carbon dioxide. When over-breathing happens hypocapnia occurs which means the body is depleted of carbon dioxide and less oxygen is released. This means that less oxygen is available for the muscles, organs, and other tissues because the hemoglobin will hold onto it rather than release it. Signs of this include excess yawning, sighing, fatigue, and increased stress levels. [168]

In order to achieve optimal health, we must slow our breathing and take deeper diaphragmatic breaths in and out through the nose. Think about it this way, when you're relaxed or in a state of ease have you noticed that you take deeper inhalation breaths through your nose? Look at all the animals in the animal kingdom (apart from dogs if they are hot). They all breathe in and out through their noses. The fastest land animals breathe through their noses even while chasing prey! In a state of stress our breathing becomes quickened as we breathe through our mouth and **the body prioritizes inhalation vs. exhalation**. This causes our exhalation muscles to become weak over time. With mouth breathing you also end up getting less oxygen into your body, even if you're breathing more!

According to Patrick McKeown, author of the book *The Oxygen Advantage*, children who regularly breathe through their mouth end up with structural changes to the face and jaw which impair breathing. Later in life, mouth breathing not only makes for poor sleep, but also causes sleep apnea and can lead to obesity. This is mainly due to how poor sleep negatively affects the two hormones involved in regulating appetite: ghrelin & leptin. Leptin is the hormone responsible for making us feel satiated after we eat, while ghrelin makes us feel hungry. So, a lack of sleep equates to higher ghrelin and lower leptin levels. It's a recipe for weight gain. Shifting your breathing from your mouth to your nose can make a huge difference in your health. [170]

By breathing through your nose, you can increase your O2 levels by 10-20% according to McKeown. [171] Nasal breathing also increases nitric oxide. Nitric oxide relaxes the smooth inner muscles of your blood vessels which causes them to widen, thus increasing circulation. Not only that, but nitric oxide helps blood vessels stay flexible which will prevent arterial sclerosis and plaque buildup. [172] This will allow more oxygen to get where it needs to go. When you combine nasal breathing with exercise you have nitric oxide production within your body, and thus improve oxygen transport.

To learn to breathe through your nose you need to consciously focus on it every day. You need to actively breathe through your nose more often, no matter what activity you're doing. After doing it consistently for a minimum of twenty-one to thirty days, it eventually becomes a habit. Your nasal passages will clear, and it will become easier to breathe. When I started actively focusing on my breathing, I noticed a difference in how much more relaxed I was feeling. I noticed I could put my body into a state of calm no matter how stressed I was. Breathing through my nose during exercise is a bit more challenging and it's an ongoing work in progress. What I can tell you though is that my ability to breathe has gotten stronger. You will notice an immediate difference once you start. For further and more in-depth information, I highly recommend purchasing Patrick McKeown's book, The *Oxygen Advantage*. It goes into way more detail than the scope of this chapter can offer.

There is research that shows daily exercise with nasal breathing improves oxygen transport. This is due to the increased CO_2 and nitric oxide levels in the lungs and arterial blood. [173] Breathing through your nose during exercise is like training at a higher altitude. Athletes who train at a higher altitude do so because of the performance enhancing benefits gained from exercising in an environment where the oxygen supply is less. In these conditions the body adapts by increasing red blood cells, so it becomes more efficient at getting oxygen to the tissues. When you breathe through your nose during intense exercise training you do not get an adequate amount of oxygen into your body. This is known as hypoxia. You might think this sounds a little counterintuitive, but it has some amazing benefits.

A study conducted at the Japan Institute of Sports Sciences over a period of eight weeks put athletes into a hypoxic room (a room with limited oxygen supply) and had them perform resistance exercises. During the training, "levels of plasma oxygen were lower in the [experimental group]." Yet, remarkable increases in growth hormone, capillary growth (capillary-to-muscle-fiber-ratio), and vascular endothelia growth factor, along with increased muscular endurance were seen in this group. To summarize in laymen's terms, the group training under oxygen reduced conditions (experimental group/hypoxic group) had a dramatic increase in red blood cells and "was better able to restore their oxygen supply to tissues, [even] when their circulation to [said tissues was lessened]!" [173]

THE POWER OF BREATH

It has been said that your breath is tremendously powerful because it acts as a gateway to your nerve system. **By focusing on your breathing throughout the day, you can radically decrease your stress levels.** To reiterate, you should be focused on taking deep, but light and slow diaphragmatic breaths in, and letting the natural elasticity of the lungs and diaphragm release the air naturally. Focus on breathing through your nose and slowing your breath down. Both inhalation and exhalation should be light and not forceful. Remember, this kind of breathing activates the vagus nerve which controls the parasympathetic part of the nerve system. The parasympathetic half of your nerve system is responsible for rest, digest, and repair. This allows your body to go into a state of healing. This kind of breathing also helps you to focus because blood is directed to parts of the brain that are involved in problem solving. [174]

If you were to practice regular breathing exercises daily your breathing would be much better – no matter what the exercise. One exercise that McKeown wrote about in the chapter, "Breathe Light to Breathe Right," (The Oxygen Advantage) helped to correct my over-breathing pattern. According to McKeown, when we breathe too much over a long period of time (days – weeks – months) "our respiratory center adjusts to a lower tolerance of carbon dioxide" which leads to an increased respiratory rate and "breathlessness during physical exercise." Remember, CO_2 is key to our breathing and if we breathe too much, we end up with less CO_2 overall, therefore less oxygen is delivered to our muscles, organs, and tissues. This triggers us to breathe more and take more big, deep breaths in through our mouths. What we must do is RESET our respiratory center by training it to do something different. This is why intentional breath work is so important. [168]

Here is a simple breathing exercise to get you started. To do the exercise you must start by sitting up straight and relaxing your shoulders. Keep your head and chin level or in slight extension, but never in flexion. When you flex your head forward and down it restricts breathing (see Chapter 4). Your shoulders should be back and not rounded forward so your chest is opened and your breathing is unrestricted. With one hand on your chest and the other just above your naval, take a small, light breath in through your nose and then gently let it out. As the air comes in, place gentle pressure on your chest and abdomen making each inhalation breath smaller and smaller until you feel a tolerable need for air. On the exhale, let the elasticity of your diaphragm and lungs naturally expel the air without your effort. [168]

Try to maintain this tolerable need for air for two sets of three to five minutes. McKeown states that this exercise is enough to "help you reset your breathing center and improve your body's tolerance for CO_2." You may have to start with one to two minutes for two sets and work up to more. One thing is for sure, as you practice this daily it will get easier and you will eventually notice an increase in your energy and endurance. For example, I was able to jog for a longer duration on a treadmill at a pace of 6.2, even while breathing through my nose. The big thing is to make sure your breathing never becomes erratic during this exercise.

"If your stomach muscles start to contract or jerk or feel tense, or if your breathing rhythm becomes disrupted or out of control, then the air shortage is too intense. In this situation, abandon the exercise for 15 seconds or so and return to it when the air shortage has disappeared."

Patrick McKeown

[168, Pg. 75-76]

BREATHING AND THE LYMPHATIC SYSTEM

Another benefit of deep breathing through the nose is that it has a powerful cleansing effect. Deep breathing stimulates the flow of lymph fluid which is carried into the blood stream and then metabolized by the liver. Toxins are then filtered through the kidneys and excreted in the urine. Your lymphatic system is considered the "sewage system" of the body. It's a drainage system that removes excess waste fluid from the body tissues and returns it to your blood stream. This excess fluid contains dead cells, cancer cells, dead bacteria, and toxins along with some proteins and fats. If this fluid wasn't absorbed into your lymphatic system, it would accumulate and cause swelling. In fact, if your lymphatic system completely stopped working for a mere twenty-four hours you would be dead or hospitalized. [168 - Pg. 73, 30]

Unlike the circulatory system where oxygenated blood is pumped throughout the body via the heart, the flow of lymph fluid is dependent upon the movement of the body, muscles, and the diaphragm. This is yet another reason why "motion is life" and why it's so important to EXERCISE! Exercise is powerful in this way for two reasons.

1. You must move to exercise (well duh!)

2. Your respiratory rate increases and becomes more intense (as is the case with jogging or burst training) when you exercise. [175]

HYPERBARIC OXYGEN CHAMBERS

Hyperbaric Oxygen Therapy (HBOT) has been used for centuries, but it wasn't until the 20th century that it became widely known and used. The U.S. Navy successfully used HBOT on deep sea divers suffering from decompression sickness (bubbles of nitrogen gas formed in the bloodstream causing severe joint pain). In the 1950s a cardiac surgeon in the Netherlands, Dr. Boerema, used HBOT to successfully treat children with congenital heart diseases like pulmonic stenosis. Dr. Boerema is credited with being the father of modern-day hyperbaric medicine. Later it was realized that HBOT could help speed up recovery from injuries, bone infections, chronic wounds, neurological conditions, and even carbon monoxide poisoning. [176] It has even been used to experimentally treat cancer. By 1999 the FDA recognized the value of HBOT. Many hospitals today contain HBO chambers. [177]

Athletes like Lebron James and Tim Tebow use hyperbaric oxygen chambers to help with performance and recovery. So, why am I including information about HBOT in a chapter on exercise? Because it's all about getting oxygen into your body. The reason HBOT is so effective is because it involves breathing in pure oxygen in a pressurized environment. The air pressure is increased 2.3 to 4.5 times more than normal air pressure. This forces oxygen deep into one's body. With HBOT, the volume of oxygen is increased in the blood and the red blood cells become more malleable which increases their ability to deliver oxygen to tissues. [178, 179]

The brain is the largest consumer of oxygen – consuming an average of 20% oxygen. When performing different activities oxygen supply is shifted from one region of the brain to another via a complex mechanism known as blood perfusion modulation. In oxygen depleted environments our ability to perform complex activities is hindered. This is based on the hypothesis that getting more oxygen into the brain could simply make the brain work better. [180]

Thus, a double-blind, randomized controlled, crossover study was conducted at the Israel Rehabilitation Center for Stroke and Brain Injury on twenty-two healthy individuals twenty-two-years of age and older. What they found was that HBOT "significantly enhanced BOTH cognitive and motor performance." People were able to not only do single tasks better, but they were able to perform multi-tasks better. What's cool is that many studies have derived the same findings! The researchers stated in conclusion that this study supports the hypothesis that oxygen is a "rate limiting factor for the brain." [180]

When oxygen is delivered at an increased atmospheric pressure your body can absorb more of it. This means more oxygen is absorbed into the red blood cells, blood plasma, cerebral spinal fluid, and the brain. Similar to water – oxygenating your body has to do with how much you absorb, not just how much you take in by breathing. As said previously, if we breathe too shallow and too rapid, a sign that we have increased stress in our life, we end up limiting our body's intake of oxygen. When it comes to cancer, however, it's anaerobic. This means that cancer thrives in a low oxygen environment (hypoxic environment). [181]

Therefore, some outside-the-box thinking doctors have used HBOT as part of their protocol to successfully treat cancer patients. Because HBOT increases the amount of oxygen in the blood plasma and RBCs, more oxygen is delivered to all tissues, including tumors. [178] Since cancer cells are cells that have gone rogue, they refuse to die because they do not "innately" know they are part of a greater whole. The theory is that when these rogue cells start getting oxygen, it causes them to switch on apoptosis, which is their programmed cell death. In a sense, it's like they begin to recognize the bigger picture and can see they are part of a greater whole. It's also important to include here that HBOT along with a ketogenic diet (low carb, high fat diet) has shown to significantly slow tumor progression and increase survival time. [182]

You may want to think about including HBOT in your arsenal for achieving optimal health. To utilize an HBOT chamber there are a few options. The absolute best thing to do would be to purchase a portable one you can utilize in your home. There are several companies that provide portable, at home units. The cost ranges from $10,000 to $30,000 a unit depending on what you buy. If that's not a good option for you, there are plenty of outpatient clinics that have units for about $100 to $350 per session. Several of my colleagues utilize portable HBO chambers in their practices. The good news is that your health insurance may cover your HBOT sessions, or at least a portion of. Ask your insurance provider if you are covered. However, there are some contraindications to using HBOT, especially if you have a medical condition. I suggest speaking with your primary care physician to make sure the therapy will be a good fit for you.

EXERCISING WITH OXYGEN

Exercising with oxygen (EWOT) is something a ton of athletes are doing now. Everybody from Tiger Woods, Michael Phelps, and several athletes from the NBA, NFL, MLB, and MMA use certain types of oxygen therapy to help enhance their athletic abilities. [183] EWOT is done using supplemental oxygen which fully saturates the red blood cells with oxygen. You also end up with dissolved oxygen in the blood plasma. The increased oxygen allows for increased work output and endurance. A German doctor by the name of Manfred Von Ardenne conducted twenty-five years of research on oxygen and exercise. He discovered that using exercise while breathing supplemental oxygen did "increase oxygen utilization at the cellular level." He had great success with treating disease conditions like arteriosclerosis, hypertension, hypotension, and other disorders. [178, 184]

In his research Dr. Ardenne discovered that most people had a condition where the capillary beds were inflamed, swollen, narrowed, and thickened. This reduced blood flow and oxygen delivery to the tissues. He found that this condition was reversible with his "oxygen multi-step therapy." His therapy involved patients working out for eighteen days with oxygen. To help the body utilize oxygen they would take potassium, magnesium, and vitamin B6 thirty minutes before they began to exercise. Thirty minutes after taking the supplements they started exercising on a stationary bicycle or treadmill while breathing 4-6 liters of oxygen per minute through a mask. Every twenty minutes the patient would speed up the intensity of the workout to their aerobic target heart rate which is 70-80% of the maximum target heart rate. This allowed for increased blood flow and oxygen delivery. [184]

At the conclusion of the study Dr. Ardenne was able to summarize that working out with oxygen does the following:

- Gets more oxygen circulating in the blood
- Helps to restore blood flow
- Expands constricted capillaries & decreases swelling
- Improves cerebral blood flow – "Can help heal ischemic ulcerations in diabetic patients." [185]
- Increases the production of ATP
- Gets O2 into the cells which increases ATP production which is fuel for the cell
- Works faster than a hyperbaric oxygen chamber (it's a time saver)

EWOT can be a powerful way to train, but how do you do it? First off, there are clinics scattered throughout the U.S. where you can exercise with oxygen. However, I prefer the do it yourself method which involves purchasing an oxygen concentrator. Oxygen concentrators work by pressurizing the air and separating the nitrogen from the oxygen, so you get a pure, concentrated stream of oxygen. Brand new oxygen concentrators can range anywhere from $1,000 to upwards of $3,500 and usually require a prescription from a doctor. But the good news is you can get a refurbished one for hundreds of dollars rather than thousands and you don't need a doctor's prescription for these.

According to Dr. Jonathan Edwards, M.D., you want a unit capable of delivering 5 or 10 liters of oxygen per minute. [183]

You want the unit to be directly connected to a 400 to 900-liter reservoir. The reservoir collects the pure oxygen, making sure you have a constant supply of it during exercise. During exercise, your respiratory rate increases from a normal 4 to 6 liters per minute to about 60 to 70 liters per minute which is why having a direct hookup to a reservoir is essential in maintaining a constant stream of pure oxygen. Otherwise you would get a mixture of outside room air and would no longer be breathing in pure oxygen.

Once the reservoir is filled with oxygen a dual valve oxygen mask is hooked up to CPAP tubing. The mask and the CPAP tubing can be purchased from virtually any medical store. Connect the CPAP tubing to the intake port of the mask. When you exhale, air goes out the out-take port. [184] The oxygen mask should be comfortable and fit flush with your face, so it doesn't leak.

HOW TO DO EWOT

(As taken from Ben Greenfield's blog.)

What you need

1. Oxygen concentrator (5-10 liters per minute)
2. Reservoir (non-toxic, free of volatile chemicals - consists of a big bag that fills with 600-900 liters of pure oxygen)
3. CPAP tubing to attach from concentrator to reservoir
4. CPAP adapter with the ½ inch PVC cap
5. Dual-valve oxygen mask *(medical store)*

EWOT can be performed on any type of cardio equipment, i.e. treadmill, indoor bicycle, Stairmaster, etc. Before you begin the exercise a warmup of 10-15 minutes should be performed **without oxygen**. After you get your heart rate up, put the oxygen mask on and begin a burst training style workout. Dr. Edwards recommends sprinting to 90-100% of your maximum power or heart rate for thirty seconds and then resting for 1 to 1.5 minutes. He also recommends repeating the intervals 8 to 10 times. [184]

There is another form of training that involves exercising with restricted oxygen. It's often done by holding the breath during interval training or running sprints, which helps to lower sensitivity to CO_2. Breath holding stimulates the kidneys to kick out more of the hormone erythropoietin which stimulates the maturation of red blood cells in the bone marrow. With the presence of more CO_2 in the blood, the spleen kicks out more RBCs. More RBCs in the bloodstream means increased delivery of oxygen to all tissues, including muscle tissue. Obviously, this would help increase athletic performance and endurance, thus, increased VO2 Max! According to McKeown, "the concentration of erythropoietin can increase by 24% when the body is subjected to lower oxygen levels using breath-hold exercises." [168, Pg. 109] There are companies like LiveO2 that have EWOT systems that switch from oxygen concentrated air to oxygen depleted air with the flip of a switch. The key thing to remember is that breathing less and not over-breathing causes CO_2 levels to go up, and as CO_2 levels go up more oxygen is "offloaded." This is the reason it would be good to train with both increased oxygen and depleted oxygen.

STRENGTH TRAINING

It is important to note that it is good to have days where you just focus on strength training. Although you end up working your muscles and becoming stronger when you do interval training, a focus purely on strength training is good for balanced fitness levels. Strength training involves lifting heavier weights to build muscle and gain strength.

One of the biggest benefits to strength training is it builds stronger bones by increasing bone density which reduces your risk of osteoporosis. [186] Strength training also improves your quality of life because it makes it easier to *adapt* to day to day life activities. [187] Think about it, if you're stronger you will be able to perform various tasks with a lot more ease and grace. There is evidence that shows strength training can improve balance, thus reducing the risk of falls. Another significant benefit that comes with strength training has to do with the increase in muscle mass. Larger muscles require more calories to maintain. This will increase your metabolism.

A study by Harvard and the University of Denmark showed that men who lifted weights thirty minutes per day, five days per week may be able to reduce their risk of diabetes by a whopping 34%! [188]

There are several different styles of strength training you can utilize. I personally like to use free weights in my strength training routine, along with body weight exercises like pushups, pullups, and planks. I also like to use resistance bands because they add variety to your everyday free weight exercises.

Here is a simple routine you can do for strength training. I call this the *full-body training method*. Pick two exercises, one upper body and one lower body. For example, pushups and air squats. Do as many pushups as you can (flat back, tight abdominals, arms slightly wider than shoulder width apart) by slowly going down for a count of "1-2-3" (this is called eccentric contraction), when your chest gets close to touching the floor pop back up by pushing up with your arms for a count of one. Your elbows should lock as your triceps contract (concentric). Once you finish the pushups, stand up and with your legs slightly wider than shoulder width apart and do the same type of eccentric and concentric contraction with your air squats. Repeat this workout for three to four sets and then add two more exercises.

Note: Eccentric contraction causes muscles to shorten & concentric contraction causes muscles to lengthen.

I usually do this type of routine for a good six to eight exercises on average. You can combine any two, three, or even four different exercises. Make sure you rest between each set. Wait for your heart rate to get back down to a resting heart rate before doing the next set. You can combine pullups and pushups. You can combine bicep curls and leg curls. The combinations you can choose are limitless. You can also do three to four different exercises in a single circuit. When you breathe during weightlifting, inhale during the eccentric phase and exhale during the concentric phase. Try to only breathe through your nose, and if need be, only exhale through your mouth.

WHAT ABOUT STRAIGHT CARDIO?

I believe that doing pure cardio has its place. With interval training (burst training) you *can* get the best of both strength training and cardio. However, having strength training days and cardio days mixed in with interval training days allows for your body to be worked in different ways. This means your body must adapt to all the different kinds of physical stress you are putting on it. The more your body is forced to adapt, the better shape you will be in. When it comes to cardio, doing something simple like running at a steady pace on a treadmill for twenty minutes can be beneficial. Swimming is a good way to do cardio as well because it's low resistance. With cardio you want to try and control your breathing through your nose as much as possible.

Regardless of what type of exercise you engage in, don't forget the importance of stretching. Stretching should be done daily with the goal of creating flexibility and strength. We use our muscles every day which causes them to shorten and tighten. Over time this day to day stress adds up to a decrease in range of motion and discomfort. Muscles that are shortened and tight can easily be pulled and injured. So, it's very important to create a daily stretch program. Even five minutes a day worth of stretching can make all the difference in your flexibility and strength. According to David

Nolan, a physical therapist at Harvard-affiliated Massachusetts General Hospital, "You don't have to stretch every muscle you have."

> "The areas critical for mobility are in your lower extremities: your calves, your hamstrings, your hip flexors in the pelvis, and quadriceps in the front of the thigh." Stretching your shoulders, neck, and lower back is also beneficial. Aim for a program of daily stretches or at least three or four times per week." [189]

David Nolan

I recommend to all my patients that they stretch twice per day. This consists of stretching once in the morning after they have been up and moving around for at least thirty minutes and once at night right before they go to bed. Stretching is a phenomenal way to begin and end the day. I recommend five to ten minutes total to stretch the upper and lower body. To make it easier to stretch regularly, think about the different regions your body is composed of. Moreover, there are over 600 muscles in the body, do you think you need to know which specific ones you're stretching to get a good stretch? No, just stretch them region by region. Here are the overall regions.

BODY PARTS TO STRETCH

- Neck
- Shoulders
- Arms & forearms
- Upper back
- Core/Abdominals
- Lower back
- Hamstrings
- Quads
- Glutes
- Calves
- Ankles/Feet

Static stretching consists of stretching a group of muscles beyond their normal limit and holding the stretch for a few seconds or minutes. A good example of this would be yoga. The great thing about static stretching is that it lowers blood pressure, decreases respiratory rate, and generally relaxes you. It feels incredibly good! However, according to Ben Greenfield, in his amazing book *Beyond Fitness*, static stretching has its limitations. It can slow you down and detrimentally effect your performance, mainly because it does not increase mobility, it hinders it. Furthermore, it negatively impacts explosiveness because it makes muscles and tendons too loose. [190, Pg. 126-127] Static stretching is best done post workout, or at the end of your day to help relax you right before bed. In fact, I do a quick static stretch routine right before bed to help me relax. When I begin incorporating static stretching before I went to bed, I found that I slept better. It's a great way to end your day.

For a list of static stretches to do to help you sleep better go to Thrivespinecenter.com and check out my blog *on* "Five amazing stretches to help you relax before bed." Also, check out this link: *wikihow.com/stretch* for more information.[46]

I went to an As vs. Giants game a while ago and had the opportunity to watch them warmup. I saw none of the players performing static stretches. All the players were actively stretching, meaning they were doing stretches with movement – otherwise known as ballistic stretching or dynamic stretching. Studies show that stretching with movement can improve performance. As Greenfield states, "dynamic stretching can improve power, strength, and performance during a subsequent exercise session." [190] This is primarily because it incorporates so many more things than just stretching a particular muscle group. Hence, the name dynamic stretching.

Key Notes: Dynamic stretches must be performed using smooth and patterned movements within a normal range of motion. Ballistic stretches are virtually the same thing but involve going beyond normal range of motion. They also involve higher speed movements, like bouncing for example. Caution must be utilized with both types of stretches because injury can and does occur. Any dynamic stretch can be turned into a ballistic stretch by adjusting speed and range of motion. This is especially good to do after you have already warmed up using dynamic stretches.

Two of my favorite dynamic/ballistic stretches to do every morning are:

- *Frankenstein Walk*: This stretch is used a lot by mixed martial arts students to help them loosen up their lower backs and kick higher. It involves taking a step forward and with the opposite leg, swing it out in front of you with the heel flexed. The leg can be totally straight or slightly bent. I absolutely love this stretch. You want to do about 5-10 on each leg.

- *Open Crescents*: This stretch is a dynamic stretch used to loosen up the hip joint and is especially good for runners. I have used this stretch before my softball games. To do it you are going to take a step forward and with the opposite leg bend the knee up and externally swing it out to the side. Then bring the knee back to the front and repeat. This forms a half circle or crescent. Do 5-10 on each leg.

For a full list of both upper body and lower body dynamic stretches go here - > *thrivespinecenter.com Blog "Top Dynamic Stretches to do Daily."*

Utilizing muscle work is another way you can improve flexibility; this happens to be my absolute favorite way to not only increase flexibility but decrease pain and stress. When I refer to muscle work, I'm referring to deep massage work on the soft tissue. A professional deep tissue massage specialist can "attack" your tight muscles like nothing else can. Our muscles get worked daily through working out, all our athletic endeavors, while walking, running, and even sitting. As a result, our muscles, tendons, and fascia get tight and adhesions form over time. Adhesions are also known as knots (Cumulative Injury Cycle). [191] Ben Greenfield describes the Cumulative Injury Cycle like this.

> "In the cumulative injury cycle, a repetitive effort (like riding a bicycle) causes muscles to tighten (such as your hip flexors). A tight muscle tends to weaken, and a weak muscle tends to tighten, which creates a vicious, well, cycle. As the muscle becomes tighter and tighter, the area of tension experiences more and more friction and pressure, which increases the potential for injury and inflammation.... [189, Pg. 129]

Furthermore, this tightness leads to decreased blood flow to the muscles and with decreased blood flow comes hypoxia *(lack of oxygen)*, which results in more fibrosis and adhesions, which leads to more injuries and problems down the road. [189, Pg. 130]

MUSCLE TISSUE

Our muscles consist of muscle fibers that are bundled together into motor units. When you want to move your arm, the brain sends a message down your spinal cord to the motor units of your arm and your arm moves. Our muscles are meant to be soft, strong, flexible, and engaged (especially in our day to day activities). There are over 600 muscles in our body that are layered over each other, running in all different directions which allows for many different types of movement (twisting, flexion, extension, pronation, supination, translation, lateral movement, and many different combinations of each). Many muscles "fire off" synergistically, even with the simplest of movements. For example, when we bend over to pick something up, we are engaging hundreds of muscles in our body.

We put a lot of stress on our skeletal muscular system over our lifetimes. Due to bad posture (sitting at a desk for hours on end), constant use, working out, playing sports, bad nutrition, dehydration, etc. our muscle tissue loses its pliability over time and the muscle fibers start sticking together and forming adhesions. If these adhesions are never addressed, they buildup and form knots. What's more, there is an opaque connective tissue that covers, attaches, and encloses all the muscles and separates underlying tissues (internal organs) from each other. This tissue, as you might have guessed, is called fascia.

Fascia is a fibrous connective tissue made up of collagen fibers. This tissue is super flexible and can withstand lots of tension. [192] However, due to injuries, sedentary behavior (like sitting for thirteen hours per day), lack of motion, dehydration, NOT STRETCHING, etc. a "fuzz" type tissue builds up between the fascial interfaces of our muscles causing us to become stiff. Hence, why you feel a need to stretch in the morning. When we stretch this fuzz tissue "melts" away and we become loosened up. However, this fuzz tissue turns to fibrotic adhesions and "fails to differentiate the adjacent structures effectively [meaning they get glued together]. This can happen after surgery where the fascia has been incised and healing includes a scar that traverses the surrounding structures." [193] This leads to a decrease in flexibility and mobility, allowing for further injury as muscle layers become stuck together.

The good news is regular stretching and deep tissue work can break up adhesions in the muscles and fascia tissue. You can also effectively do some muscle work on yourself in the convenience of your own home with a foam roller, muscle roller stick, and a tennis ball, among other things. Foam rolling is a great way to break up adhesions and loosen muscle and fascial tissue. Greenfield recommends doing thirty passes on each muscle group at a time. [189] You can purchase a foam roller at your local Target or Walmart.

A tennis ball can be great for working on a specific area of the muscle. The tennis ball works great to roll out knots formed in the glutes, hamstrings, and between the shoulder blades. I love using a tennis ball to roll out and loosen up my glutes after a workout. Try it by placing the tennis ball on the area you want to work while lying on the ground. Use your body weight to slowly move side to side, forward and backwards to roll out the area of concern.

There is no better time than right now to start moving. The benefits of consistent exercise are huge, especially when it comes to one's overall health, mobility, and fitness. If people could see what their insides looked like due to their sedentary lifestyles, there would be a lot more people working out and exercising. Obesity has become a huge epidemic in the United States. The bad fat, known as visceral fat, is the fat that surrounds the organs of sedentary people. And when people have too much of it, it can begin to negatively impact organ function. For example, it can detrimentally impact liver function and interfere with hormones. This will inevitably lead to insulin resistance and eventually diabetes. Plaque builds up in the walls of the arteries due to sedentary behavior. All of this is primarily because we don't move enough. Therefore, lack of motion is primarily responsible for ill-health in America.

Hence, the reason I titled this chapter, "Motion is Life." If we don't move enough, it drastically decreases our quality of life. If you don't "USE IT, you LOSE IT." Is it any wonder arteries become stiff? Visceral fat builds up and muscles become tight and weak. We aren't moving enough!

Try the burst training exercise and if that's too much for you try walking regularly for a minimum of twenty minutes a day, seven days per week. Make a point to do some type of exercise a minimum of four days per week. Join a gym and make sure the gym has a sauna. I'll explain why in the next chapter. If you utilize the gym regularly, it's well worth the monthly investment. For example, I spend one hundred bucks a month for a local gym membership for my wife and me. We work out a minimum of four days per week, sixteen days per month. That's thirty-two work outs in a single month. That means I'm only spending about three dollars per day. NOT BAD! So, for less than a cup of coffee, you and your spouse can work out regularly.

It's important that you begin moving more and doing what's necessary to challenge your body. Otherwise you will face the consequences of a sedentary lifestyle at some point in your life. It's important to note that exercise alone can't make one healthy. There is also a PRESSING need to REMOVE the interference of toxicity.

"The elimination of toxins awakens the capacity for renewal."

-Deepak Chopra

CHAPTER 9

REMOVING TOXICITY INTERFERENCE

*"By cleansing your body on a regular basis
and eliminating as many toxins
as possible from your environment, your
body can begin to heal itself, prevent
disease, and become stronger and more
resilient than you ever dreamed possible."*

- Dr. Edward Group DC, DACBN, DABFM

It doesn't matter where you live in the world or what your ethnic background is. Your race, gender, and age do not matter, but one thing is for certain, we are exposed to an unprecedented level of toxins living in our modern-day world. We are constantly bombarded by toxins. Our bodies are being assaulted from the air we breathe, the foods we eat, toxic medications, toxic vaccines, the water we drink, household cleaning products, and much more. Shockingly, we are even being exposed to toxins before we are born.

One study that was done by the Environmental Working Group (EWG) in September of 2004 "found an average of 200 industrial chemicals and pollutants in the umbilical cord blood of ten babies born in August and September of 2004 in U.S. hospitals. Furthermore, tests revealed a total of 287 chemicals in the group.

They found toxic chemicals like pesticides, consumer product ingredients, and wastes from burning coal, gasoline, and garbage." [195] They even found dioxin, mercury, and the dangerous chemical found in Teflon (PFOA) that is linked to cancer. What is incredibly sad is that a baby developing in utero has far more of a health risk from toxic exposure than they do later in life. This study confirms that the toxins the mother is exposed to, either directly by choice or indirectly from her environment, negatively impact her developing child.

Yes, toxins are all around us. My hope is that this chapter will inspire you to make better decisions in your life that will decrease you and your family's exposure to toxins. In this chapter I lay out a specific method of detoxing your body as taught to me by specialists in the field. I also thoroughly summarize several different ways we are exposed to toxins and how to avoid them. And, finally, I cover a few controversial topics that are important to be aware of. I strongly encourage you to keep an open mind.

TOXINS

An important thing to understand is that your body is constantly protecting you from harmful toxic chemicals, metals, and industrial pollutants. Eventually, however, these toxins add up. They bioaccumulate in your body (adipose tissue), which certainly plays a role in the causation of disease, sickness, and possibly early death. One can argue that the bioaccumulation of toxins can be the sole cause of one's infirmity. The challenge for most people and doctors is seeing the link between a bioaccumulation of toxins and symptomatology.

For example, doctors are very apt to prescribe a drug to treat a person's symptoms rather than putting a patient through a much-needed detox program. Although the drugs might mitigate the symptoms, the drugs themselves are toxic. A 2011 article published in the New England Journal of medicine estimates that two million people are victims of prescription drug induced toxicity. With many Americans taking multiple medications on a regular basis, I wonder what this number would be today nearly nine years later. And, what will it be twenty years from now? I don't see it getting any better. [196, 197]

As mentioned above, toxins are stored in your fat cells, specifically your white fat cells. This would be the fat that accumulates around your mid-section and hip areas. Many toxins are fat soluble and therefore end up being stored in fat cells. Toxins, like heavy metals, industrial pollutants, solvents, insecticides, pesticides, fungicides, toxins from personal care products, drug residues, plastics, and food additives all get stored in fat cells. Foreign and exogenous heavy metals, substances, and chemicals that build up in the body are known as xenobiotics.

As Dan Root mentions in his groundbreaking book on detox, *Sauna Detoxification Using Niacin: Following the Recommended Protocol of Dr. Dave E. Root*, xenobiotics tend to remain stored in the fat cells for many years, unless acted upon. As a result, these toxins can induce inflammation which causes cellular damage, degeneration, and even death to all the cells that make up an organ or tissue because of "disease, injury, or failure of the blood supply." [196, Pg. 11] This makes sense as to why a bioaccumulation of toxins could possibly cause cancer, heart disease, and a whole host of other diseases – being that inflammation is the primary cause of all disease.

To detox the body, a biochemical process called lipolysis must be accomplished. Lipolysis is the breakdown of fat in the body which causes a "release of stored energy." [196, Pg. 60] Lipolysis occurs when an individual is in a fasting state and/or during specific heart rate training zones during cardio exercise. To accomplish this, I like to do some cardio training in the morning on an empty stomach. Exercise increases the body's core temperature and in effect, frees up toxins through the breakdown of fat. The toxins are then released into the bloodstream where they are processed through the liver, kidneys, and GI tract and then excreted in the feces and urine. A large percentage of toxins are also released through sweat, but mainly through a deep sebaceous sweat (sebum). Heat is the key component to getting a good sebaceous sweat. According to research, as mentioned in Root's book:

"Many heavy metals, methadone, amphetamines, methamphetamines, morphine, and other compounds appear in human sweat. Sebum-rich sebaceous sweat has been shown to contain high concentrations of PCBs. Enhancement of this elimination is a key purpose of the sauna." [196, Pg. 63]

SAUNA

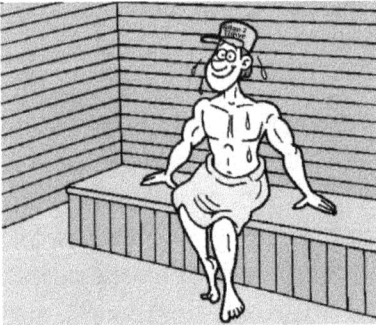

Sweating on a regular basis with exercise and sauna usage is CRUCIAL to maintaining good health. On average, I utilize a conventional sauna a minimum of 2-3 hours per week in conjunction with a full body workout and cardio. While exercise improves circulation and helps your body "mobilize" toxins (in the fluid) and get rid of them through the proper channels of elimination, the intense heat of a sauna helps your body go into a much deeper sweat (sebaceous sweat), therefore allowing your body to thoroughly detox. Root's protocol utilizes an infrared sauna which according to the research helps your body get rid of more toxins.

Infrared refers to the sun's healthiest rays. It is separated into near, mid, and far infrared waves. Each kind of infrared wave has its own benefit, but it is the far infrared that penetrates well below the surface of the skin. Far infrared waves get into the adipose tissue located in the subcutaneous layer of the skin and cause fat cells to "vibrate" and release stored toxins. [196, Pg. 64] The advantage here is that it works faster than a conventional sauna and doesn't have to use as much heat. Some research suggests utilizing an infrared sauna vs. a conventional sauna is more comfortable due to temperature and requires less time to accomplish better results.

A study done by a group of American researchers comparing the sweat of those using a conventional sauna vs. an infrared sauna found that the infrared sauna had much more of a detox effect. In fact, the sweat of those using the conventional sauna was mainly comprised of water (95-97%), while the sweat of those in the infrared sauna group was made up of about 80-85% water while the rest of it contained "cholesterol, fat soluble toxins, toxic heavy metals, sulfuric acid, sodium, ammonia, and uric acid." [196, Pg. 65] You don't find these toxins in regular sweat when you exercise.

Along with sauna use, Root's detox protocol calls for supplementation with niacin, aka Vitamin B3. Niacin primarily works because it has a rebound lipolysis effect, meaning when niacin is initially taken it inhibits the breakdown of fat (free fatty acids) and the mobilization of toxins for about 2.5 hours. After the inhibitory effect of niacin wears off, a rebound effect occurs and there is a substantial increase in fat breakdown and toxin release. According to one study, this rebound effect of niacin causes a 200% increase in fatty acid breakdown and toxin release [196, pg. 70].

Also, when niacin doses of 50 mg or higher are taken it causes a niacin flush. A niacin flush occurs when the capillaries expand and increase blood flow to the surface of your skin. The vasodilation causes the skin to turn bright red and is usually accompanied by itchiness and slight discomfort. However, the vasodilation and increased blood flow helps to enhance the body's removal of toxins through the skin, as well as through the liver and kidneys. The flush usually happens ten to sixty minutes after a high dose of niacin is taken.

Root recommended a powdered form of niacin vs. a pill or capsule. He also recommends titrating your dose up over a seven-day period to a target niacin dose (TND) for an optimal rebound effect. This is calculated at 10 mg per kg of body weight. I weigh 195 which means my target dose of niacin should be about 900 mg. Over time the body builds up a tolerance to the niacin and more of it will have to be taken to adhere to this detox protocol.

Patients treated by Root and who underwent a full two to four-week detox protocol were taking an average of 3,000 to 3,500 mg tittered up from the initial dose of 50 to 100 mg. [196, Pg. 124]

Root mastered his protocol and has step by step instructions on how to do it in his book. I will briefly summarize the protocol here, but I would strongly encourage you, the reader, to buy the book if you want a more in-depth knowledge and understanding of the protocol.

Step 1: Figure out your TND by dividing your total body weight by 2.2 and then multiply that number by 10. This represents your target dose of niacin. To start the program, you will start with 50 to 100 mg of niacin and then titrate up to your TND within approximately ten days. After your TND has been achieved, you will continue to titrate up by 50 to 100 mg doses to experience the niacin flush daily. As your body builds up tolerance you will know when you need to take more because the flush won't be as noticeable. You want to take your niacin a minimum of two hours before you begin the exercise and sauna sessions. This is to ensure rebound lipolysis is occurring to maximize the mobilization of xenobiotics and toxins. In the appendix section, I have included the niacin supplement recommendations.

Step 2: Workout twenty to thirty minutes before the sauna. The goal is to increase circulation. In the book Root recommends that cardio be performed at your training heart rate (THR) to maximize fat burn. Your body utilizes more fat for energy in this training zone vs. carbohydrates, thus releasing more stored toxins. To calculate your THR I have summarized the formula here:

220 – (AGE) = Maximum Heart Rate (MHR)

Multiply MHR by .6 or .85 to get your low and high end THR.

_____

Example for a 37-year-old
220 - 37 = 183 x .6 = 109 *(Low end)*

220 - 37 = 183 x .85 = 155 *(High end)*

A good cross training workout that blends some weight training and cardio together is also a great way to stimulate a good fat burn. In Chapter 8, Motion is Life, I talk extensively about High Intensity Interval Training *(HIIT)* and how that can get your body to burn fat while also boosting growth hormone and testosterone (two major fat burning hormones). Sprinters are great examples of this very concept because sprinters do short bursts of intense exercise followed by a brief period of rest. Sprinters have virtually zero body fat.

Step 3: Make sure you have regular access to a sauna. For a reasonable price you can purchase an infrared sauna to use in the comfort of your own home. If using an infrared sauna your total sauna time would be 75 minutes done over two sessions. The first session would last 45 minutes, followed by a 15 minute cool down session. During cool down it is recommended that you take a 5 minute cold shower to remove surface toxicants, and then, as an option, you can perform light-moderate exercises for ten minutes (resistance bands, jumping jacks, push-ups, etc.). Also, make sure to rehydrate during cool down with highly filtered water with electrolytes (salt, potassium, sodium chloride). Your second and last sauna session will last 30 minutes followed by a 15 minute cool down session. It is recommended that a calcium-magnesium (Cal-Mag) drink be consumed at this time (See supplementation below – recipe is in the appendix)

Step 4: Continue the protocol for 2-4 weeks for maximum benefit. Get lots of rest and make sure you are supplementing with vitamins and minerals, as the detox process itself can be incredibly challenging on your body. One should always look for organic vitamins and minerals that haven't been genetically modified or loaded with fillers and preservatives. A complete list of vitamins and minerals is found in Root's book on pages 118-120.

Step 5: Supplementation.

- Beginning: At the start of each session it is important to take four tablespoons of cold pressed polyunsaturated oils (organic flax seed oil, hemp, sunflower, etc.). The oils help to reduce the reabsorption of mobilized toxins.

- Middle: Drink one teaspoon of activated charcoal mixed with a full glass of water after your 20-30 minutes of exercise (cardio, HITT training). The activated charcoal works to bind to xenobiotics in the gut and safely remove them from your body via the feces. Also, after each sauna session you will replenish your electrolytes with four cell salt tablets, one tablet of potassium, and one tablet of sodium chloride mixed into one small cup of water. Drink adequate amounts of filtered water to stay hydrated.

- End: After your last sauna session is over, the protocol calls for consuming 12-16 ounces of the Cal-Mag drink to replenish electrolytes and hydrate. Calcium is critical for the proper function of the heart, muscles, and nerves. Magnesium is also needed for the nerve system to function properly. It is used in hundreds of biochemical reactions – it's essential! The Cal-Mag recipe also calls for apple cider vinegar which helps your body to easily absorb the calcium and magnesium without which these vital minerals would pass right out the other end. Because the sauna causes you to sweat profusely, a deficiency in these vital nutrients can occur if they aren't replaced. Furthermore, after you take a cold shower one tablespoon of bentonite or micronized zeolite clay mixed with one cup of water to further capture toxins in the gut is taken. It's important to note that micronized zeolite has the benefit of absorbing toxins in the blood to prevent them from being redistributed in other tissues, such as the brain.

It is important that you speak with an expert to find out if this protocol is going to be safe for you. If you have a current medical condition, it's important to speak to a licensed healthcare provider. Medical conditions such as diabetes, renal (kidney) disease, heart disease, Chronic Fatigue Syndrome, hemophilia, and hypothyroidism, among others, *can* be negatively impacted by the protocol and therefore individuals must consult and be guided by an expert in the field of detox. Other contraindications include, but aren't limited to, acute injuries if you're currently taking medications, if you're breastfeeding, if you're pregnant, or if you have a pacemaker.

Most people, regardless of their medical condition, would benefit from a detox and/or cleansing program. Due to its intensity, this detox program may need to be adjusted on an individual basis. For example, smaller amounts of niacin might need to be consumed depending on one's medical condition. Also, less time might need to be spent in the sauna, along with less time exercising. It's important to listen to your body and what it's telling you. You don't want to force your body into doing something it doesn't want to do, **BUT you also don't want to give up when the going gets tough.** As with any detox program – you will often get worse before you get better.

Possible Symptoms of Detox and Niacin Use Include

- Brain fog
- Rapid heartbeat
- Headaches
- Cramping
- Abdominal pain
- Irritability
- Hypotension (discontinue)
- Cold sweats & feeling cold
- Dizziness
- Heart arrhythmia
- Diarrhea
- Shortness of Breath
- Fatigue
- Vomiting
- Insomnia
- General feeling of sickness

- Feeling "emotional"
- Body aches
- Extreme cravings
- A yearning to sleep more

The benefits of a thorough detox program might seem a bit obvious in the sense that you are getting rid of toxins that are more than likely zapping your energy and thus your quality of life. A lot of people don't realize that their health problems are in a large part due to the bioaccumulations of toxins in their body along with continued exposure to said toxins – it's a constant barrage. Misinformation in the field of detox has led many astray, thus many Americans remain sick and their overall toxic burden increases daily. So, imagine if you were to get rid of the toxins that are decreasing your life and vitality. How do you think you would feel if your toxic burden was decreased?

Subjectively, these are some of the things people report after doing this specific detox program.

- Increased energy
- Decreased joint pain
- Decreased stress
- Weight loss
- Better cognitive function
- Better sleep
- Better sense of well-being
- Better attitude

Objective improvements include, but aren't limited to, lowered blood pressure and cholesterol. Diabetics reported a reduction or complete elimination of their diabetic medications [196].

You can order kits to test your heavy metal and toxic chemical burden before and after the detox. I think it's important to test because it can give you a stronger motivation to complete the program. Root recommends "Great Plains Laboratories" or "Doctor's Data" to test your blood, urine, hair, and feces. If detoxing from a drug, as in the case of a drug addiction, drug testing kits can be ordered off Amazon.
[196, Pg. 116]

"It has been calculated that one new industrial chemical enters industrial use every twenty minutes, and many hundreds of thousands of them are already out there. As a result, the average person living in the developed world is now contaminated with up to 500 industrial toxins, few of which have been thoroughly tested for harmful effects."

Dr. Paula Baille-Hamilton, [198, Pg. 14]

TYPES OF TOXINS

One of the best ways to detox is to never have a need to do so, which is literally impossible living in our modern world. However, we can take steps that will help to reduce our overall toxic burden. Some environmental toxins to avoid are overtly obvious, but there are also less obvious ones you need to be aware of. Following is a brief description of common toxins you need to be aware of and avoid as much as possible.

ENVIROMENTAL

There are so many "man-made" toxins we are exposed to in our environment it can be overwhelming just thinking about them all. Most of the toxins we are exposed to in the environment are breathed into the lungs and end up in our bloodstreams. These toxins end up negatively impacting all plant and animal life – making all foods (no matter how "organic" they are), toxic to a certain degree. The levels of toxins we are exposed to in our environment are unprecedented compared to any other era in human existence. One can certainly make the argument that because the world has become so infiltrated with man-made toxins in the environment, this is one of the chief reasons why we are SO SICK! This is the sole reason why I believe we should be detoxing regularly.

GEOENGINEERING PROGRAMS

Five years ago, I watched a documentary by Michael Murphy about stratospheric aerosol geoengineering called, *What in the World Are They Spraying*, and it blew my mind. This documentary explained in great depth what the long white streaks are that trail across the blue sky. I have seen these "trails" for years and hadn't a clue what was going on. Most days you can see jet airplanes laying these trails from horizon to horizon. The trails crisscross and intertwine and end up covering the whole sky in one big blanket of white which blocks the sun. It's a very big eyesore. The slang term used for these trails spoken about in many conspiracy theorist's circles and throughout the internet is "chemtrails." The scientific term used, however, is geoengineering. [199]

Geoengineering is defined as the "artificial modification of the earth's climate." [200] Many scientists, corporations, and governments want to artificially alter the earth's climate for many different reasons. "In 1961 President John F. Kennedy announced at the United Nations General Assembly a proposition to implement schemes that could effectively predict and control global weather patterns." [201] Since then advancements in technology have led to many ways of controlling and altering our weather using HAARP, satellites, cloud seeding, etc. According to Michael Murphy, in 2011 geoengineers were proposing to spray twenty million tons of toxic aluminum nanoparticles into our skies with the intended goal of cooling our planet. [199] However, according to independent research the "powers that be" have been spraying the skies with chemtrails for the past thirty years.

In fact, Raytheon, which means light from the Gods, is a technology company that describes themselves as an "innovations leader in defense, civil government, and cybersecurity solutions." They have held patents since 1991 on several weather altering and ionosphere altering technologies. [202] Raytheon's Patent # 4999637 is for the "creation of **artificial** ionization clouds above the earth." [203] But to what purpose? On top of this, **there is a list of over one hundred US held patents on weather modification**

and control. Food for thought. When you consider the fact that "they" have certainly tested their geoengineering programs in the past, you can safely assume they are still testing them to this day. The biggest difference is the programs have become more insidious.

CHEMTRAILS

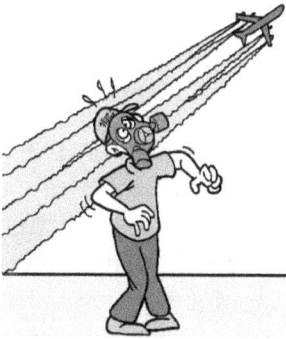

What is more insidious than a deadly combination of chemical trails that spread out to prevent us from seeing the beautiful blue sky as well the sun? We need the sun to help our bodies naturally produce vitamin D. Vitamin D is essential for our immune system to work effectively. Eventually these trails, which are comprised of several speculative toxins, trickle down to the earth's surface. They get on our skin, we breathe them in, they get into the soil, and they negatively impact all plant and animal life on this planet.

In the documentary, *Why in the World Are They Spraying?*, a group of scientists in northern California began questioning why the forest was collapsing and why people were having such a hard time growing natural organic crops. They discovered that the pH of the soil was becoming more alkaline by a factor of ten to twelve! [199] This is shocking because for plants to thrive, the soil must be acidic, otherwise they begin to die. When the scientists did further tests, they discovered incredibly high levels of aluminum, strontium, and barium in the soil, all of which work to make the soil more alkaline. These metals are considered by many researchers to be the "chemical hallmark" of aerosol geoengineering programs and have even been used by geoengineering scientists to reflect sunlight in order to cool the planet in the future. [204] Yet, all geoengineers have adamantly denied that any geoengineering efforts in the form of chemtrails are going on today.

According to independent research projects from around the world, chemtrails contain "barium, nano aluminum-coated fiberglass (A.K.A CHAFF), radioactive thorium, cadmium, chromium, nickel, desiccated blood, mold spores, yellow fungal mycotoxins, ethylene dibromide, and polymer fibers." [205] Sadly, most people think these trails are just contrails (condensation trails), but contrails usually evaporate within moments – chemtrails seem to last forever. Deniers refuse to see the obvious, and call those that question the truth conspiracy theorists.

It can't be a conspiracy "theory" if it's true...

Lastly, from an environmental standpoint, these programs are very damaging. They cause increased droughts, devastating forest fires, increased flooding, record high temperatures, ice storms, and overall weird weather patterns which have caused much alarm. However, from a human health standpoint our exposure to these toxic heavy metals and chemicals we end up breathing in is devastating as well. Independent tests done on hair follicles and blood samples have revealed extremely high levels of barium and aluminum, which can cause a vast array of problems – mainly respiratory illness and neurological disorders. [206]

Despite being called a quack, renowned neurosurgeon, Dr. Russel Blaylock, has openly talked about chemtrails and our exposure to toxic aluminum nanoparticles. According to Blaylock, these aerosolized particles travel up through the nose and along the olfactory nerve to an area of the brain called the hippocampus which is responsible for things like memory and emotions. [206] Furthermore, Blaylock states that aerosolized aluminum is one of the metals that very easily bypasses the blood-brain barrier, going directly to the brain where it accumulates. Studies in animals have confirmed that aerosolized aluminum accumulates in the brain and forms lesions, negatively impacting the animal's memory, behavior, and learning capabilities. [206] Alzheimer's Disease, which goes hand and hand with aluminum toxicity, is rapidly increasing. It is estimated that currently 5.5 million people living in the US of all ages have Alzheimer's Disease. [207] Could our constant exposure to aerosolized aluminum nanoparticles from chemtrails be contributing to the rapid rise in Alzheimer's Disease? The question remains.

One of the questions I have always pondered and many skeptics tout is, "Aren't they negatively impacting their own health as well? And, if so, why continue to spray?" If you were to Google "chemtrail conspiracy theories," there are plenty of websites, blogs, and articles debunking them as some sort of a "tin-foil-hat-wearing-crazy-conspiracy theory." The naysayers will tell you you're crazy to question reality and think that something fishy is going on. Sadly, folks working to expose the truth are usually ad hominem attacked and verbally bashed on the internet. I would encourage you to do your own research and come up with well thought out conclusions. But don't be closed minded because it's easier or because you think conspiracy theories aren't true.

If there are enough correlative things that add up and provide a plausible explanation as to what might be going on – **IT IS UP TO YOU TO SEEK OUT THE TRUTH** and turn your critical thinking skills on. Using common sense and your instincts can be your greatest ally.

Good resources to check out on this subject:

https://www.geoengineeringwatch.com
https://byebyebluesky.com
https://www.globalskywatch.com
Michael Murphy's documentaries: *What in the World are They Spraying?* and *Why in the World are They Spraying?*

HOW DO WE PROTECT OURSELVES?

The only way to fully protect us is to get the powers that be to STOP spraying the planet. However, we must assume that isn't going to happen anytime soon. Since that isn't going to happen anytime soon, we need to protect ourselves by ANY MEANS NECESSARY. Chemtrails are one of the many reasons why I feel detoxing regularly is a necessity. Below are some suggested ways to protect yourself from this toxicity.

Reduce Toxins: Focus on eliminating as many toxins in your life as possible, so you are reducing your overall toxic burden. Also, reduce your exposure.

House Filters: Purchase top of the line house filters as well as HEPA filters for all your vents. I would also invest in a good air purifier.

Eat Clean: Eat a super clean and healthy diet consisting of plenty of healthy fats and greens. (See Chapter 6)

Healthy Water: Drink plenty of purified, thoroughly filtered water that's ionized. (check out Ion Thrive System – see Chapter 5)

Supplements:

- **Vitamin C** is an antioxidant that helps to remove toxins and waste products from the body. It also helps to protect the brain. Studies show it can help prevent Alzheimer's Disease.

- **Vitamin E** is another powerful antioxidant that helps to protect the brain and remove toxins. Dr. Russel Blaylock says to take both vitamin C and vitamin E in combination. [206]

- **Chlorella** is a super food plant alga that I spoke about in the nutrition chapter. It's a potent detoxifier in that it binds to heavy metals and safely helps to remove them from the body.

- **Spirulina** is another plant alga that is packed with nutrients and protein. In fact, one teaspoon of spirulina contains four grams of protein and more protein per ounce than a steak. Spirulina is also a great detoxifier of the body.

- **Activated charcoal** works by trapping toxins and chemicals in the gut. It is negatively charged which attracts positively charged chemicals and toxins. Use activated charcoal if you're doing the detox protocol. Warning: activated charcoal can cause nausea and vomiting.

- **Bentonite clay** is recommended during the detox protocol. This powerful clay is very absorbent. It has a negative charge which attracts and binds to heavy metals, toxins, intestinal worms (parasites), pesticides, and herbicides to safely remove them from the gut. Bentonite clay is reasonably priced and affordable. [208]

- **Liquid chlorophyll** is a great supplement to add to your water. Chlorophyll is what makes plants green and it just so happens that it is a great detoxifier because it increases your liver enzymes which work to remove and eliminate waste. Chlorophyll also works to pull dioxins out of your fat cells.

- **Protandim** is a supplement I use every day because it has been clinically proven to up-regulate (increase) your body's "survival genes" through what is called the Nrf2 pathway. These survival genes radically reduce free radicals and other oxidants, thus reducing oxidative stress. I talk a great deal about oxidative stress and free radicals in Chapter 11.

Detox: Do the Detox Protocol. For more information check out the video training series created by Dan Root at my affiliate link. https://getdetoxinated.teachable.com/p/sauna-detoxification-using-niacin/?coupon_code=DETOX50&affcode=363985_ktcp3qj3

DDT

DDT is a pervasive insecticide that was heavily sprayed in military and civilian populations in the 1940's to combat malaria, typhoid, and other insect-borne diseases. Initially it had great success. However, despite warnings from investigators and doctors, it was later approved in 1945 for broad use in the United States. And, when I say broad use, I mean it in every sense of the word. DDT was infused into paint and wallpaper, trucks would drive through neighborhoods spraying huge clouds of white smoke to fumigate the area, kids were heavily sprayed while they swam, it was even considered so "safe" we were taught that you could eat it by the spoonful and put it on your food. Warnings came and researchers tried to sound the trumpet, but they were called quacks and charlatans and were quickly dismissed. [209, 210]

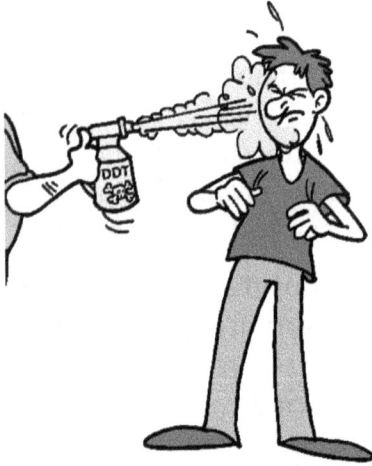

These warnings were because pesticides and insecticides were known central nervous system poisons. In fact, it was scientifically determined that DDT was harmful to all forms of life. One such "quack" trying to sound the trumpet was Dr. Morton S. Biskind, MD. This is what he had to say about what he called "X-Disease," a syndrome affecting animals and humans alike. In his 1953 article, published in the "American Journal of Digestive Diseases," he states:

"[X-Disease] ... studied by the author following known exposure to DDT and related compounds and repeatedly in the same patients, each time following known exposure. We have described the syndrome as follows. In acute exacerbations, mild clonic convulsions involving mainly the legs, have been observed.

*Several young children exposed to DDT developed a limp
lasting from 2 or 3 days to a week or more...* [209]

What was interesting is that during that time Biskind noted, "Beginning in 1946 the rate of increase [for polio] more than doubled." [209] Polio is a virus that in its most severe form may cause paralysis. [211] In 1952, 57,628 cases of polio were diagnosed in the United States. These numbers are more than double the 27,000 cases of polio diagnosed in 1916. Biskind pointed out that there were studies (Lilly, National Institutes of Health) that showed DDT "may produce degeneration of the anterior horn cells of the spinal cord in animals, [resembling those in human polio]." Biskind further tries to sound the alarm in his writings.

*"When the population is exposed to a chemical agent known to
produce in animals lesions in the spinal cord resembling those in
human polio, and thereafter the latter disease increases sharply in
incidence and maintains its epidemic character year after year, is it
unreasonable to suspect an etiologic relationship?"* [209]

It doesn't seem unreasonable to question the role that chemicals play in human health and disease. Even today these chemical technologies are rushed into use despite NOT having the long-term safety studies done to support them. We end up becoming guinea pigs and the long-term damage is irreversible. Barbara Cohn, an epidemiologist, conducted a study of 20,000 pregnant women and children exposed to DDT between the years 1959-1976. She was able to detect a fivefold increase in breast cancer in those exposed to DDT before puberty. The study also showed an increased risk of breast and testicular cancer in their offspring. [212]

Even though in the US the use of DDT was banned in 1972, it is still possible to be exposed to it today, mainly because of its resiliency. According to the CDC, "DDT and its related chemicals can remain for a long time in our environment." [213] It persists in the food chain as it bioaccumulates in the fat cells of animals which means that higher concentrations and levels are found in bigger animals of prey. Shockingly, in the study done on fetal cord blood, mentioned in the beginning of this chapter, DDT was one of the organochlorine pesticides found. This gives credence to the fact that we should all be detoxing regularly, because these toxins can affect our offspring and future generations. [195]

Polychlorinated biphenyls (PCBs), another industrial pollutant found in fetal cord blood, were massively produced in the 1920's by a company well known for destroying the environment – Monsanto. I can't even write their name without cringing. "PCBs, were used as hydraulic fluid, for cutting oil, [as well as a] lubricant for electric motors, capacitors, and transformers." [214] The first PCB plant was in the state of Illinois where it was proven that Monsanto and another company were dispelling PCBs into the sewage treatment systems. This first location coincidentally has one of the highest rates of birth defects. Monsanto has been sued for hundreds of millions of dollars because of this one chemical alone – MAINLY because they dumped it into streams and rivers, fully knowing how toxic it was. [214, 215, 216]

Here is a quick Top Three list for all the environmental toxins produced by Monsanto.

1. *Agent Orange & Dioxin*: Monsanto and Dow Chemical are primarily responsible for spraying hundreds of millions of pounds of dioxin containing herbicide onto more than 400 million acres of farmland. Dioxins are well known for being a primary cause of cancer, severe birth defects, neurological disorders, etc. Both Monsanto and Dow used this herbicide (2,4,5-T) combined with the herbicide 2,4-D to produce agent orange. It is estimated that 12.1 million gallons of agent orange were dropped onto 4.8 million Vietnamese during the Vietnam war. According to the Vietnamese Ministry of Foreign Affairs, this resulted in 400,000 people being killed or harmed and 500,000 children being born with severe birth defects. Women had higher rates of miscarriage and stillbirths, as did many

animals. American troops were also negatively affected. By the 1990's nearly 40,000 disability claims were filed by American soldiers. Many Vietnam vets suspect their cancers, thyroid disorders, and their wives' miscarriages were due to agent orange exposure. [215, 217]

2. *Roundup:* This is one of the most popular weed killers. The active ingredient in Roundup is glyphosate. For decades, the toxic effects and health risks of glyphosate contained in Roundup were downplayed and dismissed. However, most recently, Monsanto was sued for $289 million dollars because it was proven that Roundup caused plaintiff, Dewayne Johnson's, (age 46) terminal cancer. As a groundskeeper for a San Francisco school, Johnson would spray the herbicide 20-30 times per year. According to Johnson, sometimes during windy days his face would end up covered in the herbicide. At the age of forty-two he developed a rash which was later diagnosed as Non-Hodgkin's Lymphoma. Sadly, Roundup has gotten into everything. So, regardless of whether you use the herbicide outside of your house or not, odds are you have been exposed to it many times during your life. You might be astonished to learn that roughly **75 % of the food you buy in a grocery store contains genetically modified ingredients** which probably contain glyphosate residue. For a list of foods that contain the highest levels of glyphosate, go to my blog titled, "Foods High in Monsatan's Glyphosate." What's even more astonishing is that glyphosate residue was found in several childhood vaccines. Dr. Stephanie Seneff, a Microbe Inotech Laboratories scientist, explains that certain vaccine viruses, including the MMR (measles) and flu (Influenza) vaccine are grown on gelatin derived from the ligaments of pigs fed **GMO** feed. The GMO feed contains a heavy amount of glyphosate and some of it ends up bioaccumulating in the collagen containing ligaments used for making gelatin. Founder of the Center for Disease Prevention and Reversal and co-producer of the movie *Bought*, Dr. Toni Bark, MD, said "I am deeply concerned

about injecting glyphosate, a known pesticide, directly into children. Neither Roundup nor glyphosate has been tested for safety as an injectable." It goes to show you how pervasive spraying chemicals on our food and soil can be. The solution here is to purchase organic food and shop your local farmer's market. By law, organic food cannot contain any genetically modified ingredients. [218, 219]

3. *Genetically Modified Food:* Genetically modifying crops has been utilized by farmers for thousands of years. When farmers wanted the best quality and yield, they would utilize what is called plant breeding. Plant breeding involves methods such as selecting plants with desirable characteristics and then crossing or interbreeding them with closely (or distantly) related plants to produce crops that are of a desired quality. For example, a farmer might breed pest resistant corn with high yielding corn to produce a high yielding and pest resistance corn crop. Plant breeding is VASTLY different from genetically engineering plants. They are two entirely different things. Monsanto just so happens to be the leader when it comes to genetically modifying and engineering foods. Genetically altering foods usually involves genetically altering the plants genetic material with the genetic material of an unrelated organism. Monsanto genetically altered corn, cotton, and soybeans so they could create their own pesticide. How they were able to do this is something straight out of a sci-fi movie. Monsanto scientists took genes from a bacterium that produces its own insecticide and implanted them into the genetic material of corn, cotton, and soy plants. Odds are you have eaten genetically modified corn and soy for most of your life without knowing it. Of course, there haven't been any long-term studies done to show how GMOs might negatively impact human health and our ecosystems. In fact, 300 independent researchers, after looking at the available research, including the research that says GMOs are safe, signed a statement which says GMOs are neither safe nor unsafe and that there is no

[true] "scientific consensus on GMO safety." *(Environmental Sciences Europe)* Would you want to ingest a GM food when the only people saying it is unequivocally safe work for the very companies that make the GM food? I seriously doubt you would. The Academy of Environmental Medicine encourages doctors to prescribe a diet consisting of no GMOs, citing animal studies showing organ damage, GI, and immune system disorders. To me, real food is the way to go vs. eating Frankenfood – don't deny your gut instinct. [220, 221, 222]

PLASTIC

There is a great documentary called *TAPPED*. The film revealed that we throw away an estimated thirty million one-time use plastic water bottles every day, most of which ends up in the Pacific Ocean. What is even more crazy is that 40% of all bottled water is just cheaply filtered tap water, and it's expensive! One of the main issues with plastic has to do with a chemical that is used to harden it called bisphenol A (BPA). BPA has been used for over forty years in the making of plastics and it's everywhere. It's used in water bottles, the lining of canned foods and drinks, and believe it or not - paper receipts! BPA has even been detected in the air, dust, and water. Due to its omnipresence, almost everybody at any given time would test positive for BPA. Odds are that you and I would even test positive, and to me that SUCKS! [223, 224]

BPA has been linked to endocrine disruption, hormone interference, fetal development problems, behavioral issues, cancer, cardiovascular disease, and child development problems. So, the question remains, "Should you just buy BPA free plastic?" Sure, you can buy BPA free, but other chemicals used in the making of plastics are harmful as well. Chemicals like polyvinyl chloride [which by itself] "releases dioxins, phthalates, vinyl chloride, ethylene dichloride, lead, cadmium, and other toxic chemicals." Here's the kicker, when plastic is exposed to heat it breaks down – meaning these toxic chemicals are released into the water you're drinking, into the air you breathe from the plastic that off gasses in your car, and it can even get onto your skin where it is eventually absorbed into your blood stream. Cheryl Watson, a professor in the biochemistry and molecular biology department at the University of Texas Medical Branch in Galveston, strongly advised people not to store their bottled water in hot places. She said heat causes the molecules in the plastic to speed up going from one phase to another so that these chemicals used in the making of plastic eventually leech into the water you're drinking. [225]

You might be surprised to find out that most receipts are lined with BPA that gets onto the palm of your hand when you crumple them up. Once the plastic gets onto your skin it will eventually be absorbed into your blood stream. [226] I opt out of receipts, but if I need a receipt for my business, I leave it in the bag and eventually transfer it to a folder I use for tax purposes.

Avoid plastic water bottles by buying a stainless-steel container to keep your filtered water in. Don't ever leave your plastic containers in the heat, always keep them in a shaded area. And, NEVER heat up any plastic container in the microwave. If you still use a microwave, STOP NOW! Third, always park your car in a shaded area or use a sun visor for your windshield. Also, leave the windows in your car slightly cracked so that some of the off gassing that may occur exits your car. It's really that simple.

INSIDE THE HOME

Have you ever walked down the cleaning isle of a grocery store and smelled the off gassing of all those wonderfully toxic chemicals? At that point you are essentially breathing in a vast array of toxic and harmful chemicals that are carcinogenic. Here are a few you should be aware of: phthalates (fragrance), triclosan (antibacterial soaps), ammonia, and chlorine.

Anytime a product has "fragrance" on the label, phthalates are usually the culprit. The issue with phthalates is they can be inhaled, and they can also be absorbed through the skin. Phthalates are also known endocrine disrupters. Anything that is absorbed through the skin goes right to your organs via the bloodstream.

Triclosan is used as an antibacterial in hand sanitizer. It's also a probable carcinogen. Tests have shown that quite a bit of it has polluted our streams and rivers. America's obsession over toxic hand sanitizers is an oxymoron. On one hand we want our hands to be clean, but on the other hand we are using a toxic substance to do it! Does that make any sense whatsoever? No, it doesn't! Non-toxic soap works simply fine for cleaning your hands.

Ammonia is found in cleaning products like Pine-Sol. I can still remember my mom cleaning the linoleum floors in the kitchen with Pine-Sol and I can still remember the feeling of my lungs burning when I would breathe in. Listen, if the off gassing burns your lungs when you breathe, it's usually toxic. Ammonia is going to irritate anybody who has lung issues – especially those with asthma and COPD. Yet, all and all, it's toxic regardless of whether you have lung issues. Use an organic, non-toxic floor cleaner or make your own. In our office we use a non-toxic cleaner composed of thieves and filtered water.

Thieves is an essential oil concoction made up of clove, lemon, cinnamon, eucalyptus radiata, and rosemary blends. It gets out tough stains and leaves a good scent behind. Most importantly, it's completely non-toxic and can be used for a variety of different cleaning purposes. [228]

I wrote extensively about chlorine in Chapter 5. Chlorine is used in a lot of bathroom cleaning products. It is absorbed rapidly through the skin – some say in as little as twenty-six seconds! Studies show it can disrupt the function of the thyroid. Because chlorine is very reactive it reacts to organic matter and forms disinfection byproducts which are known carcinogens. It isn't good to breathe in chlorine, and like ammonia, it irritates the bronchioles of the lungs and causes inflammation. [227]

You can make your own all-natural (organic) cleaners at home. It's as simple as that, really! Vinegar is a great cleaner if you can get over the smell. Combine a little vinegar and lemon and mix with filtered water and you have made yourself a great all-purpose cleaner. Here is a quick all-purpose cleaning recipe I found on the internet.

3 parts filtered water

1-part vinegar

1-2 tsp lemon juice

5-7 drops of lemon essential oil or thieves essential oil

Add to spray bottle and fill remaining amount with warm water. [228, 229]

Your carpet is composed of a ton of toxins that you probably don't want to hear about. Most carpets are loaded with volatile organic compounds (VOC's) – like fire retardants which are carcinogenic. These chemicals in carpet create a gas which eventually gets into your respiratory system. They also are absorbed through your skin when you walk around your house barefoot. Older carpets also contain a ton of dust mites, dust, dirt, pesticides, and other various toxins that are brought in from pets and shoes. These microscopic toxins get trapped in the carpet fibers and are kicked into the air whenever we vacuum or scuffle our feet. The best thing to do is remove your carpet and install tile, bamboo, or wood flooring. But if you love carpet like I do and prefer your rooms carpeted – make sure to buy natural wool carpets or rugs. These natural "green carpets" don't contain all the harmful chemicals that store-bought carpets contain. [230]

PERSONAL CARE PRODUCTS

My heart goes out to women who have grown up in this matrix system where using toxic products to make themselves look beautiful is considered "normal." Women use makeup, perfumes, deodorants, shampoos, and soaps that are loaded with numerous toxins that bioaccumulate in the body. There are too many toxins to mention here, but I will name a few.

Parabens

Parabens are used in many cosmetic products as a preservative. Although this preservative works to slow the growth of bacteria and make the product last longer on the shelf, some alarming studies show that it may be linked to breast cancer. Parabens penetrate the skin and mimic estrogen. A rise of estrogen in the body causes an increase in cell division in the breasts and possibly the growth of tumors. The cosmetic products themselves only contain trace amounts of parabens, however these bioaccumulate in the body over time, which can potentially lead to problems down the road. Females typically start wearing makeup when they are teenagers and continue to use makeup consistently (almost daily) throughout their lifetime. It's very important for girls and women of any age to buy organic, non-toxic products that contain NO parabens (read the labels). Parabens can be labeled under several different names: butylparaben, methylparaben, propylparaben, etc. so be aware. [231. 232]

Formaldehyde

Formaldehyde, like parabens, is used as a preservative in many cosmetic products to kill off microorganisms. In fact, the FDA estimates it is used in one out of every five cosmetic products to prolong the shelf life. If exposed to large amounts of it over time, it can be a potent carcinogen. It's important to note that we are exposed to formaldehyde from a variety of different sources (car exhaust, secondhand smoke, gas stoves) in addition to cosmetics. Don't buy products that contain formaldehyde.

Look for these formaldehyde releasing chemicals on the cosmetic product label.

- DMDM hydantoin
- Imidazolidinyl urea
- Diazolidinyl urea
- Quaternium-15
- Bronopol (*2-bromo-2-nitropropane-1,3-diol*)
- 5-Bromo-5-nitro-1,3-dioxane
- Hydroxymethylglycinate

[231]

Aluminum

Aluminum salts have been used in deodorant since the early 1900's to stop unpleasurable odor, yet we now know through science that aluminum is a potent neurotoxin.

Aluminum has been linked to Alzheimer's Disease, bone disorders, and breast cancer.

Despite this knowledge, product manufacturers continue to use trace amounts of aluminum in their products because it works great as an antiperspirant. Personally, I would much rather sweat and stink.

According to a 2005 article written in the Journal of Inorganic Biochemistry, there is a high incidence of breast cancer in the upper outer quadrant of the breast, as well as "reports of genomic instability in outer quadrants of the breast" which seems to correlate with locally applied cosmetic chemicals. The article further states that aluminum can cause "both DNA alterations and epigenetic effects" which could play a potential role in breast cancer. [233]

The solution is to buy organic, aluminum free deodorant, but when doing so make sure the product doesn't contain triclosan for reasons mentioned above. Some deodorants also contain propylene glycol which is a liquid alcohol used in some anti-freeze. It is considered less toxic than ethylene glycol but has still been linked to disrupting the endocrine system. When in doubt, always go with a non-toxic version or make your own with coconut oil and baking soda. You shouldn't have a hard time finding an effective brand of non-toxic deodorant at a Whole Foods, Sprouts, or your local health food store.

Many shampoos and body washes contain several of the toxins listed above including parabens, triclosan, and phthalates. Two other common ingredients used in shampoos and body wash that we should be concerned about are sulfates and polyethylene glycol. [234]

Sulfates are a chemical detergent that may possibly cause an imbalance in our hormones. Even more concerning is the fact that sulfates contain traces of dioxane, a well-known carcinogen.

California has classified polyethylene glycol as a developmental toxicant which means it is harmful to babies, children, and pregnant women. It also contains traces of dioxane.

Seeking out organic shampoo and body washes that are truly *natural* can be a very daunting task. As a consumer you must understand that organic doesn't truly mean ORGANIC! This is because manufacturers get away with loopholes in the labeling laws. I found a great article titled, "The 20 Best Organic Shampoos that are Actually Non-Toxic," by Skincare Ox, a website that focuses on making the world of skincare a bit easier for the consumer. I have included the link in the reference section. [234]

I will not go into detail about filters here since we already discussed them in a previous chapter. Buying a shower filter is a very affordable way of keeping toxins out of your body. As mentioned in the chapter on Water (Chapter 5), chlorine is a toxin you want to keep from getting into your body. Unfortunately, for us, we absorb much more chlorine through our skin than we do from our drinking water. When you take a hot shower the pores in your skin open and chlorine is rapidly absorbed. Also, when the water begins to steam you are then breathing in chlorine in its gaseous form. [235]

Name brand toothpastes are the worst to use to clean your teeth – mainly because these brands contain fluoride which is a known neurotoxin. Refer to our discussion on fluoride in Chapter 9. Fortunately, you can easily make your own toothpaste, but if you're like me and you're looking for something convenient, any health food store will have fluoride free, non-toxic toothpaste. I personally use Tom's "fluoride free" Toothpaste.

It's odd that a toothpaste tube has a warning label that says to call poison control if swallowed because of the toxicity level of fluoride, YET fluoride is dumped into the drinking water supply of almost every city throughout the country. This is what makes fluoride one of the most **unregulated** drugs on the face of the planet. As a rule of thumb, always drink filtered water. See Chapter 5 for more information about fluoride and water filtration.

I was debating writing about tampons as a man, but I must speak the truth on the matter. You want to go as NON-TOXIC as possible and here is why.

> "The vaginal tissue is lined with permeable mucous membranes which protect the body from bacteria, but which can also easily absorb or be irritated by other chemicals. Vaginal tissues are filled with blood vessels and thus have a near direct route for chemicals to be absorbed into your bloodstream. Studies have shown that hormone chemicals, like estrogen, will be absorbed vaginally at 10-80 times the rate that the same dose would be absorbed orally. So, there is real concern about the potential for chemicals associated with tampons affecting women's health." [236]

Tampons contain a toxic barrage of chemicals known to cause cancer and disrupt hormones. Dioxins, pesticide residues, and UNKNOWN chemicals used for fragrance are just a few of the toxins found in tampons that are linked to a multitude of health conditions in women. The good news is that there are feminine care companies who list out all their ingredients in their products and are also committed to going "ALL-NATURAL." For a list of these companies visit the website listed here: *https: www. womensvoices.org.* [236]

You probably haven't considered the fact that the lovely fragrance you smell after you wash and dry your clothes with synthetic chemicals is toxic. We have been hardwired into thinking that when something smells good it equates to that item being clean. This couldn't be any truer than when it comes to the wonderful world of laundry. Name brand laundry detergents are packed with upwards of 15 to 20 different chemicals that have been proven to cause hormone imbalances, cancer, dermatitis, and several other problems. The laundry detergent you choose to wash your kid's clothes with could be causing ADHD and flares of their allergies. The bad news is that most name brands you're familiar with are toxic. There is absolutely nothing to be cheerful about using Cheer! The good news is that there are a ton of non-toxic, safe options you can purchase online or from your local health food store. You should also purchase fabric softener and dryer sheets that are non-toxic. Look for the "Made Safe" website in the blog titled: "Is your Laundry Detergent Killing You?" (https://www. thrivespinecenter.com) [237]

MEDICAL PROCEDURES

This is always one of the most controversial topics to talk about as many in the medical field say that the "benefits always out-weigh the risks" for most medical procedures. There seems to be an overwhelming consensus that we should just listen to our doctors or our governing authorities when it comes to health care despite our apprehensions and unanswered questions. The problem with this argument is the fact that all medical schools are heavily funded by the pharmaceutical companies which have a vested interest in making sure the masses seek out medical care. So, of course the information taught at the medical institutions will always downplay the adverse reactions that may occur because of the medications, medical procedures, and vaccines. Also, our politicians who work to pass legislation that would call for "forced" medical procedures, as is the case with vaccines, are "SPONSORED" by pharmaceutical companies. The pharmaceutical companies line the very pockets of the politicians who are passing legislation that heavily encroaches upon our freedoms as Americans. I find it sad and downright, WRONG!

There are three things I want to touch upon in this section: mammograms, prescription medications, and vaccines. All three have been proven to be highly toxic to humans and yet the risks are downplayed by the medical community.

MAMMOGRAMS

In 2012 the British Medical Journal reported that mammograms can increase a woman's risk of getting breast cancer, especially if they have the BCRA 1 & 2 gene mutations. In his book, *Preventing Breast Cancer*, Dr. John Gofman reports that "75% of breast cancers are caused by radiation, primarily medical x-rays." [44] Mammograms use high dose ionizing radiation while compressing the breast tissue. In fact, one mammogram can have the radiation equivalent of 1,000 chest x-rays. The other issue with mammograms is that when the breasts are compressed at 42 lbs. between two metal plates, this makes for a very painful procedure for women. Shockingly, it only takes 22 pounds of pressure to rupture the encapsulation of a cancerous tumor which can spread malignant tumor cells into the bloodstream. [238, 239, 240]

Sadly, women go through this torture year after year while also increasing their accumulative exposure to radiation. This is despite the fact that in 1995 "The Journal of the American Medical Association reported that there is no evidence that breast X-ray exams significantly reduce breast cancer deaths among women in their forties. In 1993 the National Cancer Institute stopped endorsing mammograms for women in their forties." [44] There are also a high number of false positives (6%)

that occur which lead to further screenings (more radiation), and other unnecessary invasive procedures like biopsies, surgery, radiation, and chemotherapy. [240]

The absolute best thing to do to ward off breast cancer is to focus on prevention. According to breast surgeon, Susan Love of UCLA, "at least 30% of tumors found on mammograms would go away if absolutely nothing was done." [240] If we understand the basic premise that the body has an amazing ability to heal itself NO MATTER WHAT, then we can understand that even in the worst of circumstances the body can still heal itself.

> *How many people completely heal from cancer DESPITE*
> *the highly invasive medical treatments rather*
> *than because of them?*

According to Mercola, "the strength of your immune system is a major factor in determining whether or not you beat cancer." [240] Furthermore, nearly everyone has cancerous and pre-cancerous cells in their body by the time they are in their forties, BUT NOT EVERYONE DEVELOPS CANCER. [240] So, what is the difference that makes the difference?

> *It all comes down to removing interference and*
> *adding good things into your life.*

If we work to remove the things that prevent our bodies from functioning properly and add in things that support our body's own natural healing systems, like our immune system, then we are more likely to prevent sickness and disease, INCLUDING cancer! This is the power of epigenetics (Refer to Chapter 3: The Power of Your Mind).

If you want to have your breasts safely screened, thermography is the way to go. Thermography uses infrared technology that detects temperature changes on the surface of your skin. The images are computerized and displayed on a screen to show a heat map of the breasts. A provider can look for significant temperature changes that usually occur with cancerous growth and make recommendations accordingly. The temperature change occurs because when a breast tumor forms extra blood vessels also form with it. In effect, tumors have their own blood supply. This not only increases blood flow, but it can also cause inflammation, as is the case of inflammatory breast cancer. This in turn raises the skin temperature which is easily detected with thermography. Once these changes are detected, further testing would be needed to confirm a diagnosis of breast cancer. [241]

The major benefit of thermography vs. mammograms is thermography uses no radiation which makes it much safer. Thermography can also detect vascular changes due to breast cancer many years in advance, making the cancer (possibly) easier to successfully treat. [241] Every year more and more health centers are adopting thermography as a safer way to screen breast tissue. If you're looking for a safer approach, a simple search on www.duckduckgo.com (a better search engine than Google) can help you find these places.

PRESCRIPTIONS

In the very first chapter of this book I pointed out that statistically adverse drug reactions are the fourth leading cause of death in the United States. There is reason for that. I will boldly say it again right here for you to read: YOU CANNOT POISON THE BODY BACK TO or INTO HEALTH. All drugs act like a poison in your body – tricking it into doing something it wouldn't normally do. A drug for example, might block pain or stop your liver from producing cholesterol. It might work to force your body into producing more of a certain chemical or stop your body from "up-taking" a certain hormone or neurotransmitter (SSRI's). Over the long run this could potentially cause your body great harm. As stated in Chapter 1, a reported **200,000** people die of adverse drug reactions every year in the US.

In an article about drug toxicity titled, "When Medicine Makes You Sick," Mukaila A. Raji, M.D., Chief of Geriatric Medicine at the University of Texas Medical Branch in Galveston states that drug toxicity is "a major public-health issue even for people in their 40s and 50s." Furthermore, he states that "most drugs are eliminated from the body [via] the kidneys and liver but starting around the fourth decade we start accumulating fat and lose muscle mass. This is accompanied by a progressive decline in the ability of our kidneys and liver to process and clear medications." [242] This would of course lead to the buildup of toxins and make a person more prone to drug toxicity. What makes this issue even more problematic is that the symptoms of drug toxicity are often more subtle than you'd think. They may show up as confusion, dizziness, memory loss, balance issues, brain fog, fatigue, etc. Doctors can fail to see the symptoms as signs of drug toxicity and end up "attributing them instead to a new medical condition," thus a new diagnosis is made. A new medical condition leads to more prescriptions and the patient ends up worse. [242]

It was said by a colleague of mine, Dr. Billy Demoss, D.C., that "M.D." stands for "more drugs/more dope." It's hard to argue with this point because when you go to a "regular" doctor you usually come away with a prescription. There is never really any coaching or any good advice on how to take better care of oneself. How many times have you been to the doctor only to come away with yet another prescription and no real answers? Dr. Raji says, "There is a tendency for physicians to prescribe a medication for every symptom, and not every symptom requires a medication." [242] I would make the argument that most health problems require serious lifestyle changes and not merely "management" via prescriptions.

If most people would focus on being proactive rather than reactive with their health, they would be less likely to ever have the kind of health problems that would require medications.

This is the underlining message in this book!

BE PROACTIVE WITH YOUR LIFE!

VACCINATIONS AREN'T IMMUNIZATION

This last medical procedure I chose to write about is the most controversial, especially in this day and age and with our current political regime (Democratic Party) trying to strip away every available freedom we have. This includes being able to opt out of having to get the CDC recommended vaccines. This comes at the hands of a supposed measles outbreak in which the mass media and the CDC told us there are over 1,000 confirmed cases of measles with no reported deaths. Might I add that the **only** photo produced of one of these supposed 1,000 cases was proven to be photoshopped by CNN and was taken down [243]. Yet, due to the overwhelming amount of fear pumped out by these pharma backed media sources, many people, including unknowledgeable and misguided politicians, are jumping on the band wagon of forced vaccination programs. In the state of California, for example, all exemptions have been removed except for a medical exemption. This means a person cannot opt their kids out of vaccines for religious, philosophical, or personal reasons if they want their child to attend public school. Sadly, most states have already followed suit, and the ones that haven't are well on their way.

As I write this section, the current legislation being proposed in California, SB276, would severely restrict a doctor's ability to write a medical exemption as a proactive way of preventing vaccine injuries in their patients. The physicians would be restricted to writing only five medical exemptions per year. All medical exemptions would be reviewed by a state appointed, licensed physician, surgeon, or registered nurse in order to be approved or deemed inappropriate. [244] What's important to note is these state appointed officials will have absolutely ZERO contact with the patients. This means that a child's fate will be left entirely in the hands of an official who will have no interaction with them.

So, the only thing left for a parent to do is homeschool their children. But even that option will soon be heavily regulated by the state. And, it isn't just about the kids either. Adult mandates for vaccinations are right around the corner – it is only a matter of time before legislation on this front is proposed.

Therefore, I believe we need to become knowledgeable about these medical procedures and not just assume they are safe because it's what we have always been told. Just because the governing bodies and authorities say that vaccines, or any medical procedures, are "safe and effective" doesn't make it so. There was a time when cigarettes were backed by the CDC as safe and effective. Not surprisingly, brave doctors who spoke out and said smoking was not safe were called quacks. Thus, we MUST question the so-called SETTLED SCIENCE and be open to the fact that conspiracies can and do exist.

What I have written about in this section will hopefully inspire you to do your own investigation and begin to question this matrix in which we live in. What you need to know regarding vaccinations is based on the hidden, censored, and suppressed science that "they don't want you to know about" as well as *common sense*. I have used resources in this section that come from medical doctors and knowledgeable sources who have bravely spoken out against the tyrant that is BIG (P)harma. Might I add that all these doctors have been labeled quacks by the medical establishment and have practically been disbarred from the medical profession. This means they were willing to risk their livelihood for the sake of the TRUTH. I find that admirable and downright courageous, especially when compared to the rest of the medical profession which is SO RIDDLED with conflicts of interest.

For this reason alone, one should begin to question the whole vaccine program. Two questions come to mind:

1. Why are these doctors who question the vaccine program in its entirety and vocalize their concerns in a professional manner shunned, censored, and ad hominem attacked?

2. Why are we told not to question vaccines, despite the overwhelming evidence that vaccines do cause injury?

Common sense says injecting toxins is potentially bad for one's health, especially for an infant who has an underdeveloped immune system.

Within this section I'm primarily focusing on three issues regarding vaccines: #1 Toxicity (toxins in vaccines), #2 Vaccines are not adjusted by weight, #3 The vaccine schedule and the timing in which they are given.

*"No child is born with an intact immune system. During the first two years of life the immune system is literally struggling into existence. Despite extravagant claims by the medical community, how that immune system is assembled by the body is still largely unknown. What is known for certain is that subjecting the infant's immune environment to an array of manmade pathogens, suspended in a **toxic solution of preservatives and adjuvants, absolutely can have a detrimental effect on the formations of the child's brain and nervous system.** All scientists – including the vaccine manufacturers – admit as much."* (Dr. Tim O'Shea – *Vaccination Is Not Immunization.*, Emphasis mine). [245, Pg. Intro]

"Vaccines are like the training course for the immune system" touts one website, supposedly dedicated to science. [246] This is what most of the medical profession believes. It is also the "settled" consensus of vaccinologists and most scientists across the board. The idea of vaccines isn't necessarily a bad one, it's quite admirable; the problem is the application. First, vaccines supposedly work by introducing a dead or weakened pathogen into the bloodstream, so the patient gets a "mild" case of the disease (i.e. Measles, Polio, Influenza, etc.). The idea is this dead or weakened pathogen causes the body to produce antibodies to the vaccine and immune cells, which remember the pathogen and theoretically protect you for life. [245] However, if vaccines guarantee immunity for life, then why are multiple doses given? Why are booster shots needed? These are only the "tip of the iceberg" questions.

OUTBREAKS, GERMS, and PLAGUE

Immunology as it turns out isn't as simple as the antigen/antibody paradigm. There is a lot more to the story then we hear about. In fact, natural immunity involves other organs and systems in the body that invaders must go through before ever entering the bloodstream. The gut, for example, is thought to play a huge role in our immune system. It was proven that a healthy gut contains up to three pounds of flora, all coexisting in harmonious balance within our bodies. [245] Vaccines bypass all the protective barriers our bodies have set up to fight off disease. Dr. O'shea says it well below.

"Natural Immunity. With the actual disease, the organism must pass through many of the body's natural immune defense systems in the nose, throat, and lungs before it ever gets as far as the bloodstream. It's likely that the organism slowly triggers many unknown biological events, essential in building true natural immunity, before it ever reaches the bloodstream."

[245, Pg. 41]

Think about it this way, if you were in a castle and the enemy was coming, would you let down the castle gates and allow them to come right in? Would you put a bridge over your mote so they could march over it? Would you tell your archers to take the rest of the day off? Vaccines are like a Trojan Horse, regardless of whether the viruses in them are "weakened" (attenuated) or dead, they will never be as good as natural immunity. When I was a kid, I got chickenpox. It is likely that I will never get it again.

But multiple shots and boosters are needed because a person's immunity wears off. In communities of FULLY vaccinated (vaxxed) individuals, which means they received all their shots plus their boosters, they still have large outbreaks. This means the kids and/or adults still get the very diseases they were vaccinated for.

The CDC reported "Measles Outbreak in a HIGHLY Vaccinated Population – Israel." In July and August of 2017, nine measles cases were reported among fully vaccinated Israeli soldiers. [247]

Westlake, Massachusetts prides itself on having high vaccination rates among its students. In fact, "98% of 7th graders had all of their shots according to state data." Despite having all their shots, including their booster shots, 30 students were diagnosed with whooping cough. According to the CDC the booster shot for whooping cough protects "70% of people in their first year after receiving it and 40% four years after receiving it." [248] The question for you is how do they come up with these seemingly arbitrary percentages?

"Twenty-five sailors and marines aboard a ship were diagnosed with parotitis, a disease very similar to mumps, in December." U.S. soldiers receive every single dose of every single vaccine there is, including the measles, mumps, and rubella vaccine (MMR). [249] Parotitis is not a disease, it's a painful swelling of the parotid glands and it's caused by the virus mumps, herpes, or Epstein-Barr. [250]

The Germ Theory, which was introduced by Louis Pasteur, says certain diseases are caused by microorganisms (bacteria), essentially, germs cause disease. This set medicine with the job of coming up with the right drugs and vaccines to kill off the offending pathogens, but not the patient. The problem with this is well stated by O'Shea below.

"Rarely is nature so black and white about things, ever notice that? For one thing, bacteria and viruses tend to be picky about their environments. That's why some people get colds and others don't [it isn't just about exposure]. That's why some survived the bubonic

plague. That's also why some doctors and nurses seem to be
immune to disease, even though they're surrounded by it every day."

[245, Pg. 32]

Did the rats cause the trash or did the trash bring the rats? Watch any episode of "Hoarders" on TV and you will understand that the environment the hoarders have created in their home attracts rats, mice, and disease carrying bugs. The environment was conducive for bug life. Similarly, disease happens when our bodies are starved of nutrition and weak. When our bodies can't function at their optimum capacity because of interference, we are more susceptible to disease.

"Low resistance, filth, toxic diet, bad lifestyle [and] weak
immune system[s] [cause disease]. Such imbalances
render the blood a hospitable medium in which
opportunist organisms may be cultured."

[245, Pg. 33]

Having suffered two strokes that left him with some paralysis on one side of his body and then a severe bout of uremia, Pasteur, while lying on his death bed said something like this, "Bernard was correct. I was wrong. The microbe (germ) is nothing. The terrain is everything." Basically, Pasteur admitted his germ theory had been wrong all along. [251] Sadly, the entire theory behind the vaccination program is based on Pasteur's idea that he admitted was wrong. The germ theory perpetuates a false sense of fear that microbes are going to kill us all, and that without vaccines we would all perish. And yet, we have survived through eons of time without the advent of vaccines and modern medicine. We find a way to survive.

If you were to study the history of disease you would find that the 1800's and early part of the 20th century were plagued by a variety of insidious diseases. People got sick and they died, especially in impoverished areas. The industrial revolution brought more factories into the cities. The factories motivated people to move from the countryside to the inner cities to find work. This gave way to overcrowded conditions as housing was inadequate to accommodate the influx of people. As the population was confined to these small areas called slums, disease flourished. [252]

"Clean water, proper sewage treatment, and fresh air did not exist in these areas. [Inadequate ventilation left the air stagnant and un-breathable]. Without any sanitary infrastructure, human and animal waste would flow into the streets, ending up in local streams and rivers which happened to also be the people's primary water supply. Sanitary facilities designed for smaller populations failed. Cesspools [would] overflow and seep into the local water supplies."

[253]

(A cesspool is an underground container for temporary storage of liquid waste and sewage. [254])

Along with these disgusting and inhumane living conditions, there were no zoning laws which meant factories could be within proximity to where people lived, all the while spewing out toxic smoke and dumping their chemicals next to crowded tenement housing. Improper sewage and waste management led to deplorable conditions which allowed vermin to flourish. In these poor and impoverished areas pigs and rats ran rampant in the streets while disease carrying bugs flourished. People threw their trash in the streets with buckets of their own waste. The dead and rotting carcasses of horses, dogs, and other animals lay in the streets for days to weeks at a time. The food people ate was often contaminated with bacteria and was of extremely poor quality. In fact, milk was so bad it killed an average of 8,000 children annually. [252] Combine all this with the unbelievable long hours people would endure working in coal mines, mills, glass factories, etc. and you can understand why people suffered from disease. A lot of the workers were children averaging seven to nine years of age. They would sometimes work up to sixteen hours per day!

People were overworked, malnourished, and exhausted which created the perfect conditions for disease to thrive. [245]

But all the infectious diseases people died from were not the issue. These were merely the symptoms of a greater problem. It was the environmental factors that allowed the right conditions for disease to manifest and flourish. Thus, the greatest thing done to drive down disease rates was improving living conditions. This included proper sewage and waste disposal management, clean drinking water, proper zoning laws, comfortable, safe housing, cleaner streets, worker age restrictions, and believe or not, doctors washing their hands. [245] A CDC scientist confirmed this in a 2000 article published in the Journal of Pediatrics in which he stated that 90% of the mortality rates due to infectious disease in the 20th century declined before vaccines were even available!

"Thus, vaccination does not account for the impressive declines in mortality seen in the first half of the century...nearly 90% of the decline in infectious disease mortality among US children occurred before 1940, when few antibiotics or vaccines were available." Dr. Suzanne Humphreys

For obvious reasons, most medical doctors have probably never heard of the people I am going to mention now. None of these people agreed with the Germ Theory made popular by Pasteur. First, Dr. Bechamp was a renowned French biologist who, along with Claude Bernard (renowned French Physiologist), believed that microorganisms within the body changed or pleo-morphed based on the inside environment. Bechamp discovered that microorganisms exist within the body and theorized that these organisms become dangerous when the body is unhealthy. In other words, it wasn't the germs that caused the disease, it was the terrain that allowed the germs to take over. Bechamp strongly disagreed with Pasteur as can be seen in the quotes below. [256]

"Bacteria do not cause disease, and therefore serums and vaccines can neither prevent nor cure disease."

Dr. Bechamp

"The most serious disorders may be provoked by the injection of living organisms into the blood... into a medium not intended for them may provoke redoubtable manifestations of the gravest morbid phenomena."

Dr. Bechamp

Harvard graduate and president of the Infectious Diseases Society of America, Dr. Edward H. Kass, gave a speech on October 19, 1970 that probably would have resulted in the loss of his license today. During his speech he produced charts on measles, pertussis, and scarlet fever that showed these infectious diseases were already dramatically declining before the advent of any vaccines! No vaccine has ever been produced for scarlet fever, yet how often do we hear about scarlet fever now? We never hear about it anymore because it's virtually gone! Dr. Kass had this to say during his speech.

*"This decline in rates of certain disorders, **correlated roughly with socioeconomic circumstances**, is merely the **most important happening in the history** of the health of man, yet we have only the vaguest and most general notions about how it happened and by what mechanisms socioeconomic improvement and decreased rates of certain diseases run in parallel."*

Dr. Edward H. Kass

What's most important to note here is that Dr. Kass never denotes vaccines as mankind's great savior from infectious disease despite the fact that he was a medical doctor and President of the Medical Society for Infectious Diseases! [257] This would be considered heresy by today's standards! He told the un-watered-down TRUTH. Of course, you will never hear this information from the "lamestream media." And your doctor has probably never heard of Dr. Kass. I'm assuming this information isn't in the syllabus of any medical class taught at any medical college, go figure.

Rudolph Virchow was a Polish pathologist who authored "The Cell Theory." He was one of the first to recognize the importance of the cellular makeup of the body, declaring, "The body is a cell state in which every cell is a citizen." He also was first to correctly identify that cancers came about from healthy cells and theorized that cancer was caused by irritation in the tissues. This is interesting because we know inflammation is a primary factor in most diseases. Virchow strongly opposed Pasteur's germ theory and proposed instead that **"germs seek their natural habitat: diseased tissue, rather than being the cause of diseased tissue."** If Virchow were alive in the 70's he would have agreed with Dr. Kass because he thought that socioeconomic factors were the major cause of disease and that the way to health was more political than medical. [257, 258]

TOXINS IN VACCINES

The toxins in vaccines are vast. There are a multitude of toxins in vaccines that are neurotoxic and are poisonous to every system in the body. In fact, nobody in their right mind would take the ingredients listed in a vaccine, put them into a glass of water, and then drink them. Yet, we have blindly accepted that *injecting* these toxins into our own as well as our children's bodies is somehow safe and benign.

When talking about the toxins in vaccines, proponents of vaccines always use the words "trace amounts." They use this argument to defend the use of heavy metals, chemicals, aborted fetal cell DNA, or animal cells used in the manufacturing process of vaccines. Their argument is, "We needn't worry because the toxins in vaccines are in ridiculously small amounts and are virtually insignificant as a whole." Thus, the words "trace amounts." The problem with this argument is twofold: A lot of these toxins bioaccumulate in the body, especially in the brain, liver, and kidneys because the body can't get rid of them fast enough. Eventually they will cause a tipping point which may cause many health issues to ensue. Second, the toxins are injected. **One should never underestimate the potency of toxins when injected vs. ingested.** Think about snake venom, two drops of venom from the deadly Black Mamba snake is enough to kill a person. But, if you take this same deadly venom and drink it (ingested), it wouldn't do a darn thing. This is because the venom would be broken down in the stomach and eventually filtered out of the body. Let me give you a major example of how this works regarding vaccines. [259]

Available Pub Med studies on aluminum, which is an adjuvant used in many vaccines, demonstrate that the human body absorbs most of the aluminum and struggles to get rid of it when it is injected. In one such study it was shown that only about 0.3% of aluminum is absorbed when administered orally to healthy individuals. However, when aluminum bypasses the GI tract and is administered intravenously (into the bloodstream), 40% is absorbed in healthy adults and "up to 75% is retained" in newborns. Furthermore, the study goes on to show that if the body's ability to eliminate aluminum is exceeded it will accumulate in the brain, heart, liver, kidneys, and other organs causing health problems, including death.

"If a significant aluminum load exceeds the body's excretory capacity, the excess is deposited in various tissues, including bone, brain, liver, heart, spleen, and muscle. This accumulation causes morbidity and mortality through various mechanisms." [260]

Aluminum is a known neurotoxin that has been placed on two federal regulatory lists. As mentioned above, aluminum is an adjuvant. Because vaccines bypass the body's natural immune reaction pathway, a **toxic adjuvant** needs to be used to stimulate an immune response. A 2013 study published in the Journal of Immunology Research concluded that the available scientific and medical literature shows a clear link between neurodegenerative disorders and aluminum in the vaccines. The authors of the study stated:

*"In young children, a **highly significant correlation exists between the number of pediatric aluminum-adjuvanted vaccines***

administered and the rate of autism spectrum disorders. Many of the features of aluminum-induced neurotoxicity may arise, in part, from autoimmune reactions, as part of the ASIA. [261]

"ASIA" refers to an aberrant autoimmune/inflammatory condition caused by adjuvants used in vaccines. Of course, this happens. To reiterate - you're injecting a toxic, heavy metal intramuscularly which eventually gets into your bloodstream. It doesn't belong there. Therefore, the body goes into a full-blown inflammatory response.

Sadly, I'm sure this condition goes underreported by the Vaccine Adverse Event Reporting System (VAERS).

For many different reasons, it is estimated that only 1 to 10% of all adverse vaccine reactions ever get reported.

This ultimately means there are a lot of adverse reactions happening because of vaccines, that sadly never get reported. This leaves the general populous in the dark and perpetuates the myth that vaccines are "completely safe and effective." [262]

Lastly, manufacturers of certain drug products (Parenteral Drugs used in TPN therapy) are required by the FDA to label their package inserts stating the drug contains "no more than 25 mcg of aluminum per kilogram of body weight." This is because aluminum is toxic, and it's especially toxic for premature babies whose kidneys aren't working at 100%. Furthermore, the FDA has also stated that the maximum amount of aluminum a person can receive must only be 5 mcg per kg of body weight but should not exceed 25 mcg. **However, when it comes to drugs vs. vaccines, the FDA requires no component safety testing for vaccines and vaccine schedules.** This means vaccines can and do have well over the maximum dosage amount of aluminum. [263]

The Hepatitis B vaccine (HEP B) given on the first day of a baby's life contains 250 mcgs of aluminum per shot. This is fourteen times the amount of aluminum in the FDA approved maximum dosage amount! In addition, at "Well-Checkup" visits at two, four, and six months, babies often receive up to eight different vaccines that add up to over 1,000 mcgs of aluminum! According to the FDA, this amount wouldn't be safe for a 350-pound adult. [264]

As a Christian and "Pro-Lifer" I am appalled that there are more than twenty-three vaccines that contain cells, cellular debris, protein, and DNA from aborted babies. [265] Regardless of mine or anyone's moral position on abortion and aborted fetal tissue used in the making of vaccines, the primary concern should be placed on the cross contamination of DNA that occurs and the potential for health risks. There was a large cohort study done on all children with vaccination records born after 1969 in the USA, Western Australia, the UK, and Denmark, who later developed a diagnosis of autistic disorder. It was determined that there was a "highly significant association" of these children being vaccinated with vaccines manufactured using human cell lines containing fetal DNA and retroviral contaminants. The science seems to show that "human fetal DNA fragments can induce autoimmune reactions which provoke genetic mutations." [266]

Injecting the foreign DNA of another human being into an infant can cause a cross reaction with the child's own DNA, as the body can have an immune reaction to the foreign DNA.

> "Administration of fragments of human fetal (primitive) non-self-DNA to a child could generate an immune response that would also cross-react with the child's own DNA, since the contaminating DNA could have sections of overlap very similar to the child's own DNA." [267]
> Dr. Theresa A Deisher, Ph.D., founder, and lead scientist at Sound Choice Pharmaceutical Institute

Common sense alone tells you this is weird science and to precede with caution. According to Deisher, the amount of foreign DNA contamination in the MMR II, Chickenpox, Pentacel, and Hep A vaccines is significant enough to be concerned. This level of contamination is enough to activate a receptor (Toll-like Receptor

9 – TLR9) and induce autoimmune attacks. [267] Autistic children have antibodies against human DNA in their bloodstream, which children without autism do not have. This may explain the autoimmune attacks. [268]

Formaldehyde is best known as an embalming fluid used to preserve dead bodies for open casket burials. It also can be found in trace amounts in furniture, building material, and animal and plant-based foods. [269] It is even produced in the body as a natural byproduct when we metabolize foods. [270] What isn't well known about formaldehyde is that it's used in the production of vaccines to inactivate viruses so that they don't cause the very disease the vaccine is to prevent [271]. Formaldehyde, to put it bluntly, is toxic and has been studied extensively for its ill effects due to ingestion, inhalation, and direct contact exposure with the skin or eyes. Formaldehyde is so potent that if enough of it is inhaled or accidentally ingested it can cause acute damage to the liver, kidneys, pancreas, brain, and several other organs. It has even been classified as a probable cancer-causing agent or known carcinogen by several agencies including the American Cancer Society, the FDA, and the National Cancer Institute, etc. [272]

Yet, little is known about injecting small amounts of formaldehyde into the body. Like aluminum, formaldehyde is used in trace amounts (micrograms = mcgs) in several vaccines, including the Hep B vaccine which is given on day one of life. Dr. Sherri J. Tenpenny, D.O., author of "Saying No to Vaccines: A Resource Guide for All Ages," stated, "By the time a child has turned five years of age, he or she has been injected with a total of 1,795 mcgs or 1.795 milligrams of formaldehyde [272]." Not to mention that in the first five years of the child's life his/her brain, organs, and neurological system is doing a tremendous amount of growth and development.

Proponents usually combat this argument by saying the small amount of formaldehyde used in vaccines is so minute that it likely wouldn't cause harm. And, the body naturally makes formaldehyde as a byproduct of digestion, so it can't be harmful, right?! The rebuttal to this is simple. Our body can handle anything better via natural exposure. For example, when formaldehyde is ingested, produced in the body, or inhaled in small amounts, it's rapidly and safely broken down in the body and then easily eliminated. However, little information is available to address exactly what happens metabolically in the human body when formaldehyde is injected.

Nor is there any available information that discusses how a child's body handles formaldehyde vs. an adult. Although 1.8 milligrams over the first five years seems like a small amount, there is a vast difference between ingestion compared to injection, which the science has yet to conclusively say is safe. Furthermore, this amount doesn't account for future shots containing formaldehyde between the ages of five and eighteen. Food for thought.

POLYSORBATE 80

According to the FDA polysorbate 80 (P-80) is used in vaccines as an emulsifier to prevent ingredients from separating. [273] In pharmacology, P-80 is used to enhance the delivery of chemicals (chemotherapy) and certain drugs into the brain because it allows them to cross the blood brain barrier. [274] The reason we have a blood brain barrier is to protect us from toxins entering our brain. The brain is separated from the circulatory system by this barrier which prevents chemicals and toxins from entering our central nerve system. However, this barrier is particularly weak in infants and older people which means that it's more penetrable for these vulnerable age groups. [275]

The concern is that P-80 might be making it easier for the other toxins in vaccines to cross the blood brain barrier. There is a glaringly obvious lack of basic scientific studies regarding the safety of using P-80 in vaccines.

Mercury is the MOST toxic, non-radioactive element on planet earth! Mercury poisoning, for example, causes immune, sensory, neurological, behavioral, and psychomotor dysfunctions which are all traits that define Autism-Spectrum Disorder, interestingly enough. In the 1800s a syndrome known as "Mad-Hatters Syndrome" was coined after the hatters started developing severe neurological symptoms because of the mercury solution they were using to turn fur into felt. The mercury fumes would off gas, therefore, breathing in the mercury vapors was slowly poisoning them over time. [276]

Does injecting any amount of mercury, even if it's just a fractional amount, make sense on any level?

Mercury has been used and is still used in some vaccines in the form of Thimerosal. Thimerosal is 50% ethyl mercury which according to "hundreds of peer reviewed studies by leading government and university scientists, is extremely toxic to the brain and neurological system." As of 2003, due to much controversary, the drug makers (pharmaceutical companies) removed most thimerosal from vaccines. "However, during the same year the CDC added flu shots containing massive doses of thimerosal to the pediatric schedule." [277]

There is also scientific evidence to suggest that aluminum greatly increases the toxicity of mercury. Given that the influenza shot (Flu Shot) contains 25-50 mcg of mercury, what happens when it's given in conjunction with aluminum containing vaccines, as is the case with a typical baby well-visit? [276]

FDA LOOPHOLE

As long as thimerosal is not used as a preservative, the FDA has given the vaccine makers an out and they can label their product as thimerosal free. The DTaP, DT, Hib, and meningococcal vaccine still contain mercury, as well as multidose flu shots. [278]

TOXINS IN VACCINES: A QUICK LIST

- Thimerosal
- Borax (sodium tetraborate decahydrate)

- Aluminum
- Anti-Freeze (Ethylene Glycol)
- 2-Phenoxyethanol
- Phenol
- Methanol
- Neomycin sulfate
- Sorbitol sweetener
- Beta sropilactone
- Amphotericin
- Large foreign proteins
- Animal viruses
- Mycoplasma
- Foreign DNA [279]

- Glutaraldehyde
- Monosodium glutamate (MSG)
- Sulfate and ghosphate compounds
- Ammonium sulfate
- Gentamicin sulfate
- Tri(n)-butyl phosphate
- Polyribosyiribitol
- Beta propiolactone
- Animal organ tissue and blood
- Latex
- Human viruses
- Genetically modified yeast

For a complete list of excipients, check out this link http://www.vaccinesafety.edu/components-Excipients.htm from the Institute of Vaccine Safety at John Hopkins University.

NO LIABILITY FOR VACCINE MAKERS

The year was 1986 when President Reagan passed the National Childhood Vaccine Injury Act. The name sounds very admirable, but I assure you that it isn't admirable at all. The vaccine injury act came about because parents were filing multimillion-dollar lawsuits against the vaccine makers due to the irreparable damage vaccines had caused their children. Rather than admit blame, the medical establishment, along with the vaccine makers, denied any causal link between vaccines and the damaged child. Instead, they blamed the parents and chalked up their all too willing suspicions of vaccine injury as nothing more than delusion brought about by distress. Afterall, "correlation doesn't equal causation" in the minds of the vaccine makers and the lined pockets of politicians.

What the childhood vaccine injury act really did was remove liability from the vaccine makers, giving them a free pardon to continue making their vaccines without any proper recourse. It's annoying getting sued all the time and having to deal with those distraught and "crazy" parents who claim vaccines killed their kids or caused them serious harm. So, the government chose to subsidize vaccine production, meaning awards from lawsuits were now going to be paid with a tax added to every vaccine administered (tax dollars paid for by the vaccine recipients) and not big pharma money. [280] If their petition is approved by health and human services, a court appointed special master determines whether they will get compensated. On the Health Resources and Services Administration website it states this:

"The National Vaccine Injury Compensation Program is a NO-FAULT (emphasis mine) alternative to the traditional legal system for resolving vaccine injury petitions. It was created in the 1980's after lawsuits against vaccine companies and health care providers threatened to cause vaccine shortages and reduce U.S. vaccination rates which could have caused a resurgence of vaccine preventable disease." [281]

When money gets involved with politics and healthcare it doesn't matter what's right, it only matters what's going to maintain the status quo. Afterall, if the vaccine program were to fall, the entire house of cards would fall with it. The vaccine program is the cornerstone of modern medicine. It is their "holy, sacred cow" and if the truth were to come out, the system would be turned upside down! Can we trust that the vaccine makers would make a reliable and safe product if they can't be sued? If there's no recourse?

"To date over four billion dollars has been awarded to families with vaccine injured children through the compensation program."

https://www.hrsa.gov/vaccine-compensation/data/index.html

No safety studies have ever been done on giving multiple vaccines at once, so how do we know it's safe? At a routine infant well-check visit multiple vaccines are administered at once on different limbs. In a single visit an infant can receive up to six shots! [282] For example, at the two month checkup a baby receives the DTaP, Hib, IPV, PCV, and the RV. Shockingly, if a parent happens to miss their child's two month checkup, the pediatrician will play catch up on their next visit and will inject between twelve and fifteen vaccines. Where is the science to show that's safe, let alone scientific? Many of these shots contain multiple viruses. For example, the MMR shot contains *live* measles, mumps, and rubella viruses. The TDaP contains tetanus, diphtheria, and pertussis viruses. The flu shot can contain multiple viruses in one. Each vaccine also contains several known toxins and carcinogens. So, where is the science to show injecting multiple vaccines with multiple live and attenuated viruses, along with toxins, is even remotely safe? There are absolutely ZERO safety studies.

Where in nature do you get exposed to multiple viruses at once that bypass the body's natural defense mechanisms and end up directly in your bloodstream?

Section 13.1 of any vaccine package insert states, "Has not been evaluated for its carcinogenic or mutagenic potential or impairment of fertility." Drug manufacturers use the package insert as a legal document to help buffer them from litigation. The package insert protects the drug maker if a doctor prescribes the drug to a patient that may be contraindicated for a vaccine. It's a legal document that the FDA requires. However, in the case of vaccines, they are considered so safe that carcinogenicity is considered implausible and therefore the vaccine makers feel no tests are necessary. [283] Afterall, there are only trace amounts of formaldehyde and other carcinogenic compounds in vaccines, therefore they probably won't have any adverse effects (insert sarcasm here with eyeroll).

The obvious hole in this argument which "pro vaccinators" fail to acknowledge is that cancer takes decades to manifest. It's not something that happens overnight. And, as Dr. O'Shea points out in his book, they use immortal cell lines in the production of vaccines.

"The use of continuous cell lines or immortal strains to maintain continuity of a vaccine year after year, standard within industry since [Edward] Jenner, has been extensively criticized. A possible correlation is obvious between culturing cell lines that cannot die and the creation of cancerous tumors." [245, Pg. 45]

If cancer happens to develop ten, twenty, or thirty years later as a result of a vaccine, would there be any way to prove it? The answer is an obvious, no. According to the American Cancer Society, cancer is the second leading cause of death in children between the ages of one and four. This just so happens to correlate with an ever-increasing vaccine schedule. Furthermore, we see a simultaneous increase in pediatric cancers along with chronic neurological and autoimmune disorders. [284] It's important to note there have been absolutely zero studies on the current CDC vaccine schedule. **NONE, ZILCH, NADA!!!** If there have been no safety studies on the collective schedule, how can we know for sure vaccines don't cause cancer, or mutagenicity, or impairment of fertility?

"I have no hesitation in stating that in my judgment the most frequent disposing condition for cancerous development is infused into the blood by vaccination and re-vaccination."

Dr. Dennis Turnball (thirty years as a cancer researcher) [285]

I will quote my good friend and "self-sabotage coach," Jason Christoff, on this one.

"If we are supposed to listen to doctors who present the science regarding vaccines, what are we supposed to do with these medical

doctors who present the hard science, proving vaccines aren't safe or effective? How do we decide between the two sides? One side saying poisons hurt children and the other side saying poison is healthy for children? If science is the unbiased pursuit of truth, why is the science these doctors present not included in the material [pediatricians and other doctors] provided for parents? Why is the hard science proving vaccines don't provide immunity and that they're dangerous not presented to the public by the mainstream media or the medical profession?" [286]

In the appendix I have included a list of medical doctors who have courageously spoken out and continue to speak out against the vaccine industry machine and the current narrative. There is also a list of questions for you to read through, ponder, and possibly ask your doctor about.

A study done prior to the 2002 vaccine schedule compared the brains of fully vaccinated (US vaccine schedule) infant macaque primates to that of saline injected macaques (a true controlled group and a true placebo). Both groups underwent PET and MRI imaging at four and six months of age "which represents very specific time frames within the vaccine schedule." The researchers discovered that the vaccinated group showed the same brain changes as those of autistic children. The editor of the journal stated:

"An alarming finding is reported by Hewitson and coworkers showing that in infant monkeys who were immunized, the amygdala does not show the normal pattern of maturation but is hypertrophied. Although these are only preliminary data, given the well-known role of the amygdala in generation of fear and other negative emotions, they support the possibility that there is a link between early immunization and the etiology of autism. [287]

Using the macaque monkey is a good animal model to study because there are similarities between the human brain and the macaque brain. [288] However, further investigation is still warranted. This study should have sparked further study and investigation, instead it just led to more skepticism by the medical community.

So, why hasn't the CDC done a study on vaccinated vs. unvaccinated children? Afterall, the CDC does own "more than fifty patents connected to vaccinations." [289] Wouldn't they want to put the "nail in the coffin," so to speak and prove once and for all that vaccines are the be-all and end-all to preventing illness and show that they are 100% safe and effective? Why haven't they done a study like this to show unequivocally that vaccinated children are healthier on all levels?

Just a thought, maybe they don't have to. The vaccine industry already makes thirty billion dollars in profit every year, so why would they want to even attempt to do a study that could potentially tarnish their profits and turn the medical world upside down? [289] This is what the medical establishment states as a reason why those studies haven't been done. Because "withholding vaccines from children (control group) would be unethical." What they are saying is they don't want to let the children be exposed to potentially deadly infectious diseases without protection. It seems admirable, but at the same time I can't help but think that it's a very convenient cop out.

DRUG TESTING

In phase two drug testing, clinical controlled trials are done to compare patients receiving the actual drug to people who are treated with an inactive substance like a sugar pill. This is done to test the effectiveness of the drug. Both the control and the test group have no idea whether they are taking the actual drug or if they are taking the placebo, this is known as a single-blind study. [290] Sometimes double blind controlled clinical studies are performed when both the examiner and the participants do not know who is getting the drug and who is getting a placebo.

This level of scientific testing has not been performed on the current vaccine schedule. Vaccines are tested one at a time, but no safety studies have been performed on the CDC schedule in its entirety. Also, none of the vaccines on the current US childhood schedule have ever been tested against an inert placebo. Instead a different vaccine is used OR they will do an injection of a noxious substance such as aluminum. Why not take several parents throughout the United States who aren't going to vaccinate their kids and compare them to the same number of parents who wish to fully vaccinate (CDC schedule) their kids and see what their health outcomes are over twenty to thirty years or so? It seems like a reasonable study if the socioeconomic factors are relatively the same.

When researchers want to test a new vaccine to see if it causes an increase in neurological disorders, they only compare it to the general populous. The problem is most of the population is vaccinated, at least 90%. If you aren't taking a good look at the vaccinated vs. the unvaccinated, then you are only testing the study group against itself and the results can be flawed.

A pilot study to establish overall health outcomes between fully vaccinated, partially vaccinated, and completely unvaccinated homeschooled children was published in the Journal of Translational Sciences. Six hundred and sixty-six homeschooled children, ages six to twelve, across four different states were assessed "based on their mothers' reports of vaccinations and physician diagnosed illnesses." Out of the 666 children, 261 were unvaccinated and 405 were fully or partially vaccinated. The results of the study showed a clear difference between the health outcomes of the two groups. [291]

1. Vaccinated children were four-fold more likely to be diagnosed with Autism Spectrum Disorder.

2. Vaccinated children were thirty-fold more likely to be diagnosed with hay fever.

3. Vaccinated children were twenty-two-fold more likely to require allergy medication.

4. Vaccinated children were fivefold more likely to be diagnosed with a learning disability.

5. Vaccinated children were 340% more likely to be diagnosed with ADHD.

6. Vaccinated children were 5.9-fold more likely to have been diagnosed with pneumonia.

7. Vaccinated children were 3.8-fold more likely to be diagnosed with a middle-ear infection.

8. Vaccinated children were 700% more likely to have had surgery to insert drainage tubes in their ears.

9. Vaccinated children were 2.4-fold more likely to have been diagnosed with any chronic illness.

This study concluded that, "the extent to which these findings apply to the population of homeschooled children as well as the general population awaits further research on vaccinated and unvaccinated children." Investigating and understanding the biological basis of these unexpected nonspecific outcomes of vaccination is essential for ensuring evidence-based vaccine policies and decisions." [291]

"No vaccine safety reports have been filed with the U.S. department of Health and Human Services (HHS) in 32 years as required by Federal law. If the Government can't enforce vaccine manufacturers to ensure the safety of their products then something is very wrong!"

Basically, the vaccine makers need to do more research and this study should have inspired them to do so. However, like Galileo in his day, it was met with hostility. Why is it that any good study speaking to the contrary of the current vaccine narrative is met with hostility, like it was heresy or something? I like what J.B. Handley says in his book, "*How to End the Autism Epidemic.* He states:

*"The vaccine makers have PR budgets and PR firms, and any vaccine study that shows vaccines **don't** cause autism makes the national news. Every single one, every single time. Where are the studies that compare vaccinated versus unvaccinated children?*

> *They don't make the news because their answers implicate*
> *vaccines. They hide in plain sight, are shared widely in the*
> *autism community [and natural health communities], [but]*
> *are ignored by the mainstream press.* [292]

Vaccines are never adjusted by weight. A full grown 180 lbs. male receives the same MMR shot that is given to a toddler at 12-15 months old. Same for the Hep B shot given to an infant on their "birth" day. According to Dr. Boyd Haley, "A single vaccine given to a six-pound newborn is the same as giving an 180-pound adult thirty vaccines on the same day." [245] The question then becomes, "How much toxicity can an infant take in a single visit?" Furthermore, how many vaccines will be enough? Where are we going to draw the line?

The American vaccine schedule is a one of a kind. We receive more vaccines than any other country in the world and yet remain one of the sickest. This should make our children the healthiest on the planet, right?

With the ever-increasing vaccine schedule, we have seen the correlation of ever-increasing childhood illnesses/diseases. Autoimmune disease has become a household name. More and more Hollywood movies feature autistic actors in them. Teachers express concern over rising numbers of kids with autism, food allergies are on the rise, attention deficit disorder is a common diagnosis we hear about, and so on, and so on, and so on.

Below you can see the rising rates of vaccines given per year.

1986: Twenty-three doses of seven vaccines
1997: Thirty-three doses of nine vaccines
2016: Sixty-nine doses of sixteen vaccines
2017: Seventy doses of seventeen vaccines
[293]

"In 1953 health officials at the U.S. Centers for Disease Control told doctors to give children 16 doses of four vaccines by age six.

In 1983 it was 23 doses of 7 vaccines by age six. In 2013 it was 69 doses of 16 vaccines by age 18, with 50 doses given by age six. With infants and children in America getting four times as many vaccinations as their grandparents, how healthy are they?" [294]

- Today one in six children is learning disabled. In 1976 it was one in thirty.

- Today one in nine children has asthma. In 1980, it was one in twenty-seven.

- Today one in fifty children develop autism. In the 1990s it was one child in 555.

- Today one in 400 children have diabetes. In 2001 it was one in 500. [294]

A picture says a thousand words: *"Enuf said."*

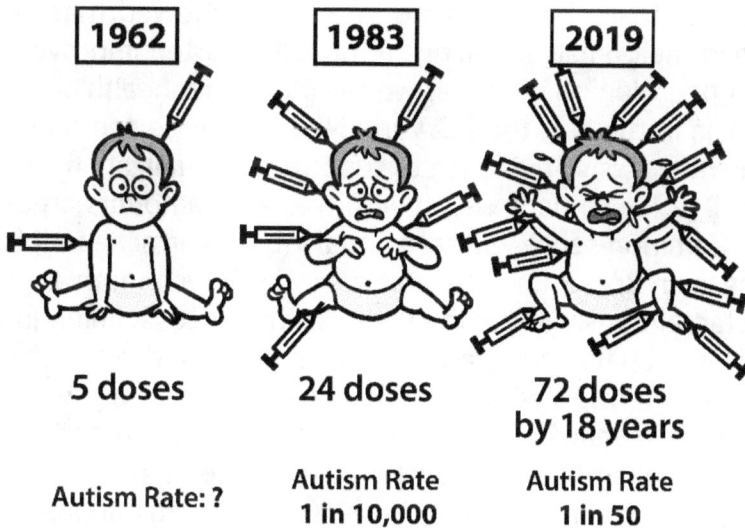

1962	1983	2019
5 doses	24 doses	72 doses by 18 years
Autism Rate: ?	Autism Rate 1 in 10,000	Autism Rate 1 in 50

Mercury in the teeth, what's my beef? Amalgams, also known as silver fillings, contain mercury. What's surprising is that many people don't realize their old dental fillings contain mercury. Mercury fillings off gas and create mercury vapors that you can't see, detect, or perceive. Mercury vapors are in fact odorless. This creates an even bigger problem when you consider the fact that the mercury in a person's mouth is off gassing daily. According to the WHO, mercury vapors are created by grinding the teeth, gum chewing, and drinking carbonated beverages. Brushing your teeth probably causes the mercury to off gas as well. [295]

There is a great film called, *The Beautiful Truth*, about a well-known holistic method of treating cancer called, "Gerson Therapy." In the movie, two doctors wearing gas masks hold an amalgam filled tooth with a pair of plyers in front of a phosphorescent screen and light. They brush the tooth and lo and behold you can see the black smoke created by the mercury off-gassing. With a special device nicknamed the "mercury sniffer," they were able to measure the mercury gas at 191, which according to one of the doctors, Dr. David Kennedy, D.D.S. "OSHA would have people exit out of the building." [296]

Mercury is toxic. Studies done in Sweden showed that people who had their amalgam fillings removed reported improvements in their neurological issues, as well as their other health problems. However, in the U.S. the FDA and NIH have reported that there isn't any conclusive evidence to support that amalgam fillings are harmful. [295] So here we go with the trace amounts argument again. Common sense will save you a lot of heartache in this life. Having mercury, a known neurotoxin, in your mouth that can be instantaneously absorbed through the mucosal lining in your mouth is probably NOT a good thing. The good news is there are holistic dentists who specialize in removing amalgam fillings. Try using the search engine www.duckduckgo.com and type in "dentist amalgam filling removal specialist." See what comes up and investigate further. There is a technique in dentistry appropriately called the Safe Mercury Amalgam Removal Technique (SMART). Ask your dentist if he has heard about it. I had mine safely removed by a dentist specializing in this technique.

The first step to detoxing your body is avoiding or severely limiting the amount of toxins you're exposed to. We are exposed to a tremendous amount of toxins on a regular basis, but don't let that scare you. The body has an amazing ability to detox itself, even without the use of a sauna and niacin. Over time however, the detox mechanisms in our body get worn out and we eventually end up suffering from the bioaccumulation of toxins in our system. So, therefore, we need to remove the interference of toxicity regularly.

The sauna has been a godsend for me in that I use it regularly to help minimize the amount of toxic burden in my body. For years it has been my go-to to help me sweat out the toxins. When sweat has been tested, it was found that it had things like lead and arsenic in it. An article in the New York Times reported that, "The body does appear to sweat out toxic materials, such as heavy metals and BPA." [297] However, the article goes on to say that the amounts are irrelevant. But this is merely describing regular sauna use. According to the research, infrared saunas do appear to facilitate a much deeper sweat. When combined with the lipolysis rebound affect created by the niacin, you will get a much better detox.

In fact, in Root's book he described protocols he has used to successfully treat September 11 first responders and ground zero workers who were exposed to a variety of toxins by breathing in all the dust, metal and chemical particulates in the air. I vividly remember the huge clouds of grey dust that came billowing down the streets and alleyways of NYC. Could you imagine breathing in all of that and expecting your body to naturally detox itself without assistance? Needless to say, one should focus on detoxing regularly and avoiding toxins as much as possible.

"It is health that is real wealth and not pieces of gold or silver."

-Mahatma Gandhi

CHAPTER 10

VITAMIN "S" FOR SLEEP

Sleep is an essential nutrient,
It is the Vitamin "S" that many
people don't get enough of.

- Dr. Jay

In the constant hustle of life, people are simply not getting enough sleep. I see more and more people who seem to be chronically tired, despite having plenty of caffeine circulating through their blood stream. In this chapter I will attempt to not only explain the importance of sleep, but I will also explain how to get more **quality** sleep. I emphasize the word "quality" here because you can sleep forever and still wake up tired. So, lets dive into the most important ingredient you absolutely need, what I like to call, "Vitamin S!"

Sleep plays a critical role in your health and healing. Getting a good night's sleep can be like hitting the reset button. This is because during sleep your body works to balance itself. The science showing what sleep can do for your brain and your body is profound. In doing my research on sleep I was pleasantly surprised to find that your brain undergoes a detox as cerebral spinal fluid (CSF) flow is increased. This increase in CSF flow helps your brain rid toxic proteins like beta amyloid which is found to accumulate in the brains of Alzheimer's patients. [298]

Sleep helps to build your body up, assists the body in repairing itself, and helps to recharge your batteries! Sleep is so vital for the body, yet so many people neglect it. There is this pervasive thought in our culture that sleep is a *waste of time*, especially among entrepreneurs. Jokingly people say things such as, "I will sleep when I'm dead." I'm certainly guilty of saying things like this. It's a lie though because you cannot live your best life while cheating yourself out of sleep.

Optimal sleep for most people is considered seven to nine hours of sleep per night. I bet you, like many others, simply aren't getting enough sleep. According to a CDC report written in 2006, the number of Americans sleeping six hours or less per night has increased since 1985. [299] While the immediate effects of sleep deprivation, such as feeling tired and having brain fog, can be noticeable, other symptoms are subtler and deadlier. It is paramount that you make sure you regularly get a good night's sleep.

Although we spend most of our lives sleeping, getting quality sleep ensures we will be more productive throughout the day. A 2010 study observed that out of 4,000 employees at four large American corporations, the ones who suffered from insomnia or sleep deprivation were far less productive than the employees who slept well. The study showed that the employees not only suffered from productivity losses, but also had trouble with memory and time management skills, among other things. [300] Sleep helps us to live our lives more *thoroughly*. Meaning, we aren't like zombies mindlessly going through the day; trying to get through it or possibly even suffer through it.

I'm sure you can attest to the difference you feel when you get a good night's sleep vs. only sleeping four to five hours. During finals weeks of chiropractic college, it was not unusual for me to stay up until one or two in the morning, cramming multiple days during the week. I always woke up feeling punch drunk. But here's the thing, I'm not talking about one or two nights of not getting enough sleep. I'm talking about the health consequences of not getting enough sleep for years.

SLEEP CYCLES

There are four stages of sleep we go through to complete what's called a sleep cycle. A complete sleep cycle is between 90 and 120 minutes. The cycle repeats itself about four to five times a night with normal sleep. The first three stages are called non-rapid-eye-movement (NREM) stages and the fourth stage of sleep is called rapid eye movement (REM). Stage three sleep is the most restorative stage because your body is in a deep sleep. In fact, it is awfully hard to wake somebody up during this stage. [301]

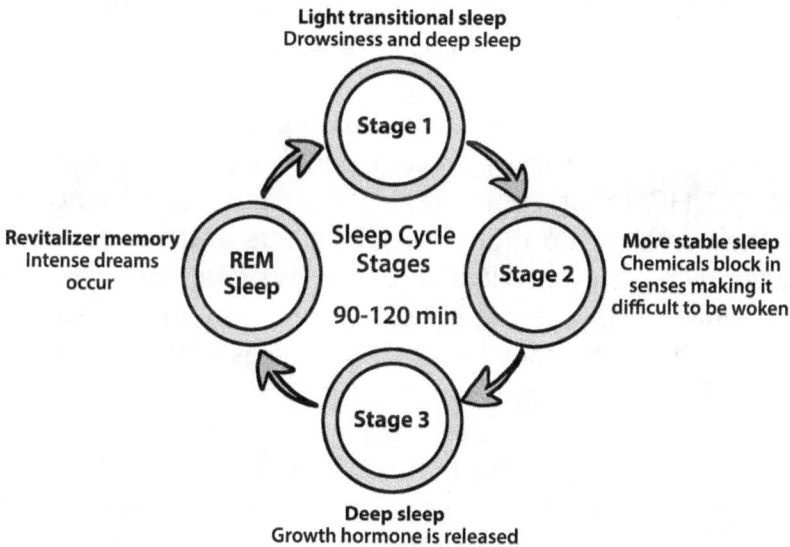

Light transitional sleep
Drowsiness and deep sleep

Stage 1

Revitalizer memory
Intense dreams
occur

REM Sleep

Sleep Cycle Stages
90-120 min

Stage 2

More stable sleep
Chemicals block in
senses making it
difficult to be woken

Stage 3

Deep sleep
Growth hormone is released

During stage three your brain waves are in a delta state which is 0.5Hz - 4Hz, a slow brain wave state. During this stage, your body releases a hefty amount of DHEA which is a precursor for male and female sex hormones, human growth hormone, and serotonin. In the REM stage, or stage four, you dream. It's important that we get a minimum of four to five complete sleep cycles per night for optimum health. This is what it means to get a *"good night sleep."* If you wake feeling groggy, it is likely that you woke in the middle of a sleep cycle. [302]

HUMAN GROWTH HORMONE, CORTISOL, AND METABOLISM

One of the biggest "get more quality sleep motivators" involves one of the chief hormones released by your pituitary gland, human growth hormone (HGH). Some researchers estimate that up to 75% of human growth hormone is released during sleep. HGH is an anabolic hormone, meaning it works to build things up in your body. HGH is essential for your health because it plays a role in healthy metabolism and energy levels. It also helps to maintain your lean body muscle mass. Some studies indicate it may prolong your life. It is considered the fountain of youth hormone.

HGH is released the first couple times you cycle through stage three sleep, but the majority is released about an hour after you fall asleep. [302]

Sleep deprivation has been shown to negatively affect the release of HGH because it changes your body's natural sleep cycles. It isn't that HGH stops being released because of a lack of sleep, but the overall amount of HGH that is released decreases. Thus, your body ends up producing less of this vital hormone overall. And, while HGH decreases, a catabolic hormone (breaks stuff down in the body) called cortisol increases when you are sleep deprived. [303]

Cortisol has always been one of the hormones that get a bad rap, but the reality is, if your body produces it there must be a good reason for it. Cortisol plays a key role in several different processes, mainly metabolism, blood sugar control, immune system regulation, and decreasing inflammation. Despite all of this, it's still called the stress hormone because your body releases it during periods of stress. But, as it turns out, it too has a natural circadian rhythm.

The circadian rhythm of cortisol peaks and dips. It is lowest around 3:00 am and then gradually starts to rise with a peak around 8:00 am. The reason for this early morning peak is because cortisol will elevate your blood sugar levels in the process of waking up. In a normal functioning body, it will gradually taper off from 8:00 am on and decrease as evening approaches because your body is preparing you for sleep. [304]

When you are sleep deprived and overstressed there is no longer a nice, natural release of cortisol in the body. Instead, cortisol is increased and decreased; it goes up and down throughout the day like a roller coaster.

As cortisol stays elevated at night it suppresses melatonin, thus making it harder for you to get a good night's sleep.

Ultimately, sleep deprivation leads to increased stress levels and a prolonged elevation of cortisol. It's a vicious cycle that keeps repeating itself over and over again. If this negative cycle continues for months to years without change, health consequences will surely follow. [304]

The consequences of prolonged levels of cortisol are vast. It can result in decreased growth hormone, as well as other major hormones like testosterone and estrogen. Your immune system is also suppressed making you more susceptible to getting colds and flus. When cortisol goes into overdrive it causes chronic inflammation in your body. Chronic inflammation is the number one cause of the top diseases that kill in the U.S., including cancer, heart disease, and diabetes. The great thing about getting more quality sleep is that it will help balance your cortisol levels. It can even help you lose weight!

Sleep loss has been found to impair insulin sensitivity which leads to a decrease in your body's ability to metabolize glucose. Insulin is needed by the cells in your body to absorb glucose. When your body becomes less sensitive to it your pancreas must produce more of it. This, of course, can lead to Type II Diabetes. Researchers at Cedars-Sinai Medical Center in Los Angeles, CA conducted a study on canines in which they discovered that one night of sleep deprivation decreased insulin sensitivity by a whopping 33%. They concluded that sleep could be a more critical factor for insulin sensitivity than a high fat diet. The major issue with insulin is that it is considered a fat storage hormone, so when your body is producing more of it you are more likely going to pack on the pounds. What you want is for your cells to be very responsive or sensitive to insulin. [305]

Sleep loss has also been shown to affect two major hormones when it comes to your appetite: leptin and ghrelin. Leptin is a hormone released by your adipose tissue (fat tissue) which suppresses appetite. Ghrelin is a peptide produced in the stomach which stimulates appetite. In a study done on 1,024 participants it was concluded that short sleep (less than 8 hours) led to a decrease in leptin and an increase in ghrelin. [306]

So, staying up late and shortening your sleep can lead to an increase in appetite and negatively affect your ability to control your impulse to eat. Researchers involved in this study reported that "changes in appetite regulatory hormones [that come] with shortened sleep may contribute to obesity." Here's the real kicker, when you're super tired and exhausted, what foods do you tend to go for, super healthy foods or processed "C.R.A.P" (carbonated, refined, artificial, processed) foods? Nine times out of ten you are going to go for that bag of chips or the cookies in the cupboard. By getting enough quality sleep you can help take back control of your appetite, make better food choices, and lose weight!

MELATONIN AND SUNLIGHT

We can't talk about sleep without mentioning melatonin, your body's powerful antioxidant like hormone. This powerful hormone plays a role in regulating glutathione and super oxide dismutase, two of your bodies most potent free-radical fighters. Amazingly, melatonin, unlike other antioxidants, can cross the blood brain barrier where it accumulates in the central nerve system at much higher amounts than in the blood. This offers strong neuroprotective effects, especially under elevated conditions of oxidative stress or intensive neural inflammation. According to some experts, melatonin is more powerful than Vitamins A, C, and E! When it comes to your health and getting quality sleep, you need melatonin. [307, 308]

Melatonin is made from serotonin in the pineal gland. It is also found in small amounts in many plant-based foods. According to Shawn Stevenson, author of the book *Sleep Smarter*, tart cherries contain the highest amount of melatonin. Pineapples can boost your body's ability to make melatonin. [309]

Melatonin follows a natural circadian rhythm that is opposite of cortisol. Where cortisol is higher during the day and lower at night, circulating melatonin is lower during the day and highest at night. This is because the two factors that play an important role in the circadian rhythm of melatonin are light and darkness.

By design our bodies secrete more melatonin as dusk approaches, preparing us to get a better night's sleep. What's amazing about this is that the whole process is regulated by your nerve system. The retina of your eye relays information about light and darkness to an area of your brain called the hypothalamus, which eventually tells your pineal gland how much melatonin to release. The more darkness detected, the more melatonin is produced and then released. Low levels of melatonin along with elevated levels of cortisol during the day help us stay awake. It's called the "sleep-wake-cycle" and it's a dance your body innately does on its own. But we can help it or severely hinder it based on our lifestyles. [310]

When it comes to sleep, we are like the employees at a major business and the product we are selling is sleep. If we do a good job for the business, business is good, it runs well, and we get adequate amounts of sleep. However, if we start showing up late to work, not listening to the boss, and we don't do what we are supposed to do, the business will soon go south. When this happens guess what product fails to sale, SLEEP!

You might be surprised to hear that one of the things you need to do for the sake of your sleep is to make sure you get adequate amounts of sunlight every day. The reason for this is that the light receptors in your eyes cause the center of your brain to produce more serotonin – the precursor for melatonin. The problem is most of us tend to be bad employees and we don't get enough of the full spectrum light our bodies need to produce enough serotonin. [311]

According to an article written about sleep on Howstuffworks. com, 6:00 am to 8:00 am gives you the most beneficial exposure to sunlight. Your body is most responsive at this time of day. This has to do with the fact that your body has a natural biological clock built in. When you are exposed to sunlight in the morning it helps to stimulate clock genes located in the hypothalamus of your brain. These clock genes are sensitive to light and darkness and work to regulate cortisol and melatonin secretion. Therefore, getting exposure to early morning sunlight helps to regulate your body's biological clock and keeps you in sync with the earth's 24-hour daily cycle. A lack of exposure to sunlight for extended periods of time causes dramatic changes to a person's sleep-wake-cycle. The person who works in a cubicle starring at a computer screen all day is not getting an adequate amount of sunlight and more than likely struggles to get quality sleep. [311, 312]

You now know that melatonin is synthesized by serotonin in the pineal gland.

> *This means that an optimal functioning pineal gland is paramount for quality sleep and having superb health.*

There is a phenomenon, however, where this tiny pea-sized gland becomes calcified. Another term for this is "brain sand," and it isn't a good thing. One of the chief ways your pineal gland becomes calcified is from fluoride. The accumulation of fluoride forms phosphate crystals that then create a hard shell around the gland. A calcified pineal gland isn't going to produce melatonin as readily, and it impairs your sleep-wake-cycle. As mentioned in Chapter

5, our biggest exposure to fluoride is from unfiltered tap water. Toothpaste is probably our second biggest exposure to fluoride. Although, according to some research, you can "decalcify" the pineal gland. To do so, you need to **avoid fluoride at all cost.** [313]

CAFFEINE, ALCOHOL, AND SLEEP

In Chapter 5 I gave you five reasons to quit caffeine and sleep should be your number one. Aside from suppressing melatonin production, it causes an increase in adrenaline. Next, cortisol puts your body into fight or flight mode. This is how it gives you the illusion of having energy, but it's not "real" energy. It's fake energy because it leaves you at a deficit, meaning you end up crashing. When this happens, most people feel the need to run to the coffee shop again and again to get their fix. And this is because caffeine is an addictive drug. But, it's not just the caffeine in coffee that's bad, it's all the other toxins as well.

Due to modern agricultural practices, coffee is heavily sprayed with pesticides and herbicides, more so than any other food. According to Stephen Cherniske, M.S. as stated in his book, *Caffeine Blues*, "Coffee often contains a raft of pesticide residues and other contaminants such as nitrosamines, solvents, and mycotoxins. These carry well-defined health risks, some of which are carcinogenic." These toxins, along with 700 other volatile substances identified in coffee, are most likely going to negatively impact your sleep. [314]

What's surprising about caffeine is it has screwed up your sleep, even if you feel like you got a great night's sleep. Shawn Stevenson writes about a study that was done using participants who drank caffeine six hours before bed. Findings reported a measurable sleep loss of one hour. The odd thing is they didn't even feel it. This is because the objective testing showed they weren't getting adequate amounts of stage three and four in their sleep cycle. [309] Ultimately, caffeine at any time during the day may cause sleep loss.

I like coffee and caffeine as much as the next guy, but after doing the research on it, I've decided it does more harm than good. Caffeine holds you back from getting a great night's sleep and your dependency on it is nothing short of an addiction. Don't be a slave to caffeine, life can be much better without it.

Many Americans use alcohol to help them fall asleep faster, but research shows this isn't so good for your sleep. The times when I passed out from a night of drinking, I never woke up the next day feeling like a million bucks. Odds are, you have probably experienced this too. This is in large part due to how alcohol effects your brain. While alcohol might help you to fall asleep or pass out faster, it still zaps your sleep. For one, alcohol has been shown to greatly suppress melatonin which affects how your clock genes in your hypothalamus respond to darkness. This would throw off your natural circadian rhythm of sleep as well. [315]

Alcohol also negatively impacts the REM stage of sleep (stage 4). I haven't discussed this stage of sleep in great depth, but the REM stage is important for mental restoration. A reduced amount of sleep in this vital stage can impair your memories. When the REM stage of sleep is negatively impacted, it makes you more susceptible to waking in the middle of the night and the quality of your sleep goes down. [316]

If you are frequently using alcohol as a crutch to fall asleep, you should question why you feel the need to do so. That is where the real problem lies. Maybe it's the caffeine you drink in the mornings, maybe it's the day to day grind of life, maybe you're going through some deep-rooted problem and you're suffering from stress? There are so many different factors that play a role in not getting enough sleep. The positive thing is, once you reduce those factors and start utilizing the sleep hacks I have listed below, you are going to get more quality sleep and you won't be dependent on alcohol or sleep medications to do so.

I feel like this is one of the most critical things people need to focus on in their lives. As we talked about earlier in this chapter, your body does its best healing at night when you're asleep. Your body balances its hormones and you gain mental restoration from a great night of sleep. Sleep is just as important as any workout or supplement, and it should be a critical focus in any healthy living program you decide to do.

SLEEP HACKS

So, how do you get better quality sleep more often? Here are some simple, but amazing sleep hacks. I will list them here and go into detail on each one below.

- Go black
- Artificial light
- Exercise
- Stretch before bed
- White noise
- Get off your screens
- Read

GO BLACK

Black out your room with light blocking curtains or blankets. Make it a mission to block any light coming into your room. The darker your room is, the more melatonin your body releases and the easier it is to fall asleep and stay asleep. In my bedroom I have even used blankets, thumbtacks, and duct-tape to block the light from coming in. I believe this to be the number one thing you can do to get better quality sleep. So, GO BLACK! [309]

ARTIFICIAL LIGHT

Make sure all electronic lights are either covered up or shut down. For example, we run a fan in our room which has very bright blue lights on the top of it. These lights could interrupt our sleep without us even knowing it. So, I put a beany on top of it to completely black out the light. The same is true for red lights found on things like digital clocks and power cords. I also shut down our router at night for two reasons. One, the artificial light it gives off and two because of the electromagnetic radiation (EMR) it emits. I talk about EMR more in depth in Chapter 11. [307, 309]

EXERCISE

You should work out in the morning or early afternoon. Doing cardio exercises earlier in the day helps to balance your hormones and tire you out. One interesting thing about exercise is that when you burn up all that excess energy in your body, it raises adenosine levels in the brain. Adenosine is another hormone which is responsible for making you feel tired and sleepy. In Chapter 8 I talk about how incredible high intensity interval training or HIIT is for your health. This would be an example of a great exercise to do in the morning. You could also exercise outside as the sun is coming up to get your daily exposure to sunlight. Remember, you don't need a gym to workout.

STRETCH BEFORE BED

Along with exercising earlier in the day, something I found to be beneficial for my sleep is stretching. For me, stretching at night before bed creates a calming effect and I fall asleep faster. Along with the stretches I focus on my breathing. Doing deep diaphragmatic breaths in through the nose where you expand first your belly and then your chest stimulates your parasympathetic nerve system, helping to further relax your body. The average person does all their breathing from their chest with very rapid and short inhales and exhales. The problem with this type of breathing is that it stimulates the sympathetic nerve system and puts the body into fight or flight mode making it much harder to fall asleep. Just remember, *stretch and breath*.

WHITE NOISE

White noise is defined as a consistent noise that contains many frequencies with equal intensities. [317] A fan would be a perfect example of white noise. White noise is handy because it drowns out or masks any sudden noises that would cause you to awaken. I have a fan in our bedroom that sits on the end table on my side of the bed. I have a hard time sleeping without it. There are also free white noise apps you can download on your phone. Try a few and see which one works best for you. I use the white noise apps when I'm traveling and staying in a hotel.

GET OFF YOUR SCREEN

The brightly lit screens from your TV, computer, and especially your phone may be your biggest sleep deterrent. This is because the light tricks your brain into thinking it's daytime, thus it suppresses melatonin production and throws off your sleep-wake cycle. Stevenson recommends in his book, *Sleep Smarter*, to limit your screen time before bed. In fact, he suggests shutting everything off at least ninety minutes before bed. [309] He also suggests downloading a blue light blocker onto your phone and computer because blue light has been proven to interrupt sleep cycles and to affect melatonin production. A blue light blocker blocks this shorter light wave, so your screens have less of an impact on your sleep. But as a rule, it is best to eliminate screen time at least an hour before bed.

READ

Reading before bed can be an incredible sleep hack. I found that every time I do this, I begin to feel sleepy and within twenty minutes or so, I'm out! Many doctors believe that reading helps to relax your body and mind, helping to prep you for sleep. Your eyes also get tired as you read through the words on the page. I have also experimented with reading out loud. For whatever reason I have found that when I read out loud, I fall asleep faster. Make sure you read something that is relaxing or enjoyable, not something that is going to get your adrenals going! Some research has even shown that reading a fictional book before bed may help you dream.

SUPPLMENTS FOR SLEEP

One supplement I take for sleep that has helped me tremendously is full spectrum CBD oil. CBD is the main, non-psychoactive component in the cannabis plant. It has amazing anti-inflammatory properties for the brain as well as the body. CBD works on the endocannabinoid system in your body. This system works to bring the body back into balance when it is off. It is one of the major systems involved with healing your body. It's also involved in energy, pleasure, and relaxation. Research shows that CBD can help reduce anxiety and increase sleep quality and length. In minute doses CBD improves daytime sleepiness which helps with the sleep-wake cycle. Full spectrum CBD oil contains different percentages of some of the other important cannabinoids in the cannabis or hemp plant which creates a beneficial "entourage effect" within the body. [318]

I would recommend taking CBD as a supplement because the benefits are vast and wide ranging. I look at full spectrum CBD oil as adding more "greens" into my life! Of course, speak to your doctor or do some extensive research on the subject before taking CBD. But, along with sleep, full spectrum CBD oil has some amazing healing properties.

Word of Caution: Full spectrum CBD may cause you to test positive for THC, so always speak to your employer first. If it's a major concern you can always take pure CBD oil. With this you won't test positive and you still get some healing benefits. I sell CBD on my website. You can use this link to find tons of amazing CBD products: https://www.hempworx.com/spartanchiro.

Melatonin is amazing BUT taking melatonin because you're not getting adequate amounts of sleep isn't necessarily the answer. For one, if you're drinking caffeine, stressed out, if your room is too light, if you're not getting enough exercise, etc., then your pineal gland isn't going to produce enough melatonin to get adequate amounts of sleep. So, taking melatonin as a supplement is not dealing with the CAUSE of the problem.

Here is another issue I see with taking exogenous melatonin. It is never as good as the real thing. When you take exogenous melatonin vs. letting your body do what it naturally does on its own, you down regulate your body's ability to make melatonin. This is similar to what happens when a bodybuilder takes steroids and his body drastically down regulates the amount of testosterone it is producing on its own. This can leave the bodybuilder dependent on taking exogenous testosterone for the rest of his life.

However, as we get older our bodies start producing less and less melatonin and it might be important to supplement it. As explained above, melatonin is a super antioxidant like hormone and plays a significant role in regulating glutathione and super oxide dismutase. So, melatonin isn't just important for sleep, it's important for several reasons. Bottom line is you want to get your body to produce the exact, right amount of melatonin it needs by utilizing all the sleep hacks listed above.

Your body is AMAZING – it has an innate ability to produce exactly what you need at the exact time you need it, but you have to work to remove interference and add good things into your life. Basically, you must support your body's natural healing capabilities vs. interfering with them!

CHIROPRACTIC CARE AND SLEEP

Chiropractic care can have a profound effect on your sleep. One way that chiropractic care can help you have better sleep has to do with the alignment and integrity of the upper cervical vertebra (cervical = neck). The atlas (see Chapter 4: Power of The Nerve System) houses and protects the brainstem. The brainstem is the beginning of the spinal cord and it controls the communication flow between the brain and the rest of the body. It's also responsible for many of the processes that take place automatically without conscious thought. These processes include things like breathing, heart rate, and the sleep wake cycle. During the sleep wake cycle the brainstem communicates with the hypothalamus to regulate the shift between wake and sleep cycles. The brainstem along with the hypothalamus also contains cells that release GABA which reduces the activity of the arousal centers in the brainstem and hypothalamus. [319, 320]

When the atlas shifts out of its normal position, even by a few millimeters, it can cause pressure on the brainstem and inhibit its ability to function at 100%. This in turn can negatively impact your ability to sleep well. Chiropractic care works by addressing the misaligned vertebra via specific adjustments that bring the vertebra back into alignment. Therefore, the alignment of your spine is necessary for you to function at your optimum. Why? Because it houses and protects your spinal cord and the precious nerve roots which relay messages back and forth between the brain and your body. [321]

In my clinical experience I have seen a lot of patients who tell me they are sleeping better because of their chiropractic care. One reason for this is because they're in less pain, therefore they stop tossing and turning at night. But, the other more profound reason for this happening is because of how chiropractic positively affects the nerve system. Although more research needs to be done in this area, there is a lot of anecdotal evidence supporting chiropractic care and sleep.

In a 2005 retrospective study printed in the JMPT, "One third of 154 patients [struggling with insomnia] reported their sleep pattern was changed immediately following a chiropractic adjustment [321]." If you are struggling with your sleep and have tried everything, chiropractic might be the missing link.

GROUNDING

ADHESIVE BACK

18"

36"

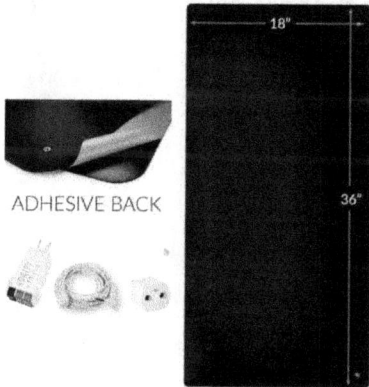

The idea behind grounding has to do with reconnecting to the earth. When your body is grounded it becomes equal to the electrical potential of the earth. This means that excess electrical charges that build up in our bodies via static electricity, EMF exposure, etc. can be balanced out by "grounding" ourselves to the earth. Research shows that balancing with the earth helps with the sleep-wake cycle because it helps to dissipate the excess stress that builds up within the body. [322] What is cool, is that you can sleep on grounding mats that plug into your wall. Many people report better sleep, less pain, and an improved sense of well-being by using grounding mats daily. You should also use a grounding mat while driving your car. In the following chapter I discuss this in more detail.

For more information about grounding mats and where to buy them, check out this link. https://www.earthing.com.

A big problem that inhibits good, quality sleep is something most people don't even think twice about. It's called electromagnetic radiation (EMR) and almost every household has a lot of it flowing through their house at the speed of light. It passes into the body and wreaks havoc on the way our cells communicate with each other. We'll discuss this in more depth in the next chapter.

Hopefully by now you understand WHY sleep is so important. Furthermore, you should understand that getting better quality sleep isn't that hard. All you have to do is follow the sleep hacks mentioned above and you will notice a difference in your sleep right away. If you're not getting enough sleep, the most common denominator is your lifestyle. Therefore, as I am prone to say, "Remove the interference and all else will follow." Simply get rid of or severely limit the lifestyle habits that are causing you to lose sleep.

"No matter how much it gets abused, the body can restore balance. The first rule is to stop interfering with nature."

- Deepak Chopra

CHAPTER 11

ZAPPED: REDUCING "EMR" EXPOSURE

*"Although we are constantly exploring the subject,
currently there is no direct evidence that
links cell phone usage to brain cancer."*

Thank You for Not Smoking, American screenplay written
and directed by Jason Reitman

We live in a technological era that has brought us wonderful advancements like Wi-Fi. This allows us to connect to the internet through our wireless devices using a high frequency radio signal. It is similar to how your car's radio tunes into a radio station signal over the airways. Your device can pick up on a signal that connects to the internet via the air. It's amazing how much these wireless devices have practically taken over our lives. [323]

As I look around the coffee shop while I'm writing this chapter, I see a couple of guys using their tablets and I see another guy who is distracted by texting on his smart phone while his buddy is trying to talk to him. I bought my non-caffeinated beverage by inserting my credit card with a circuit chip into a machine connected to a computer, connected to the internet via Wi-Fi. We can now connect to the internet whenever and wherever we are. Everything has become "smart." We have smart cars, smart homes, smart phones, smart meters, and smart TV's. We even have smart toasters and washing machines, among other things. It seems that everything can now be connected to the internet. This is great for several reasons. One, we always have access to the internet, and therefore information. Two, we can activate and monitor our smart devices via our cell phones. But what are the possible long-term negative effects of all these wireless devices on our bodies? We are only now just beginning to understand the detrimental effects of this kind of technology.

WHAT IS ELECTROMAGNETIC RADIATION?

Each one of our smart devices puts out Electromagnetic Frequency (EMF) or Electromagnetic Radiation (EMR). EMR is all around us because it is a form of energy. According to Wikipedia, "In physics, *electromagnetic radiation* (EM *radiation* or EMR) refers to the waves (or their quanta, photons) of the *electromagnetic* field, propagating (radiating) through space carrying *electromagnetic* radiant energy. It includes radio waves, microwaves, infrared, (visible) light, ultraviolet light, x-rays, and gamma rays." For the purpose of this chapter I am talking about high frequency, aka radio frequency (RF) which is non-ionizing radiation. This is the type of radiation that your cell phone, smart meters, and all wireless devices are constantly emitting. [324]

You can't see electromagnetic waves. It's invisible energy that can only be viewed with an oscilloscope or heard with an RF reader. Similar to the waves of the ocean, an electromagnetic wave starts at zero, goes up to a peak point, back down to zero, and then keeps going down until it reaches a negative peak point. Then it returns to zero. This is called a sinus wave. As the wave moves up and down it also moves forward at the speed of light. The distance

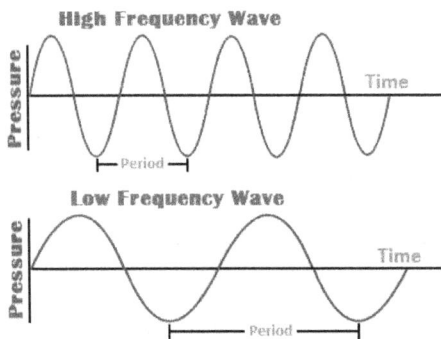

the wave travels forward is called a wavelength. Each kind of electromagnetic wave has a frequency. The higher the frequency the shorter the wavelength and vice versa. Radio waves created by your cell phone are considered high frequency. According to Dr. Jonathan Halper, PhD and author of the book, *Electromagnetic Radiation Survival Guide*, "this difference between the wavelength [frequencies] is important because it affects our ability to block and shield these waves." [325]

It is estimated that we are exposed to and bombarded by **100 million (100,000,000) more times EMR than our grandparents were.** This is shocking but makes sense because most Americans own a smart phone and other smart devices. According to Statista, an online statistic, market research, and business intelligence portal, it was estimated that there would be 248 million smart phone users in the U.S. in 2019 (latest available report). That was nearly 80% of the population at that time! Contrast this number with only 62.2 million in 2010. That's a huge jump! [326]

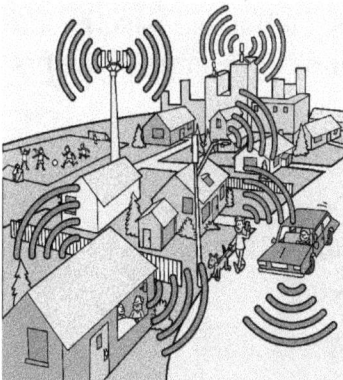

I am confident that if we could see the EMR that we are constantly being bombarded with we wouldn't want any of it.

Dr. Jay

According to Metova, a company founded in 2006 that specializes in app development, they discovered after surveying 1,000 consumers in the U.S covering a wide range of demographics that **90% of U.S consumers now own some sort of a smart home device.** According to the same study 70% of the consumers owned a voice-controlled system such as an Amazon Alexa or Google Home. Why is this a problem? Because these devices are constantly emitting EMR! Americans are increasingly becoming concerned over privacy matters because of all these smart devices, but not enough are concerned about the potential harmful effects of long-term exposure to EMR. [327]

OUR BODIES ARE BIO-ELECTRIC

Our bodies are "bio-electric" meaning all the cells within our bodies exert an electrical current and electromagnetic field. Each cell in your body is like a battery that contains a charge of 40-90 millivolts. The cells regulate this charge by utilizing electrolytes like sodium, potassium, calcium, and magnesium. This charge is crucial for the cell to perform its various functions and for your body to maintain homeostasis. The human body is constantly sending and receiving electromagnetic signals through a vast array of different cells which make up different tissues (nerve, muscle, collagen, etc.). Therefore, a cell's charge is important because it plays a critical role in cellular communication. Disruption or interference with the communication between the cells will lead to illness. [328]

Your body also receives electromagnetic signals from the outside just as an antenna does. Remember earlier when we talked about how one could use their body as an antenna with some of the first television sets?

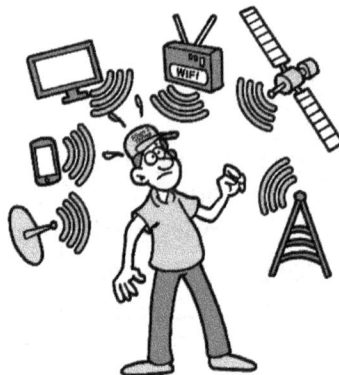

According to Ann Louise Gittleman, author of *Zapped*, this is because "[in] that moment the RF waves carrying the image are broadcasting through you." [329] The problem with EMR is that it doesn't deflect off your body like sunlight hitting a mirror, instead most of it passes into your body. Due to this constant exposure to these various frequencies we have disharmony within our body because it is struggling to communicate with itself through all these EMR waves coming into it.

EMR causes interference within our bodies. Interference leads to disharmony and disharmony leads to disease.

Since the invention of electrical power plants in 1882, the first cell phone in 1973, to today with the so called wireless revolution and the advent of the smart phone, more and more scientists and doctors have raised health and safety concerns over our increasing exposure to EMR. In 2012 the Bioinitiative Working Group, which is comprised of scientists, researchers, and public health policy professionals, published a Bioinitiative Report citing approximately 1800 studies demonstrating the negative health effects caused by EMR. [330]

These negative health effects range from childhood cancers, brain tumors, breast cancer, brain disorders, and nerve system dysfunction, among other things. The Bioinitiave report "maintains that permissible radiation levels in most countries are already 1,000 to 10,000 times too high." Even the World Health Organization in May of 2011 stated that mobile phone use may possibly be "carcinogenic to humans." "The agency now lists mobile phone use in the same carcinogenic hazard category as lead, engine exhaust, and chloroform." [330, 331]

In 2009 The European council took notice stating:

"The evidence is now strong enough, using the precautionary principle, to justify the following steps: 1. For the governments, the mobile industry, and the public to take all reasonable measures to reduce exposures to EMF, especially to radio frequencies from mobile phones, and particularly the exposures to children and young adults who seem to be most at risk from head tumors." [332]

I think the fact that the World Health Organization has expressed concern is enough for both you and me to be concerned, but let's look at this issue in more detail.

EFFECTS OF EXPOSURE

ROS molecules in excess are considered unstable and highly reactive because they strip the electrons away from stable molecules, thus creating oxidative stress. Oxygen stripping electrons away from iron to create rust is a simple example of oxidative stress that occurs in the environment. A similar thing happens in our bodies when we are exposed to free radicals or reactive oxygen species (ROS) that are normally formed as a by-product of cellular metabolism, infection, environmental pollution, and toxins.

Oxidative stress causes inflammation within our bodies. Prolonged inflammation can set off diseases such as cancer, arthritis, autoimmune problems, cardiovascular issues, and neurodegenerative diseases. There is a growing body of evidence that shows even short-term exposure to low frequency and/or high frequency EMR can cause increased ROS molecules and oxidative stress. In one such study, cells exposed to ten, thirty, and sixty minutes of 1800 MHz RF (a common cell phone frequency) increased ROS and oxidative stress. At sixty minutes of exposure the study found there was significant damage to lipids and protein. [333]

It is also important to note that the study mentioned above also showed increased glutathione levels after only ten minutes of exposure. Glutathione is a powerful antioxidant produced by the liver that can also be found in fruits, vegetables, and meats. Prolonged exposure to EMR can lower glutathione levels. Glutathione is what Ann Luise Gittleman, in her book *Zapped*, calls "a resident handyman." This is because it can "repair free radical damage on the spot as well as clean up any toxins and the injury they cause." Healthy people produce a good amount of glutathione in their bodies. People in diseased states show significantly lower glutathione levels. [329, 334]

One study published in the Journal of Pharmaceutical and Biomedical Analysis tested this theory by having twelve healthy, adult male volunteers carry their cell phones in their front pockets. The cell phones were set in the standby position with the front keypad facing the body. Results showed an increase in "lipid peroxidation" and decreased activation of super oxide dismutase (another powerful antioxidant) and glutathione. If carrying your cell phone in your pocket has the potential to decrease your bodies most powerful antioxidants, what else can chronic exposure to EMR do? [334]

The evidence for the potential negative effects of long-term exposure to EMR is overwhelming, and too much to write about in a single chapter. Suffice to say that long-term exposure to EMR has been linked to everything from sleep problems, fatigue, A.D.D in children, severe neurological impairment, infertility issues and cancer. One of the things I continually see in my office is patients who suffer from chronic fatigue or extreme exhaustion. I am convinced that a lot of their issues are due to their cell phones being attached to them. If they would minimize their RF exposure by turning their cell phones to airplane mode, there would probably be a huge difference in how they felt.

I didn't realize how pervasive my cell phone had become in my life until I started turning it to airplane mode. Once I realized the health risks, I stopped using it for Wi-Fi in my car and went back to listening to CDs. I stopped using it at the gym to listen to music and YouTube videos while I worked out. I also stopped using it in my home to check all the updates I was getting throughout the day.

Right away I noticed a difference in how I felt. It was as though I got a little more of my energy back. So, I always put my phone on airplane mode until I absolutely need to use it. And, aside from lowering my exposure to EMR, I'm not as distracted with pings, dings, email notifications, Facebook notifications, etc., etc. You can also purchase a shield for your cellphone which will minimize the intensity of the EMR. If you are feeling tired or consistently exhausted, or you have any of the problems mentioned in the previous paragraph, maybe it's time you assess the EMR in your home, your car, and your workspace. For the most part, these are the areas in your life that you can control the amount of EMR you are exposed to. I will explain exactly how you can clean up this electric noise or electropollution at the end of this chapter.

Obviously, the subject of EMR exposure has been studied extensively and the negative effects have been well documented. So, why is technology that has the potential to be so hazardous to our health even allowed? One reason is the safety standards for radiation were established in the 1950's. Researchers thought that if electromagnetic radiation doesn't ionize atoms like x-rays or gamma rays, then it can be considered safe as long as it doesn't cause a significant thermal effect upon living tissue. Their entire justification for safety is based on whether it heats up living tissue. Of course, none of the research done in the 1950's or today considers what long-term exposure to non-ionizing radiation can do to a person. We, the consumers, have become the long-term study. [325]

Also, much like tobacco science, cell phone companies fund their own studies. Some experts say that the science behind wireless technology has become the new "Tobacco Science." In fact, most industry funded epidemiological studies, unsurprisingly, show that there is no increase in brain cancer with cell phones. The problem with this lies in the way the studies were done. Internationally recognized expert on electromagnetic radiation from mobile phones, Dr. Devra Davis, M.D., Founding Director of the Center for Environmental Oncology at The University of Pittsburgh Cancer Institute and founder of the nonprofit Environmental Health Trust, states, "The way they define a cell phone user in these studies is a person making one phone call per week for six months." This begs the question, who only uses their phone once per week? [335]

According to techcrunchnews.com, an online publisher of technology industry news, "in 2016 U.S. consumers [spent] an average of five hours per day on mobile devices." Most of that time is spent on apps with Facebook taking up the largest percentage of a consumer's time, at a whopping 19%, according to the article. So, can we really trust the industry funded studies? Dr. Davis said it well when she said, "sponsored research can induce publication bias." She continues, "where you stand on an issue depends on where you sit and who bought your chair." [335, 336]

REVOLVING DOOR POLITICS AND 5G

In 2013 about $45 million was spent by major players in the wireless and telecom sector on lobbying congress. Lobbying is a nice way of saying, "corporate sponsorship." Politicians should have jackets like the NASCAR drivers, just so we can see who they work for. It's a corrupt system to say the least, but it gets even worse. In 2015 Tom Wheeler who led the two most powerful industry lobbying groups, CTIA and NCTA, became chairman of the Federal Communications Commission (FCC)! The FCC is supposed to regulate the Telecom companies, along with the FDA, to protect U.S. consumers from harm. This doesn't seem to be happening as more and more wireless technology is pushed into our lives. [337]

You've probably heard a lot about 5G, and you may even use it, but have you thought about the possible ramifications to your health when exposed to 5G? According to Fortune.com, 5G can connect 100 billion devices at speeds ten to one hundred times faster than our current fourth generation technology. To accomplish this, a new technology called beamforming will be utilized. Beamforming will "scramble/unscramble and redirect packets of data on a no-interference path back to us. This will more than likely mean an overwhelming increase in the number of wireless antennas or cell phone towers. [338]

We are talking about antennas on businesses, light poles, utility poles, homes, etc. All done for the sake of higher speed.

**Even Elon Musk has proposed a plan to beam
5G upon us from 4,000 satellites!**

So, instead of a 50-millisecond delay there will only be a one-millisecond delay. With this kind of speed, machines, like self-driving cars, will be able to "speak" to each other. According to Marcus Weldon, the CTO of Alcatel Lucent, "*Up until now, we've designed the networks for people and their needs, now we're designing it for things.*" 5G proposes to utilize frequencies above and below existing frequency bands. The inevitable problem with 5G is we are exposed to a higher and more consistent amount of dense EMR and it is extremely hard to escape it or shield ourselves from it. As a former employee of WHO put it:

"*The plan to beam highly penetrative 5G milli wave radiation at us from space must surely be one of the greatest follies ever conceived of by mankind. There will be nowhere safe to live.*"
Olga Sheean, former WHO employee and
author of *No Safe Place.* [339]

WHAT CAN YOU DO?

Remember that just because you can't see, feel, or perceive these invisible frequencies doesn't mean they aren't harming you. You have no idea what the long-term consequences are going to be for you and your family's health. Also, infants and children are more susceptible to EMR because there is more cellular activity going on within their bodies.

We tend to spend most of our time in our homes, our cars, and our workspace. Wherever you spend most of your time should be made "safe." You do have control over these areas, for the most part. What I have attempted to do below is list some quick and easy things you can do in each of those areas and ways to minimize your and your family's exposure.

Create A "Safe" Home

Go wired

Instead of utilizing wireless internet, run ethernet cables to all your smart devices, like your computers and TVs. This is what I did in my home and it decreased the EMR considerably.

Get Rid Of

Do you really need all those smart devices, like Alexa? They emit a considerable amount of EMR. I know because I have tested them with my RF Meter. You don't necessarily need all your wireless transmitting devices, but if getting rid of them isn't an option, choose to wire them. There are experts in this field, like a good, local IT person that can give you advice and even wire all your devices if you don't want to mess with it. BNI.com is a good resource to find a qualified IT person.

Put Your Phone in Airplane Mode

When you're not using your cell phone, put it in airplane mode. This shuts off the Wi-Fi function and your cell phone will cease to emit EMR. It's important to remember that radiation from your cell phone goes in all directions, but the **intensity/density of the radiation decreases "in proportion to the square of the distance from the antenna."** This means that when you need to use your phone, always hold it at least twelve inches from your body and keep it away from vital organs. According to some experts, this will decrease your exposure to EMR up to 80%! NEVER hold your phone up to your head, always utilize the speaker function. The same goes for texting, twelve inches from your body and always keep your phone at eye level so you're not looking down at it. This will help prevent "text-neck." You can also buy a good quality air-tube headset which does not conduct EMR. An air-tube headset would also increase the distance between your body and the phone.

Think Before You Make or Receive Phone Calls

When you are receiving or making a phone call, your cell phone will emit the highest amount of EMF. Always wait until you're fully connected before bringing it closer to your head or body. On a side note, it's important to know that your cell phone will emit the highest levels of radiation in areas of poor reception because it will try and utilize more power to connect. **So, either maintain a safe distance from your phone or wait until your reception is better before you use your phone.** In the back of the book I have listed some resources for companies that make cell phone shielding cases.

Move Away from Low Frequency Radiation

We spoke a great deal in this chapter about high frequency radiation in the form of radio waves, but we didn't really go into low frequency radiation. The alternating current (AC) used in American households is 60 hertz and produces an electromagnetic field. This is considered extremely low frequency (ELF). Low frequency radiation is measured in terms of milligauss (mG). The Environmental Protection Agency recommends we limit our exposure to between 0.5 mG to 2.5 mG at any given moment. The problem with ELF radiation is it's everywhere, especially in your house. Anything that is electric is going to emit an electromagnetic field, it's just at a lower frequency than the radio waves your smart devices are emitting. Examples of this include power boxes, power cords/extension cords, electrical wiring, electrical appliances, etc. The good news is distance is your friend! The intensity of the EMF emitted from your electrical sources radically decreases the farther you move away. A blender, for example, can emit up to 50- 220 mG up to four inches away and reduce to 0.3- 3 mG when three feet away [325]. I have confirmed this with my LF meter which hummed quite loudly the closer I got to the source of LF radiation and then dissipated rapidly as I moved away.

A good rule of thumb is to keep any piece of furniture you spend a great deal of time on at a distance from any strong LF emitting devices. Power strips, for example, emit a lot of LF radiation so make sure you switch them off in your bedroom, especially before bedtime. You can also purchase shielded and grounded extension cords and power cords to be used in your home. You may notice you are sleeping better once you've done this.

I would also recommend purchasing a decent quality LF meter and using it to explore all the rooms in your house. You want to use it to identify the "hot spots" in your house and work to drastically reduce them. Also, get rid of electric blankets, electric heating pads, and that waterbed from the 70's you sleep on. I have included some LF meter recommendations in the back of the book.

Shield Your Smart Meters

I interviewed the inventor of the SMART Meter Guard and asked him, "Why smart meters?" He said the reason utility companies are forcing them onto consumers is "all about the money." They don't have to have an employee come to your house every month to read the meter as with the old analog meters. This is because smart meters communicate back and forth to a central station using wireless RF technology. On top of not having to use as much manpower, these meters allow utility companies to collect more accurate information regarding usage levels. The problem is that they emit high pulsed RF waves that have been shown to cause health problems. Again, we do not know what the long-term consequences to our health will be. I always recommend taking a more cautious approach when it comes to your health.

More than likely you already have a smart meter. So, here is what you can do. **You can have it removed and pay a little extra every month, or you can work to protect yourself by blocking the RF radiation.** Pacific Gas and Electric, my utility provider, has received so many complaints regarding the smart meter that they now have an opt out option. Contact your local utility company for opt out options in your city. At the time of this writing we were renting a house, so I chose to buy guards for both my gas and electric meter. The technology utilized, a Faraday Cage, was invented in 1836 by Michael Faraday. It works "by absorbing the electromagnetic waves into the grounded stainless-steel meshing. The RF power is then shunted to the ground and dissipated." [341]

Here is a link if you want to purchase your own utility shield: http://www.smartmeterguard.com?afmc=37.

It's also important to note that smart meters may cause a phenomenon known as dirty electricity. Dirty electricity has to do with "spikes or surges of electromagnetic energy traveling along power lines and building wiring where only standard 50/60 Hertz AC electricity should be." These spikes and surges in EMR are potentially harmful, especially if you're in close proximity to an electrical smart meter or AC outlet. The reason for this potential harm is because just like any "kind" of EMR it can interfere with the electrical communication within the body leading to a wide variety of problems including, cancer, sleep disturbances, brain fog, memory issues, anxiety, irritability, fatigue, weakness, headaches, etc., the list is endless. [342]

Limit EMR From Your Computers

Computers emit all kinds of EMR. They have a Wi-Fi component, plenty of electrical components that emit LF radiation, and they can cause dirty electricity in your home. Here are some quick tips to protect you from these:

1. Connect your computer to your router using an ethernet cable and turn off the Wi-Fi component of your computer.

2. Shut off your router's Wi-Fi component (may need to contact your internet provider to do this).

3. Eliminate your wireless keyboard and mouse (think old school).

4. Situate the tower and all electrical components as far as possible from your body and where you sit at the desk.

5. Get an earthing mat to sit on and put one underneath your keyboard (more on this later in the chapter).

6. Check to see if the EMR is reduced using your LF meter.

The EMR emitted from your laptop can be extremely intense, especially if you are placing it on your lap to do your work. I would highly recommend NEVER setting your laptop on your lap. Always position it on top of a flat surface and keep your distance. I try to keep about 2.5 ft. between myself and my laptop. Remember, "Distance is your friend." The second most critical thing is to shut the Wi-Fi component off if applicable. The EMR emitted by your laptop when your Wi-Fi component is on can be strong. Either eliminate the Wi-Fi component or significantly reduce the amount of time you spend on your laptop with the Wi-Fi turned on. Laptops also emit LF radiation from the AC adapter plug and electrical components within the computer itself. Keep the AC adapter and computer as far away from your body as possible. Some laptops can also emit dirty electricity.

Eliminate Dirty Electricity

Purchase a micro-surge meter that plugs into an outlet and measures Graham-Stetzer Units (GS). A reading of fifty or above indicates dirty electricity. [325] A micro-surge meter can be purchased on this website. https://www.greenwavefilter.com

After measuring your dirty electricity, you want to neutralize it. You can buy micro-surge filters which filter out all of the surges and spikes of EMR in your outlets. These filters are simple to use.

Just plug them in your outlets. According to Dr. Jonathan Halpern, you will need an average of twelve filters for a three-bedroom apartment, most likely more for a house. [325] These filters can be purchased on the Green Wave website.

"Clean" Your Car

There can be a considerable amount of RF radiation in your car, mainly because of your cell phone and the blue tooth technology found in most modern cars. Add in GPS and other electronic components and you have a recipe for increased exposure to RF radiation. The car also acts like a metal cage (Faraday Cage) where the EMR is trapped inside and amplified.

A safe rule of thumb is to drive an older car rather than a newer one. A newer car with all the electronic bells and whistles will give off way more RF radiation than an older car. My 2017 Toyota RAV 4 LE (basic model) reads clear on my RF reader with the blue tooth off. But, a 2019 XLE Toyota RAV 4 reads high to extreme.

The other way you are exposed in your car is simply by driving through your town. The RF radiation from cell phone towers beams in through the windows as you drive. I tested this one day with my RF reader. With my cell phone and blue tooth turned off, my RF meter bounced from low (200 MHz), to high, to extreme (8 GHz) just driving down one of the main streets in the town I live in. What's even more scary is the closer I was to any cell tower, the buzz from my RF reader got stronger.

If you're driving a car with a lot of RF radiation, you can always get rid of it and buy something older. If that isn't in the cards, work to minimize your exposure. The number one thing you can do is shut off your Bluetooth on both your phone and in your car. If you can't shut off your Bluetooth, call your car dealership and see if they can.

Also, if your car has Wi-Fi make sure you can shut it off. Why do you need it anyway?

Another thing I did was to purchase a grounding mat to sit on while driving. When we drive, a build-up of static electricity occurs. This happens as our clothing vibrates and rubs against the seat. Also, the driver and passengers are exposed to voltage (electric charge in motion) and EMR coming directly off the dashboard. This increases one's body voltage which should be neutral. This buildup of static electricity causes harm and the symptoms can be vast, such as headaches, tiredness, (especially on longer drives), increased tension, etc. The mat is grounded by the metal understructure of the car. It discharges the static electricity, putting it back on the frame of the vehicle.

Grounding mats can be used in your house to sit on, lie on, exercise on, sleep on, etc. The difference being that these mats are grounded to the earth.

I have noticed a better sense of calm while driving when using a grounding mat. Others have reported feeling less sleepy.

Another thing I did was to purchase a car harmonizer on this website. https://emfsol.com/?aff=spartanchiro. The car harmonizer I have plugs into my car's cigarette lighter and supposedly works by harmonizing the damaging energetic frequencies and rendering them harmless. A word of caution, the science on this tech is still in its infancy and more research certainly needs to be done.

It's important to mention that electric cars and hybrids put out a huge amount of LF and RF radiation.

Harness Orgone Energy

Orgone, also known as Chi and Prana, is described as a universal life force that's omnipotent. Basically, it's in everything; it's in both inorganic and organic matter. Orgone energy can be harnessed and put into an energy healing pendent using orgonite. Orgonite is a compound made up of crystals, metals, and resin. According to research first explained and elaborated on by Wilhelm Reich in the 1930s, orgone has the power to attract, deflect, and hold onto energy. When it comes to EMF, research shows that orgonite can protect your body from harmful EMFs.

I have purchased multiple orgonite and shungite (a mineral, said to have strong healing powers and helps to shield a person from harmful EMFs) products from KJ Moore, a registered nurse and creator of Carpe Diem Nursing. Her website is www. carpediemnursing.org. KJ has a variety of the most creative and beautiful pyramids, bracelets, jewelry, and other healing items I have ever seen. She also will customize any order upon request. Why not wear jewelry that looks good, and serves a healing purpose?

In 1957 the U.S. federal government issued a court order unique to American history which ordered the burning of Dr. Wilhelm Reich's books. WHY?! What was the U.S. Government trying to hide?!

Understanding EMF and how to neutralize it can be daunting. If you live or work near cell phone towers, powerlines, and other high EMR producing technology, it might be time to consult with an expert. There are a lot of things you can do yourself, but making sure things are done right may take an expert. Visit this website https://www.emfexperts.com to consult with an expert in the field of EMF. The company was founded by an electrical engineer with over forty years of experience in the power and energy industry.

Web Links and Consultations

I have consulted with several experts who own companies that produce devices that protect and shield us from EMR pollution. I have spent over $600 on products from Cory Hillis, owner of EMF Solutions. I have also consulted with Michael Schwaebe, a nuclear engineer and independent expert and consultant on EMF. I have spoken to consultants from Defender Shield too. They make products for minimizing radiation from your laptop and cell phones, as well as other products. You can find them at https://www.defendershield.com. I have purchased a "xZubi," a product that sticks to the back of your cell phone and other EMF producing devices from this website, https://www.greensmoothiegirl.com. Supposedly, this device mitigates the ill-effects of EMF.

In a world that is fast tracking us toward self-driving vehicles, more wireless technology, faster speed internet, cell phone towers everywhere (churches, city parks, public schools), and more smart devices it is imperative that we PROTECT ourselves. It is my opinion that you should take immediate action to reduce you, and your family's, exposure to harmful EMF.

I'm certain that if you take action on minimizing your exposure to EMF, you will notice a difference right away. As soon as I started this journey, both my wife and I, noticed a difference in our sense of peace. When it comes to decreasing your stress and managing your peace, you must act.

What it all comes down to, and the entire purpose of this book, is two words - Full Potential. As you work towards removing interference and adding good things into your life, you will achieve better health and well-being! You will more likely achieve your full potential because better health leads to a better mind, body, and spirit.

YOUR DIVINE SENSE OF SELF
CHAPTERS 12-13

"We are not human beings having a spiritual experience; we are spiritual beings having a human experience."

-G. I. Gurdjieff

CHAPTER 12

PEACE MANAGEMENT

"You do not manage your stress; you manage your peace.
Peace is the normal, natural state God created."

- Dr. Ben Lerner, D.C.

In this last section of this book we will explore your divine sense of self. We will take a good look at your spiritual sense of self and how God ties into all of this. You are a spiritual being living in a physical body.

D.D. Palmer, the founder of chiropractic, said that the purpose of chiropractic was to "connect man the physical with man the spiritual." When I first heard this quote, I didn't fully comprehend the extent of what he was saying, but now I'm starting to get it. We have a spirit and it is our duty to fully express our spirit while we have life in our bodies.

Your body is a vessel that houses your spirit. How well you take care of your vessel directly affects your spirit. In this chapter we will look at managing your peace. This means bringing more consciousness towards maintaining a state of peace and calmness in your life no matter what is happening. Nothing could be more important to your health than learning how to manage – your – PEACE! Today, sadly, most people are worried about managing their stress. True health and well-being have a lot more to do with prevention and being proactive, rather than waiting until you're in crisis and then just managing it. Remember this discussion from

Chapter 1? Why is it that we focus so much on only managing our stress and not preventing it? This is the same as saying, "I'm just managing my disease." How lame is that statement?? There is no **power** in that! Ben Lerner articulates this very well in his book *Body by God*. Lerner stated:

> *"There is no such thing as poverty management or disease management. If you are broke or diseased, it is hard or downright impossible to manage. There is, however, such a thing as financial management or health management. By appropriately managing your finances and your health, you work to avoid the pain of poverty and disease."* [343, Pg. 239]

WHAT'S YOUR FOCUS?

First, if we only focus on managing our stress it is likely we will end up with more stress to manage. Tony Robbins said, "Where your focus goes, energy flows." If we focus on peace, then we will get more peace, unless you're the government, then peace is just a code word for "war." [344] But, that's another story in and of itself. The gurus talk about finding your "inner-peace." To me, this means you find peace in everything that is going on in your life, no matter what's going on. **Let's face it, no matter what you do the stress is always going to be there, right?** But, it's all in how you **PERCEIVE** it, keyword there.

Isn't it ironic that people who complain about their stress will always find more stress to complain about? Complainers always complain. Therefore, it's imperative that we get away from the phrase stress management. We can overcome our stress, we can do things to mitigate the stress, we can figure out new ways to tackle it, we can proactively avoid it, and we can change our thoughts, beliefs, and perceptions to make stress our companion. However, the number one rule of thumb is, don't **NUMB** yourself from stress.

Have you heard of stress eating? Many people numb themselves from the stress of life by giving in to a negative addiction that

ONLY leaves them worse! As is the case of the stress eater, the closet alcoholic, the "I 'gotta' race home from work and watch the ZILLION TV shows I 'Tivoed' person!" You simply cannot "check-out" of life as a way of managing your stress because it ALWAYS LEADS TO MORE STRESS DOWN THE ROAD. Think about it, the stress eater may end up obese, diabetic, and with high blood pressure. The alcoholic gains weight, loses his ability to think rationally, has marital issues and possible cirrhosis of the liver, bad fat around the organs, etc. etc. The chronic television watcher vicariously lives her life through actors acting out fake lives - only to look in the mirror years later and realize she hasn't done shit with her own life. What a **TIME SUCK** television is!

*It is evident that chronic stress makes us
do dumb things, habitually.*

So, what exactly is stress?

Stress is defined as, "A physical, chemical, or emotional factor that causes bodily or mental tension and may be a factor in disease causation." Stress can be a *SILENT KILLER*. [345]

Not all stress is bad, however, there are two groups of stress to concern ourselves with. One is EUSTRESS and the other is DISTRESS.

Eustress is the beneficial stress! Merriam-Webster dictionary defines it as, "A positive form of stress having a beneficial effect on health, motivation, performance, and emotional well-being." You can, in fact, "combat" negative stress with eustress. Utilizing positive stress, like exercise, meditation, and the like, is one of the most proactive ways of dealing with ongoing life stressors. [346]

Distress is the negative stress! Distress stimulates the sympathetic part of our nerve system putting us into fight or flight mode. Short-term distress isn't the problem, it's the long-term distress or chronic stress that leads to many health problems if not addressed. [347]

THE STRESS RESPONSE

The stress response is inherent to every animal in the animal kingdom, including human beings. It's a crucial response for all animals because it's part of an elaborate and wonderful inborn survival mechanism. Without our body's intelligent ability to respond to both external and internal stress, we would not have made it this far.

When it comes to external stress, the stress response begins in your head, more specifically, your brain's limbic system. The amygdala, aka the emotional center of the brain, is responsible for sensing potential threats. If a genuine threat is detected (let's say an angry dog is running straight at you full speed) the amygdala sends a signal of distress to the hypothalamus. It fires up the sympathetic nerve system, via the autonomic nerves, to cause your adrenal glands to kick out epinephrine, otherwise known as adrenaline. [348, 349]

In virtually seconds adrenaline enters your bloodstream and causes instantaneous changes to your body so you can better adapt to the perceived threat. If there's a big angry dog coming at you your heart rate increases and blood flow is directed to your limbs to prepare you for fight or flight. Digestion is restricted while your airways expand to allow you to take in more air. At the same time, your immune system releases pro-inflammatory chemicals called cytokines in anticipation of injury or possible infection. Your prefrontal cortex shuts off and your ability to think rationally goes out the window. In a moment of fight or flight you don't need critical thinking skills. [348, 349]

All of this happens in seconds and without a thought you throw up your arm and block the dog as it jumps to bite your face off! The stress response mechanism is an extraordinary example of how intelligent our bodies are! You may recall a time in your life where you reacted to an external stress and this mechanism saved your life. Maybe it helped you to swerve your car at the very last second and avoid a catastrophic accident. Maybe, you dove, superman style to catch your toddler just in the nick of time as he fell off the couch. Even when you exercise you kick this mechanism into gear! It's a good thing in the moment. But short-term stress isn't the issue, it's when the stress response becomes long-term that we have a problem. [348, 349]

There is a second mechanism inherent within the stress response, the HPA axis. The HPA axis stands for the hypothalamus, pituitary, and the adrenals. It's activated when the initial surge of epinephrine goes down. The responsibility of the HPA axis is to keep the body on high alert (fight or flight mode) until the threat passes. It does this by releasing a cascade of hormones that eventually tell the adrenal glands to release cortisol. Cortisol is also known as the stress hormone. However, it does have many benefits in the short term. [348, 349] For example, cortisol in the immediate acute phase of stress helps to decrease inflammation, rather than increase it. Cortisol tells all those excited immune cells to calm down, thus decreasing the production of cytokines which cause inflammation. Cortisol also helps to replenish energy reserves that get tapped into when the body is under stress. Furthermore, cortisol plays a huge role in the circadian rhythms of the sleep – wake cycle and appetite control (for more information on this refer to Chapter 9). So, cortisol isn't all bad. [348, 349]

The problem occurs when cortisol levels stay elevated due to chronic stress. When this happens, the immune cells become desensitized which causes the inflammation to stay elevated and possibly rage out of control. This inflammation can also block cortisol's "repair and maintenance" work. It can even bind to DNA and alter gene expression causing organs to malfunction. [348, 349]

Under prolonged levels of stress high levels of cortisol cause a yearning for foods or synthetic food-like substances that contain salt, sugar, and fat. Think "fast food" with supersized fries and a large coke, think potato chips, or ice-cream. These are all common foods that people reach for when they are overly stressed. The increased hunger we feel when we are stressed may also be due to the fact that we tend to over-breathe.

As pointed out in Chapter 8: Motion is Life, when we over-breathe, we expel too much CO_2 which increases our blood pH levels. One theory behind eating processed and acid-forming foods (bad foods) when we are stressed is that our body craves the bad foods in an effort to balance out our pH levels. Patrick McKeown points out that with short-term stress our breathing returns to normal fairly quickly, "...however, with long term stress persistent over-breathing decreases CO_2 levels for extended periods of time, meaning blood pH is not given the opportunity to normalize." [350, Pg. 178] Therefore, the urge to eat sugar, processed foods, animal products, and other acid forming foods due to chronic levels of stress may be hard to control. Many cave to their cravings, thus packing on the pounds. Certainly, chronic stress is one of the most significant causal factors for obesity.

HOW DOES STRESS AFFECT YOUR HEART AND YOUR MENTAL HEALTH?

Stress negatively affects every system in the body and over time sabotages your heart and cardiovascular system. Stress raises your blood pressure which causes your heart to work overtime. If not addressed, it can lead to a heart attack. Moreover, the over-breathing that happens because of stress decreases blood flow and oxygen to the heart, which can also cause a heart attack. Hyperventilation also negatively impacts the electrical activity of the heart and can lead to heart arrythmias. This too may lead to cardiac arrest. If one undergoes a dramatic increase in their stress levels via a crisis, stressful event, or even during exercise that too may lead to a heart attack. The inflammation created due to prolonged stress causes damage to the inner lining of the arterial walls which causes plaque to buildup. [350]

If you don't do anything to mitigate the stress, your mind will constantly stay on high alert until you're exhausted. In effect you become hyperresponsive and overreact to the smallest things.

You may find yourself snapping at your spouse or your kids. You may find that your driving becomes more aggressive. Because the prefrontal cortex is no longer working at its optimum, creative thought, multi-tasking skills, and your ability to make rational decisions becomes impaired. [349] Take, for example, the parent who must take their child to the hospital for whatever reason. Going to the hospital is a stressful event. Not only that, but the environment inside a hospital is typically stressful. Doctors and nurses sometimes use language that belittles parents and puts the fear of God into them. They can make the parent think the worst possible scenario stuff. This state of fear that the parent is in suppresses the parent's ability to think because it shuts down the prefrontal cortex. Therefore, what often happens in these terrible situations is that the parent makes irrational decisions regarding their child's health because they are in a state of fear (high stress). They have lost the ability to think rationally and ask the questions that need to be asked. Inevitably, rather than taking a more conservative approach to their child's health, they put the power into the hands of the doctor and may end up doing something highly invasive that might be completely unwarranted.

"Stress makes us do funny things that don't make NO sense."

Dr. Jay

RECOGNIZE YOU'RE STRESSED

When it comes to managing your peace, you must recognize that you're stressed. Recognizing that you're stressed can help you to accept responsibility for it and then take positive action. What this means is that you act in a positive direction as a means of dealing with your stress, versus doing something negative that would mask the symptoms of stress. Recognizing you're stressed takes recognizing the symptoms of stress. Because stress can be silent, sometimes the symptoms aren't obvious.

Below I have listed the top eight mental/emotional signs of stress. If you find that you have one or more of these common issues associated with stress, it's time for you to start working on your PEACE!

Top Eight Mental/Emotional Signs of Chronic Stress

1. *Depression*
2. *Anxiety*
3. *Anger*
4. *Low or no libido*
5. *Forgetfulness*
6. *Poor concentration*
7. *Addiction*
8. *Fluctuating Emotions*

[351-352]

If you have one or more of these mental/emotional issues going on, you're probably suffering from chronic levels of stress. Once you recognize that you're stressed out, you need to accept responsibility for it.

First, **YOU ARE NOT A VICTIM!** Feeling sorry for oneself has never gotten anyone anywhere. The victim mentality only leaves you stuck in the mud of self-pity. It's disempowering and a pervasive disease of the mind in our culture. Too many people want to play the blame game in their lives. Thus, they never accept responsibility for the stress in their lives. The tragedy is the stress only gets worse and ensuing health problems are the result.

To manage your peace, you must put yourself into the driver's seat of your life. You must quit blaming your stress/problems on things, people, and events outside of you. All issues we deal with in life have one thing in common, **our self**. Therefore, we must look to self as the primary cause of our stress. But when we are living in our own little box it can be awfully hard to see things differently. Essentially, it's hard to see outside the box when we have been living in it for such a long time!

A STORY ABOUT STRESS

As a chiropractor and business owner I have always dealt with a lot of stress. When I first opened my business, I would wake up early in the morning because I thought if I was going to be successful, I had to wake up super early. So, every morning I would get up at 4:00 am to make it to work by 4:45 am. Even on my days off I would get up at 4:00 am. As the months went by, I felt the sleep deprivation insidiously taking over my life. On top of the sleep deprivation, I was stressed over finances and I would often lay awake at night riddled with anxiety about how I was going to make ends meet for the month. Instead of being grateful and excited for what I did have and what I was going to achieve, I felt a huge sense of lacking in my life.

Unfortunately, as my stress grew my relationship suffered as a result. I began to have marital issues which perpetuated the stress. I found myself getting upset over the littlest of things, certainly a tell-tale-sign of stress. I became addicted to coffee; I used it to compensate for the adrenal fatigue I was beginning to feel. As the months went on physiological changes began to happen. I began to have heart palpitations, I started over-breathing, and I would wake in the morning with a dry mouth on most days.

I became hyper- cynical of everything. I certainly wasn't living my life in abundance. I certainly wasn't living "my best life ever." I can remember focusing on all the bad things. I focused on all the things that weren't working in my life. If a patient dropped out of care for whatever reason I would obsess over it, instead of focusing on the patients who were still undergoing care. The sad part was **I couldn't see my problems for what they were. I saw them worse than what they were.** I also couldn't see how stressed I had become. My entire self-worth was tied up in the success or failure of my practice, and I couldn't help but think about how much I sucked because things weren't going the way I wanted them to.

One day, sitting in my office alone, I began to cry. I cried out to God for His help and guidance. I was tired of the struggle and I needed to get out of my funk. Everything was crumbling around me, and I needed some help! That very day I reached out to a few of my chiropractic buddies from school who were knocking life out of the park. My friends helped to re-ground me and gave me the inspiration I needed to pull out of the fog I was in.

I immediately took righteous action! The first step was to shift my perceptions about my life. Instead of seeing my life as one big ball of lack I began to be grateful for all the good things in my life. After all, my heart was still beating, my lungs were still breathing, my mind was still working – I was still healthy. Along with my health, I still had my wife. I also had a family that had my back. I had a plethora of mentors and colleagues too who I could reach out to and get ideas from. Along with shifting my perceptions I began to see my problems for what they were, problems most business owners suffered from in the first years of business.

When I began to see my problems for what they were, instead of bigger than what they were, my anxiety levels went down. As a result, the creative juices started flowing again and I was able to come up with solutions to my struggles. I started to meditate for fifteen minutes every morning. During my workouts I stopped listening to music and started listening to self-help and informational audio that inspired me to be better and do better. I also quit drinking coffee and as a result started to experience more energy and mental clarity! How ironic since I had been drinking it for the energy! My relationship with my wife got better and eventually we became pregnant. I am blessed with a beautiful daughter who just turned one! Although I still get stressed over running a business, I don't wallow in it. Overall, I started managing my PEACE instead of just dealing with my stress. I now know what I need to do to effectively mitigate my stress and perpetuate my inner peace. You can do the same!

Peace management begins with shifting our beliefs about what's really going on in our lives. Our problems and our stress often perish in comparison to the stress that others may endure. Yet, for some reason we BLOW our stress up, we make it worse than what it is, and that makes it overwhelming. We say things like, "I'm broke," "I just suck," "my life sucks," "nobody will ever love me," "I will never get it right," etc. etc. And, we say all these things with *emotion*. Adding emotion to what we say is like pouring gasoline on a fire! Whatever your negative self-talk is, it isn't true. We make up a horror story in our minds about what's really going on. When we make our problems overwhelming, we end up stagnant and don't take the action needed. Our energy is low, and we attract more negative things into our life. Inevitably our stress gets worse.

How often have you said to yourself or heard other people say, "When it rains, it pours?" When we focus on our problems and the things that are stressing us out, we often get more of the same. And, let me clarify something here, it's not a bad thing to get pissed off about your circumstances. It's not a bad thing to experience depression because of where you are in life. It's when we stay stuck there and wallow that creates a problem. Sometimes, hitting rock bottom and your lowest of lows is the BEST possible place to be, because you can only move up from there. It's humbling, unless you choose to play the victim card.

BE THE HERO

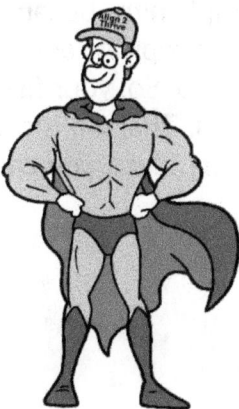

So, instead of playing the victim in the movie called, "Your Life," why not play the HERO?! All it takes is the choice to do so. That is the beginning of it. It's saying, "Enough is enough," or "I'm done with this shit," or "I'm not going to live this way anymore." You make the choice to live a better life. Once the decision is made, all it takes is action. Proactively, you focus on your peace and you take the appropriate action.

Two people can see the same accident and see it differently. This is called perception. Perception is the key to peace management. See everything as an opportunity to better your life. As the old adage goes, "You can see the glass as half empty or half full." You can even see the glass as being FULL, full of half water and half air. However, the way you choose to perceive your reality will influence the decisions you make about your future.

When it comes to stress, if we think about all the perceived bad in our lives, it will only make our stress levels worse. To quote Wayne Dyer, "When you change the way you look at things, the things you look at will change." Let me give you a practical example. If you "HATE" your job it will raise your stress levels, correct? Instead of hating your job, name five things you're grateful for about it. Because of your job, have you not acquired some beneficial knowledge? Have you not acquired some skills you can take with you and use for the rest of your life?

I hated working at Big O after my fourth year there, but I am grateful that I acquired some amazing skills, such as the art of the sale and a strong work ethic!

Here's another example. Say you're stressed about finances, is it beneficial to think about how shitty your financial situation is? Won't that add to your stress? When it comes to peace management, be grateful for what you have and then come up with action steps to get yourself out of the financial hole you're in. It makes sense, right? What if we stopped complaining, became grateful, shifted our perspective, and then took appropriate action steps? Wouldn't our lives be a lot better? I think so. So, your first step is to **shift your perspective and be grateful.** That's a more EMPOWERING STATE! *From a more empowering state, you can better do what needs to be done.*

PEACE HAS NOTHING TO DO WITH BEING HAPPY

Ask any young person what they want out of life and they will often tell you they just want to be happy. If you ask them to define what happiness is, they most likely will struggle to give you a meaningful definition. What is happiness? Is it a feeling of bliss? Can we just be blissed out twenty-four/seven? Absolutely not! Could you imagine if everybody was in a state of bliss twenty-four hours a day? Nothing would ever get done or accomplished. When I smoked marijuana, I was in a state of bliss and the only thing that was accomplished was me munching through a bag of potato chips! Life is not about being happy twenty-four/seven; it's not about being content at all times. The stress of life will happen; you will get angry, you will get sad, and you will experience anxiety from time to time. **LIFE DOES HAPPEN.** It's about KNOWING that no matter what happens in your life, it all happens for a reason! **But the secret is, believing it happens for a reason.**

Think about it, you can find **MEANING** in everything – if you choose to look for it. If you're depressed, rather than judging why you're depressed, take a step back and choose to be an observer. Think about *why* you're depressed, instead of thinking your depression sucks. Thinking about how much our life sucks gets us nowhere. **If we can focus on the WHY, we can find the SOLUTION!** The solution will always involve one potent ingredient, and that's **CHANGE!**

Change involves changing our perspective or shifting our actions. We can change the way we think about something. We can take massive action and change our life. We can work on changing our environment if we don't like it. Change always has to do with our why. We must figure out the why behind the emotion and fiercely work to change it. If you can't figure out why you're depressed, stressed, or riddled with anxiety, I suggest FOCUSING ON YOUR

HEALTH. Remember my quote: *"Focus on Your Health and All Else Will Follow."* Why? Because physical health dramatically effects your peace!

The second, but major, aspect to managing your peace involves your physical health. **The healthier you are, the better your thoughts become.** Eating a healthy diet, exercising regularly, and drinking more water has been proven to affect your psychology in a positive way. To reiterate, in Chapter 1 I said, "Your *physiology* dictates your *psychology*." Your overall health plays a significant role in your stress, especially your mental stress levels, as well as your **behavior**.

We know that caffeine, sugar, processed foods, and a sedentary lifestyle can trigger anxiety and effect our ability to respond well to our environment, but did you know that numerous studies have been done linking crime to diet? Researchers at Oxford University conducted a double-blind study on 231 violent young adult prisoners (age 19-21) and determined, conclusively, that nutrition played a significant role in behavior. The study showed that prisoners who were given nutritional supplements had 26% fewer offenses and 37% fewer violent offenses when compared to the placebo groups. The researchers summarized that good nutrition plays a critical role in human behavior and **could be a recipe for peace.** [353, 354]

The healthier you are, the better you will handle the stress in your life. Being an effective peace manager in your life involves proactively working on your health. When you are healthier, you can better adapt to both internal and external stress. Working out, for example, helps to balance your blood sugar levels which will help balance your energy levels. Working out also helps to increase your energy levels and decrease your stress levels because it balances hormones involved with stress, like cortisol. This happens while simultaneously boosting your testosterone levels, which is the hormone involved in MOTIVATION! When testosterone is good, you have a higher level of motivation. [355]

MEDITATE AND FEEL GREAT

A major action step you SHOULD take in managing your peace is to meditate every day. A lot of people misunderstand what meditation is. I used to think meditation was sitting for hours on end and humming like a monk in the Himalayan mountains. I was wrong! Meditation can be done in five minutes or less, although I would highly recommend meditating for a minimum of fifteen minutes every morning. The form of meditation I recommend is sitting, with good posture, in silence or with instrumental music playing through headphones or in the background.

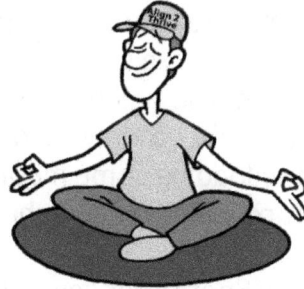

I always meditate while listening to instrumental meditation music set to the frequency of 432 Hz. This means that a meditation track has been tuned to this frequency.

Some of the greatest classical composers and musicians ever to exist tuned their instruments and based their music on the natural vibration of the note "A" tuned to 432 Hz. This frequency is said to resonate in harmony with the universe because it is thought to be mathematically consistent with nature. It is said that 432 Hz is connected to the construction of ancient works and sacred places, such as the pyramids of Egypt. Even the radius of the sun is 4,320 X 10, which equals 432,000. **Biblically, God spoke the universe and mankind into existence.** [356, 357]

There is an optimum range of vibration for every living and non-living thing on the planet. This is called resonance. When our bodies are in resonance, we are balanced. Every single tissue and organ in our body resonates at a certain frequency. This means every cell emits its own frequency or sound while also absorbing sound. This is how our cells communicate with each other. Unhealthy cells struggle to communicate and begin to "tune in" with harmful frequencies, like that of your cell phone (Chapter 5). [356]

When you meditate to 432 Hz it is thought to help balance both hemispheres of your brain. Scientists call this brain synchronization. This means both hemispheres work together in harmony, allowing for more creative thought. Unfortunately, most music has been tuned to the frequency of 440 Hz, which is thought to only resonate with the left side of your brain. Try downloading some meditation tracks set to 432 Hz and see if you notice a difference in how you feel. [356]

Note: Spotify has several meditation stations, where the music has been set to 432 Hz. Search Meditation 432.

The second biggest component to meditation is breathing. There are so many ways to breathe during meditation, as expressed by many meditation gurus. For the purposes of this chapter, I'm only going to discuss one way. In Patrick McKeown's book, *Oxygen Advantage*, he talks about utilizing an exercise he coined as, "Breathe Light to Breathe Right" during meditation. [350, Pg. 181] If you'd like to try this meditation technique, start with the instructions below.

Breathe Light to Breathe Right Meditation

(To be done 15 minutes daily)

- While sitting up straight or lying down, place one hand above the naval and one hand on your chest. Lightly compress your chest and abdomen.

- Focus on your breathing. In and out through your nose, making sure it stays nice and light. You should feel a tolerable need for air using this technique. This is contrary to what we have been taught about breathing. We have been taught to breathe deeply, in and out, trying to take in as much air as we can. While you might feel a head rush using this method, you're purposefully over-breathing and causing your body to absorb less oxygen.

- As you continue to lightly breathe in and out, you will experience a feeling of relaxation throughout your body. Feel your body release any bound-up tension.

- Think empowering thoughts *(my personal thing)*.

Along with your meditation, say positive affirmations to yourself. You can be in a state of gratitude and visualize all the wonderful things you have to be thankful for. Doing this in the morning is a tremendously powerful way to start your day! During my morning meditation I have a list of positive affirmations I say quietly to myself. I have said them so often and for so long, I have twenty-five of them I've completely memorized. Most of my affirmations consist of "I AM" statements that are said in the present tense.

Positive affirmations are the training of our subconscious mind using positive affirmation statements said out loud or silently. This is done with the intent of changing behavior and thought patterns and manifesting goals. Affirmations need to be personal, positive, semi-specific, and said in the present tense. [358]

AFFIRMATION EXAMPLES

(Feel free to use as a framework)

- I AM manifesting the life of my dreams.

- I AM a person to be admired. I AM a person to be followed because my actions are louder than my words. I exude confidence, I AM confident. I exude love and the fruits of the spirit because I AM!

- I AM so happy and grateful that money comes to me easily and effortlessly. I AM a magnet for success and prosperity.

- I AM directed by the infinite spirit within me, and I have faith in God's great and glorious plan for my life.

- I AM living my life in abundance. I have incredible health. Every single organ, cell, and tissue within my body is functioning at 100%, and I *AM* Thriving!

When saying these affirmations to yourself, it's important you believe what you are saying. Feeling inspired while you meditate is empowering. This means that your thoughts are beginning to create the feelings you would feel if you were to manifest the life of your dreams. Said differently, it's like you're beginning to feel the reality in which you wish to live! Good hormones are being released when you feel inspired and stress dissipates. Below I've included a helpful exercise you can use to reduce anxiety.

BREATH EXERCISE TO REDUCE ANXIETY

- Breathe in, breathe out.
- Hold breath for 2-5 seconds while pinching your nose.
- Breathe normally for 10-15 seconds.
- Hold breath for 2-5 seconds while pinching your nose
- Do this for 3-5 minutes total.

[350, Pg. 248]

GET OUTSIDE, GET SOME SUN!

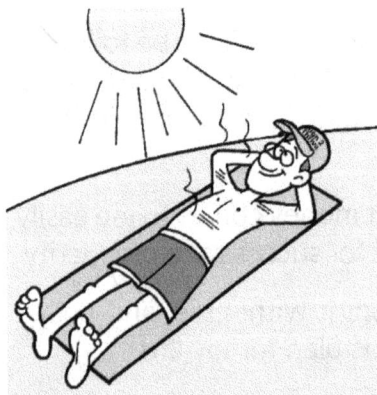

Getting out of your house and getting natural sunlight is vital. We tend to be cooped up inside buildings all day, whether it's our house or the place in which we work. We are bombarded by lighting that isn't natural. The main reason unnatural lighting is unhealthy is because it doesn't contain the full spectrum range of visible and non-visible light that natural sunlight contains.

Sunlight is powerful and it's energizing. In fact, natural light can boost energy production by stimulating the mitochondria to create ATP. This means that any cell that ramps up ATP production will be able to perform better. For example, liver cells will better be able to perform their job of detoxification. [359]

Sunlight exposure also helps us sleep better! Better sleep means less stress and more peace in your life. I spoke a great deal about how sunlight can help you sleep better in Chapter 10. To reiterate, the reason you need your daily dose of sunlight is because there are light receptors in your eyes that when exposed to sunlight cause the center of your brain to produce more serotonin, the precursor of melatonin. Unfortunately, most of us are stuck inside a building for most of the day and are exposed to long hours of fluorescent and LED lighting which is both harmful and energy zapping!

It has been proven that LED lighting can be very harmful to your eyes because of the excess blue light. The blue light causes increased oxidative stress and has been linked to accelerated macular degeneration and blindness. [359]

I recommend downloading a blue light blocker app for your phone if your phone doesn't already have one built in. There are also programs you can download onto your computers. This is critical if you find yourself using your devices for hours every day, like I do. You can also get special blue light blocking glasses that work well.

Vitamin D is the sunshine vitamin and has many amazing health benefits. One benefit is it helps the immune system work properly, which reduces the risk of autoimmune diseases which seem to be so rampant these days! Vitamin D is a hormone your body makes from cholesterol when you expose your bare skin to the sun's ultraviolet rays. It is recommended that a fair skinned person get between five and thirty minutes of natural sunlight exposure to their unprotected arms, legs, neck, back, etc. for a minimum of three to four days per week between the hours of 10:00 am and 3:00 pm. For a darker skinned person, it's going to take longer to create the same effects. A healthy body will produce between 10,000 International Units (IUs) to 20,000 IUs in thirty minutes! [360]

One of the main reasons sunlight boosts your feelings of well-being is because of the increase in serotonin. Along with being the precursor to melatonin, serotonin plays a significant role in well-being and happiness.

Sadly, one in six Americans take a psychiatric medication, most of which are anti-depressants. Of those, SSRIs, like Prozac and Zoloft, are among the most prescribed medications. These medications come with some severe side-effects, including the surprising risk of suicide, hostility, and agitation in children, teens, and young adults. In 2004 these side effects prompted the FDA to put a black box warning on all SSRI drugs. This is the strongest warning a drug or product can receive. [361, 362]

What is even more surprising when it comes to antidepressants is that most mass shootings seem to have a connection to anti-psychotic medications. "Since the increase in SSRI antidepressants being prescribed, the rise in mass shootings has increased right along with it. Evidence shows that many mass shooters were either taking or had recently taken SSRIs." [363]

The Columbine mass shooting is probably the most well-known, in which twelve students and a teacher were killed, and twenty-six others were wounded at the hands of two teenaged boys (Eric Harris, Dylan Kiebold). Both boys were taking antidepressants. [364, 365]

It's important to make sure you and your kids are getting plenty of sunlight and "good-ole" outdoors. Limit the amount of time you and your kids spend indoors. GET OUTSIDE, go for a hike, smell the fresh air! It's good for the soul. For an added bonus, take off your shoes and feel the earth beneath your feet. This helps to ground you to the earth. For more information on grounding, see Chapter 10.

LIFE IS A BEACH!

Have you noticed that being around the ocean energizes you? Have you ever thought about why that is? There is a lot of science behind why this happens. The ocean taps into all your senses! First, you're outside, so you've got the sun beaming down on you. Second, just putting your feet in the sand elicits a feeling of relaxation. The hit *Third Eye Blind* song, "Semi-Charmed Life," written by Stephen Jenkins, describes this sensation well.

> *"I believe in the sand beneath my toes.*
> *The beach gives a feeling,*
> *an earthy feeling."* [366]

This earthy feeling you feel when you take off your shoes, that feeling of relaxation, it has a lot to do with grounding and the energizing effect it has on your body. Third, staring at the ocean can bring a feeling of peace and calmness. This is primarily due to the blue color of the ocean. The color changes our brain waves and puts us into a meditative state. [367] Blue is also an inspiring color. This is why I chose it as one of the primary colors for my office.

According to "Color Wheel Pro," an online website where you can create color schemes and preview them on real world examples, the meaning of the color blue is:

"Blue is the color of the sky and sea. It is often associated with depth and stability. It symbolizes trust, loyalty, wisdom, confidence, intelligence, faith, truth, and heaven.

Blue is considered beneficial to the mind and body. It slows human metabolism and produces a calming effect. Blue is strongly associated with tranquility and calmness. In heraldry, blue is used to symbolize piety and sincerity." [368]

The sound of the waves calmly crashing on the beach while breathing in the fresh ocean air can also make you feel more alive! In fact, when the waves crash against the sand, "it stretches the water surface area, reducing the water's surface tension. Because the surface tension of the water is lessened, the water now easily absorbs oxygen from the air." This same thing happens when a waterfall crashes over the rocks. [369, Pg. 35]

The next time you are at the beach, pay attention to people's energy around you. Notice the children playing by the water's edge, watch the adults throwing a football or frisbee. You'll notice that everybody is happy and energized! Surfers get what is known as a surfer's high. The ocean is a great healer. Get out of your house more often, go outside, and find a beach.

PEACE BY GOD

The peace of God surpasses ALL understanding! In a world gone mad it is good to have a sense of peace, to know that no matter what happens, it's all going to be *good*. As a Christian, I'm taken aback by the Bible verse below.

"And the peace of God, which surpasses all understanding will guard your hearts and your minds in Christ Jesus."

(ESV, Philippians 4:7)

Often, we get so stressed with what is going on in our personal lives and with what is going on in the world, it's hard to find our sense of peace in it all. When we are worried about politics, finances, relationships, work-life balance, our kids, crises, our jobs, businesses or whatever else is going on in our lives and the world at large, we feel stuck. This is where having a peace beyond worldly understanding is needed.

As humans we are geared toward thinking worse-case scenarios. We constantly think of the worst possible outcomes, only to later realize it didn't turn out as bad as we thought it would. And, at the very least, we have the choice to **decide** to be peaceful even in the midst of chaos. We *choose* to get stressed out, frustrated, aggravated, and angry. I do it too.

I still find myself getting caught up in all those emotions when nothing seems to be going right around me. But later, when the dust settles, I realize it was all a blessing in disguise. What I mean by this is that it was all for a greater purpose because it helped me in some way shape or form. Often, we get caught up in our perception of things going on around us and we can't see the light at the end of the tunnel. We can't see the bigger picture.

> *"Peace I leave with you; my peace I give you. I do not give to you as the world gives. Do not let your hearts be troubled, do not be afraid."*
>
> (NIV, John 14:27)

See, God's got your back. God knows where the puck is going and because He does, we can be confident in the future outcome. Is it necessarily a bad thing to get stressed out in the moment, to worry, to get depressed, to have anxiety, etc.? No, I don't think it is. It's only when we choose to get stuck there that it becomes a problem. In other words, if we choose to prolong the emotion and make the choice to suffer, it becomes problematic.

Jesus was fully human and fully God. Therefore, He experienced the same emotions and stressors that we do. He experienced struggles, sorrow, heartaches, anger, worry, pain, joy, bliss, happiness, and other emotions that we experience. But Jesus didn't dwell in those emotions. He didn't let these things take him off course and away from his mission work.

Jesus, knowing He was to be persecuted and eventually crucified, was greatly troubled. In Luke 22:44 it states that Jesus was anguished.

> *"And being in anguish, he prayed more earnestly; and His sweat became like great drops of blood falling down to the ground."*

> (NIV, Luke 22:44)

Jesus didn't let his distress dictate his actions. With faith, he let what was to come, come. In Luke 22:42 Jesus kneels in prayer and prays.

> *"Father, if you be willing, remove this cup from me: nevertheless, not my will, but yours, be done."*

> (NIV, Luke 22:42)

How many times do you let your distress control the decision making in your life? Do you make empowering decisions when you're in a weakened state or disempowering decisions? We can't let fear or any other negative stressor dictate our lives. We must continue onward in life by making responsible and rational decisions from a place of empowerment, **NOT from a place of FEAR.**

Therefore, I choose to have faith that all things are going to work out exactly as intended. And, if things aren't working out as intended, I choose to believe that it's not the end of the world. From this positive mental place, I can make responsible decisions on how to move forward. All you have to do is change the way you look at things, take positive right action and ultimately have faith that it is all going to work out for the best! **BECAUSE IT WILL!**

We can also look to others for inspiration. Everybody has an inspiring story to tell!

Nick Vujicic is a Christian evangelist and motivational speaker; however, Nick's life has not been without anguish, suffering, stress, anger, and depression. You see, Nick was born without arms or legs due to tetra-amelia syndrome. He has a foot where one of his legs should be. Doctors told his parents he would be a vegetable. However, through shear willpower and tenacity, Nick learned how to do most everything using his toes, including operating and using his electric wheelchair and computer! In the motivational videos I have watched about Nick, he often shows the audience how he can get up from a fall and into an upright position. This is miraculous considering he has to use his head for leverage. [370]

Instead of sending him to a school for the disabled, Nick's parents sent him to a regular public school where he was continually bullied and picked on for looking so different. His parents encouraged him, telling him that he was beautiful just the way he was. Regardless, however, and understandably so, he became extremely depressed and hopeless. He thought about his future and what kind of life he was going to have with his disability. He thought about things like, "What girl is ever going to want to marry me?" "How am I going to hold her hand?" "If I have a child, how can I hold him?" This feeling of utter hopelessness and resentment for getting the short end of the stick led to Nick attempting suicide multiple times. What eventually stopped Nick from trying kill himself was the thought of what his parents would have to go through if he were to succeed in ending his life. He would often cry out to God, "Why did you make me this way?" [370]

"I don't need hands to hold [my wife's] hand, I only want to hold her heart. And, how am I going to hug my kids? So many kids come up to me, and it's amazing, they put their hands behind their back and hug me with their neck. And I have realized in life that even the worst parts in my life can be turned into good." Nick Vujicic [371]

Nick came to Jesus at the age of fifteen, after reading about how He cured a blind man to show the wonderful works of God. Nick thought, "If God had a plan for the blind man, He certainly has a plan for me." [30] When he was seventeen a janitor at his high school told him he would become a motivational speaker. That is exactly what he became, and so much more. Nick said in an interview,

"I was speaking in front of 300 sophomore public high school students and three minutes in half the girls were crying. One girl in the middle of the room started weeping, she put up a hand and she said, 'I'm so sorry to interrupt, but can I come up there and give you a hug in front of everyone?' She came up, she hugged me, she laid her head on my shoulder, and she whispered in my ear, 'No one has ever told me that they love me, no one has ever told me that I'm beautiful just the way I am.' I couldn't believe it; it changed my life. That's when I knew I was called to be a worldwide evangelist." [372]

Today Nick has a phenomenally successful non-profit organization, "Life Without Limbs." He has spoken around the world to millions and has inspired tens of thousands of people to come to Christ. He has also led successful anti-bullying campaigns. He has multiple best-selling books. He is married to his beautiful wife and they have four children.

Would you say that Nick has a peace that surpasses all understanding? I would. **This is the kind of peace we can have if we just decide it to be so.** We can find the good in the perceived bad. We can choose to find our peace when life isn't going our way. And, if you believe in the same God I do, then you know He is right there. You know He has your back in all of it. Have faith that as bad as life can get, that it is **ALL** for the best. Even though it may not seem that way in the midst of it – it's all for the best. There is a saying worth concluding with and that is, *"Let go and let God."*

You can't control it all, the stress will come. Adversity is going to be a part of your life – it's a part of everyone's life. Sometimes the best thing we can do is let "Jesus take the wheel," as said by Carrie Underwood.

YOU ARE NOT AN ISLAND

The last thing I want to touch upon in this chapter is something I need to scream through these pages! I have preached this one to myself many times before! We MUST begin to learn that we aren't islands! Too many times we isolate ourselves for the sake of not burdening others. This is a problem and here's why.

We are relational "BE-ings." We are designed by our *designer* to have relationships. Humans have all kinds of different relationships. We have relationships with our spouses, families, friends, kids, co-workers, neighbors, pastors, mentors, customers, clients, patients, etc. Whatever the case may be, we are supposed to interact, have conversations with, give and receive from others, and most importantly, we are to *love* other people! However, there is a weird thing that humans do. **WE ISOLATE OURSELVES WHEN THE GOING GETS TOUGH!** We act as if everything is going A-OKAY, even if it might not be. We don't reach out and ask for help. Help could mean somebody to vent to. Help could mean somebody to lean on and get advice from. An effective thing to do when it comes to managing your peace is to vent your frustrations to someone who can listen (like a good friend or your spouse) and offer you sound advice. Instead of trying to figure things out on your own, sometimes it's best to seek the advice of others because they have a different perspective than you do. This can help guide you in the right direction. I learned in life that I don't have all the answers – especially if I'm stressed out!

Unfortunately, I had to learn this the hard way. I have let myself reach the breaking point before I sought advice from my wife, friends, colleagues, pastor, and even God. Instead of taking that first step back, I wanted to try and come up with a quick fix. Pause, and ask others for their advice and help. That's what taking the first step back is all about. We become reactionary instead of responsive. Most of the time this leads to further chaos.

So, **YOU ARE NOT AN ISLAND!** Your problems aren't left entirely up to you to resolve. God tells us to call out to Him in our times of darkness. Let God Inspire you in the right direction.

"Cast your burden upon the Lord, and He will sustain you; He will never allow the righteous to be shaken."

(NASB, Psalms: 55:22)

Being around good people makes you a better person. Being in a community of likeminded individuals helps to make you healthier overall. One of the key factors of longevity is having a sense of community and a sense of belonging. People who live their lives in isolation don't fare the same health wise. When it comes to mental, physical, and spiritual health – you are better off when you belong to a group.

Take the Hunza Tribe, mentioned in Chapter 1 of this book. One of the KEY factors that makes the tribe healthier than the average American is their sense of community. Their community shares the same values, morals, ethics, and social responsibility. In fact, they teach their kids to do what is good for all. The tell-tale sign of this is that there is virtually zero crime! [373]

Studies also show that people who participate in a religion live longer, which, hypothetically could be partially due to the community aspects of belonging to a church or religious group. [374] A stronger word for community, would be connectedness. We need to feel connected to one another. Part of the reason we feel so isolated from each other is that there is, arguably, a strong sense of disconnect in the world. This, despite billions of people that are connected via the internet. We have access to billions of people, and yet we still feel disconnected culturally. I think it's because we aren't socially interacting with people in an authentic way.

According to Dr. Lisa Dunne, author of the book *Multigenerational Marketplace*, Generation Z's spend 64% of their social time with friends online, which has a dramatic impact on their face to face communication skills. More time on social media also has a direct correlation to adolescent depression. [375] For further information you can check out her website at https://www. drlisadunne.com where you can purchase a copy of her book as well.

You could be anybody you want to be on the internet. So, rather than getting the true version of people, we mostly get a highly edited version. When on social media we get the feeling that everyone is doing phenomenal, but it's mostly fake. This, in and of itself, brings about depression and anxiety, especially when we become envious. We need true interaction. More face to face conversations! You know old school style!

One of my favorite shows of all time is the *Andy Griffith Show*. The show took place in the fictional small town of Mayberry where everyone knew everybody. It depicted a community bonded by their morals and values. One of the things that made this show so popular was its portrayal of community and American values.

The show ran from 1960 to the end of the 1967-1968 season. To this day it has NEVER been taken off the air. Don Rodney Vaughan in his article titled "Why the Andy Griffith Show is Important to Popular Cultural Studies," states,

> "The serenity of Mayberry was seemingly uninfluenced by hard news. In this respect, Mayberry is like the eye of the hurricane, a

place of tranquility in a world of anything but that. Mayberry's problems and stressors were anything but the problems and stressors that most faced in the 1960s: unemployment, overcoming obstacles to voter registration, the quest for civil rights as Americans, sons fighting in a no-cause war [Vietnam], the uneasiness over the risk of nuclear war—the list could go on." [376]

It still surprises me how much this show was able to shine at a time in our history when there was so much stress and turmoil. Maybe the show was so popular because deep down we all longed to be part of a community like that. We want to know our neighbors, we want to share the same values, we all want to live in a world that does what's morally right.

We can all start by getting to know our neighbors. All you need to do is walk next door, knock on your neighbor's door, and begin with an introduction. How is it that we can live next to people our entire lives and never get to know them?

When we moved into our first rental, we introduced ourselves to our neighbors and have been friends with them (and all their friends) ever since – and we are talking years. We watch each other's dogs when we go out of town, take each other's trash to the street on trash day, we talk and have conversations! And again, it all started with a friendly introduction.

As you can see, with a little focus you can manage the peace in your life. Rather than focusing on all the stress in your life, you can be the eye in your hurricane. You can have a strong sense of peace in the middle of your storm. I do VERY MUCH believe that **WITH God anything is possible.** What gives you a peace beyond all understanding is KNOWING that God has your back!

"I can do all things through Christ, who give me Strength."

(NIV, Philippians, 4:13)

A large part of managing peace has to do with managing your mind and changing your thoughts and beliefs. Remember the principles laid out within this chapter. They will help you mentally shift your perspective, which is going to be THE biggest component to managing your peace.

If you were to apply the principals laid out in this chapter and shift your thought process from managing your stress to managing your peace – **YOU WOULD ACHIEVE MORE PEACE IN YOUR LIFE!** You will get better at not wallowing in your problems and your stress. You will BE able to focus on the solutions and be in a state of gratitude versus lack. From a place of peace, you can better serve the purpose for which you were designed.

Next, I will tie all these chapters together and help you bring more attention and consciousness to your purpose. I want to help you cultivate your BIG WHY. What is the point of being healthy? In other words, what is the purpose of doing all of this, what is the point of life without a purpose?

"The Purpose of life is a life of Purpose."

-Robert Bryne

CHAPTER 13

DESIGNED TO THRIVE

"We were all created on purpose for an incredible purpose."

- Dr. Jay

Do we have a designer? Were we indeed "Designed to Thrive?" For some, this question is perplexing. For me, it's quite simple. Every day I am given evidence there is a God. I just know what to look for. And when you know what to look for you begin to realize that the TRUTH is undeniable. This belief has dramatically affected the course of my life and how I live. This is the premise I have based this entire book on, that *we were designed, and that we were designed to thrive!*

I don't believe you and I came about by random chance. The odds of either one of us being born at this current time, right now, are virtually impossible, yet here we are. **In fact, statisticians estimate that the odds of you and I being born are 1 in 400 TRILLION or more!** So, did we just get lucky? Or, were we put here for a reason, a purpose? In fact, I bet you're wondering about the purpose of this chapter.

I'm going to give it to you straight, the purpose of this chapter is to CONVINCE you that **there is a higher calling in your life.** If we were indeed designed to thrive, then certainly we are here for something other than just to be born, live, and then die.

That part between birth and death we call living means something, don't you think? Or, is it all for naught? Look at some of the famous composers like Mozart, Beethoven, Brahms, Bach, and Vivaldi. They clearly had a purpose that was up to them to fulfill. Imagine if Mozart stopped playing or if Beethoven gave up after he couldn't hear anymore. The world would be a much different place without their incredible music to listen to.

"Our greatest fear should be dying with our music still within us."

Wayne Dyer

WHAT IS PURPOSE?

Having a purpose is the most critical component when it comes to living the life of your dreams. The online Oxford Dictionary defines purpose as "the reason for which something is done, or created, or for which something exists." [377] Think about it, without purpose nothing happens, nothing is created, life becomes mundane. Lack of purpose leads to sickness, it is death to the human spirit! There are two core beliefs I hold when it comes to purpose.

1: *WE WERE ALL CREATED ON PURPOSE FOR AN INCREDIBLE PURPOSE*

This means that we are here for a reason that is greater than ourselves. We are here to live our lives to their fullest capacity – soaking up every ounce of opportunity, fulfilling dreams that God has placed in our hearts. We are to be healthy, vibrant, and optimally functional. Why? Because the world needs to experience the best version of ourselves! Tony Robbins says, *"Life deserves for more of you to show up."* [378]

2: *WE MUST DISCOVER OUR PURPOSE*

Having a purpose INSPIRES us to act and make decisions. The sum of our life is made up of a collection of outcomes that were created by various actions. These outcomes define our life. Knowing your purpose leads to purposeful action and better outcomes. Conversely, not living out your purpose can lead to a very dismal and depressing life because the actions you take are misdirected – they aren't purposeful. Often a person will sabotage themself due to a complete lack of purpose.

When you wake up each day without a purpose, it leads to sedentary behavior and spiritual death. When I was struggling with alcohol and drug addiction, as well as seeking miserable relationships that didn't serve me, it was because I had no real purpose in my life. I was depressed and the only way I could numb out the pain of living a life without purpose was to sabotage myself with alcohol and drugs. I had no clue who I was and the potential I had within myself.

As I write these sentences, I think of the homeless person who lost their way. How can a person let themselves get so far off track? How can a person merely survive when they have a life worth living? Why?! Because they lack a strong sense of purpose that inspires them to do something better with their lives.

I acknowledge the fact that there are events and circumstances in life that throw us off track and can work to hold us down, but only if we let them. So, the question becomes: *How long will it take before we realize that our past does not dictate our future and that we have the power to change our current circumstances?*

How did Chris Gardner go from being broke and homeless, sleeping in subway restrooms with his infant son to a multi-million-dollar stockbroker? This was a guy who endured physical and verbal abuse from his alcoholic stepfather when he was a boy. At one point in his boyhood he was raped by a gang member. He endured all these things and clearly had several valid excuses for being homeless. He could have felt sorry for himself for the rest of his life, but instead he didn't let his past dictate his life. He had a profound desire to make something of his life for his son. He used the adversity to empower himself. He wasn't going to let anyone, or anything hold him back from achieving his purpose. If you haven't already seen it, I recommend watching the movie *Pursuit of Happiness*, starring Will Smith for inspiration about what it means to live a life on purpose.

How do we go about discovering our purpose? Trying to figure out what your purpose is can be one of the most challenging endeavors you will ever face. Discovering your purpose in life can take time, but it will change the course of your life forever. To be clear, when I talk about purpose, I'm talking about the reason why you do what you do? What do you want to do in life that makes an impact, and what are the reasons you want to do it? Once you've answered these questions you can start living your life on purpose. And when you live your life on purpose, nothing can stop you!

I became a chiropractor at the age of twenty-six because I realized my purpose in life was to inspire people to live healthier lives. When people live healthier lives, I believe they think better thoughts. I believe that your physiology, in a large part, dictates your psychology, which I discussed heavily in the first section of this book.

This world could be a much better place to live if everybody was healthier. I saw chiropractic care as the missing link to help people achieve optimum health!

I would have never gotten to where I am today if I hadn't discovered my purpose many years ago. I'm thankful that I didn't settle for a job that was outside my *soul-purpose*. I didn't give in to fear. It takes guts to follow your purpose. It takes courage!

Finding Your Purpose

I want you to think about why you do what you do? Do you feel like you're living out your soul purpose? Do you feel like you are living the life of your dreams? If yes, how can you do what you do even better than you're doing it now? How can you home in on your purpose and improve upon it?

If no, here is your action step: write down all the things you love to do, write down all your ambitions in life, write down all of your talents, your life goals. Do you want to travel? Do you want to spend more quality time with your family? Do you want to help people? In what capacity do you want to help them? Do you want to pursue athletic endeavors? Write it down!

Most people don't know why they do what they do. They get the job to pay the bills and as the years go on, they get depressed because their purpose is to make ends meet. They aren't going to work with a profound sense of purpose in mind. We were created for so much more. Sadly, most will never discover their true purpose in life. All it takes is intention and action, and you can discover your purpose. It takes a conscious effort to know what it is you want.

With a little focus you can figure out what it is you really want out of your life. We can have success in every area and aspect of our lives, but we must KNOW WHO we are! Your purpose must fit and be congruent with who you are! As you work to figure out your purpose, know change is going to happen. Out of change, you grow! The growth is part of the game! From this growing that happens you discover more about who you are! When growth happens, adversity happens, challenges arise, and resistance happens. If change were easy no one would ever fall back into old habits and ways. But, the only path to growth is through some level of adversity. So, you must know that it's going to get tough.

Spiritual growth happens along your journey towards purpose. However, if you're not living out your purpose there are some tell-tale signs. Spiritual strife happens when you live your life void of purpose.

Living a life without purpose causes you to feel lost. If you feel lost, know that you're not alone. Many people feel lost in life. If you don't know the direction you're supposed to be heading and you feel stuck and hopeless, this is a sure sign you're not living your life on purpose. As mentioned above, a lot of people move endlessly through life, like mindless drones. They end up working a job for most of their lives that they don't love because they need to pay their bills. Let me ask you something, is the purpose of your life to work a job you hate so you can just get by and make ends meet? Certainly, we were designed for something better. What about those who end up on welfare for decades and never do anything with their lives? I have never met a happy person, fulfilling their God-given purpose, who was living off welfare.

And, hear me out, I'm not saying that people living on the system are inherently bad. I'm saying they must feel stuck. Lost in a sea of television watching, possible drug abuse, and a lack-luster life. With all that time, why not spend hours every day learning a craft? Why not learn a foreign language to make oneself more valuable in the workforce? When you don't know your purpose, you get lazy and look for things that keep you sedated and distracted. Whether, its alcohol, television, drugs, junk food, or getting involved in other people's drama – it's all a distraction to keep us from feeling the consequences of living a shitty-life. I know because I have been there.

Living a life without purpose leaves you sad and bored most of the time. Complacency in life is death to the human spirit. One of the worst feelings in life is complacency. Just being okay means, you're not growing. Water that remains stagnant and doesn't move becomes a cesspool. In a sense this is what happens to us as human beings. If we don't strive towards better versions of ourselves, we rot. I'm not saying don't feel grateful for everything that is in your life. You can stop and smell the roses and be satisfied with all your achievements and accomplishments, but don't let yourself get so okay with everything that you stop growing as a person.

Garret J. White, creator of Wake-up Warrior, states that the purpose of life is to EXPAND. I love this concept! We should never stop expanding in life. Within this concept he talks about The CORE 4. The CORE 4 stands for Body, Being, Balance, and Business. Just to briefly explain The CORE 4:

- **BODY:** This is about your physical health. You should always want to expand on your health. If you have read through the middle section of this book, you are given the tools you need to live out a life of robust health. Therefore, never stop growing in this area of your life. Don't just do the same old workouts forever, mix it up – try something new! Remove the interference and add good things into your life.

- **BEING:** This is about your spiritual connection with God. Are you doing things regularly to expand your relationship with your higher power? How about prayer? How about reading a spiritual book to expand your thinking about your creator? Why not read the Bible?

- **BALANCE:** This is about your relationship with your family and your spouse. How often are you putting focus and energy into being the best husband or wife you can be? Are you spending more quality time with your family? I see too many parents handing their kids their smart phones to watch YouTube videos. The electronic devices have become the primary influencers for kids. To me, being a dad and an awesome husband are two of the most important roles I need to do REALLY, REALLY, WELL! I'm not letting my kid be raised by electronics and I don't want my wife to feel like my number one priority is my business. Does this make sense? Why wouldn't you want to be the absolute BEST in these categories?

- **BUSINESS:** If you have your own business, you know as I do, that you can't get complacent with your business. You know that you need to always hustle. A lot of people call this hustle the grind. If you get complacent in business, it is likely that your business will die. Look at what happened to Blockbuster, they didn't expand, they got complacent, and they went out of business. They were taken out by younger companies who were able to see the changes in the marketplace and come up with an effective strategy. [379]

If you don't own your own business, then you should start considering how you can work your way to the top of the company you work for. If reaching the top isn't possible because of corporate bureaucracy, you should consider ways you could make extra money outside your job. Of course, these extra ways should fit within the confines of something you're passionate about and want to expand on. What is a skill set you have that you want to expand on? Let's say you love playing the piano, could you teach piano? Could you create a YouTube channel and gain lots of subscribers by giving people the gift of being inspired by your music? What if you volunteered to play piano at a retirement home? There isn't a lot of money to be made in volunteering of course, but you cannot out-give what you gain in the process of doing so. I know because I have done it before.

Tony Robbins says that one of the Six Human Needs is Contribution. We must give something of value back. More on this in a minute. [380]

If you focus on expanding all these areas in your life you will never feel complacent and you will never get bored.

Living a life without purpose leads to selfishness. One of the number one tell-tale signs that you're not living a life on purpose is that you only think about yourself. It's this attitude of it's all about me that is pervasive in our culture right now. The "me" attitude will not serve humanity in a big way. Your purpose will always involve other people. God created us to be relational human beings. We are meant to live together in peace and harmony. We are meant to serve each other. This is why one of the chief commandments written in the Bible is, "To Love thy neighbor as ourselves." We are to love our neighbors as well as we love ourselves.

In direct contrast to being selfish, when you are living out your soul-purpose it will have a positive impact on others. Let's say you own your own business. In order to make money you are going to have to help others. Zig Ziglar states,

> **"You can get everything in life you want if you will just help enough other people get what they want."** [381]

In other words, you are selling value FIRST. You must provide a quality product that is genuinely going to help people. As a chiropractor I help people to live the life they were designed to live by helping their body to heal. What's even more important is I work relentlessly to inspire them to shift their paradigms, so they change their lives. My goal is to help them see the potential within themselves.

It's amazing how living out our purpose can make us more selfless. Once we realize the potential within ourselves, it is natural for us to want to express more love to others.

GRATITUDE

Do you live in a state of gratitude? Do you express gratitude? Do you stop and notice all the wonderful things that surround you every day, or are you oblivious to all the beauty that is in your life? When you're living a life on purpose you appreciate all the beauty that is in your life. You appreciate your family, your spouse, your kids, and yes, even your relatives. A life on purpose means that you always find the good in your life every day.

I like to ask people, "What is good today?" I'm always surprised that some people immediately go to the negative or they will say nothing is good. This is certainly not true! There is always beauty to be seen and good to be noticed. For starters, you woke up today! That's an amazing thing in and of itself! A lot of people didn't wake up today.

As I'm writing these words right now I'm listening to some beautiful piano music. I appreciate that my ears can hear and that my heart feels a deep sense of AWE for all the beauty in my life.

Don't ever stop appreciating all that LIFE has to offer. Make sure you are experiencing regular moments of awe in your life. You have numerous moments in your life that you can sit and ponder on and experience a sense of awe. I often will put my headphones in and listen to the instrumental music that was playing during my daughter's birth. I close my eyes, and like a movie I can vividly remember the wonderful, awe-inspiring moments of my child's birth. I remember the first time I held her in my arms and when I looked into her eyes. In fact, as I write these words my eyes are full of tears. Thinking back to this most incredible experience always puts me into a state of awe.

Another word for awe, is bliss. What "blisses" you out? What are the moments that have already transpired in your life that put you into a state of gratitude? I remember when I looked at my wife for the first time in her wedding dress, I remember our first dance, I remember my pastor praying with all us grooms' men before the ceremony. See, there are many moments in your life to be thankful for, but we tend to forget because our lives get stressful.

I think we forget what living means. I think we forget how fast time flies and we lose track of what's important. Feeling a state of gratitude means that you are in line with God's purpose for your life. If you're constantly worried, in doubt, confused, anxiety ridden, and depressed – you're not in-line with His purpose for your life.

CHECK YOURSELF BEFORE YOU WRECK YOURSELF

STOP!!! If you find yourself always complaining and never in a state of gratitude – STOP! Find a minimum of one thing to be thankful for every single day. This one thing will change your life!

Below is a poem recited by Robbin Williams at the beginning of the movie Patch Adams. It is something I have found meaningful and wanted to share with you.

"All of life is a coming home. Salesmen, secretaries, coal miners, beekeepers, sword swallowers, all of us. All the restless hearts of the world, all trying to find a way home." [382]

Your purpose is all about finding your *center*. You will find your home right there in the middle; it's who you are. I believe that it's who you were born to be. The Bible says, God has known our purpose even before we were born. He knows the number of hairs on your head and he knows your divine purpose.

"For you created my inmost being you knit me together in my mother's womb. I praise you because I am fearfully and wonderfully made; your works are wonderful; I know that full well." [383]

Wherever you are in your life right now is due to the choices you have made up to this point. The perceptions you have regarding your life right now are also your own choices. Are you lost in life because you lack purpose? Do you lack purpose because you have not a clue? You have the power to change anything about your life. If you feel like your life is shit right now, if you feel stuck, if you feel cheated, if you absolutely KNOW you're not where you want to be – you have the power to change that.

Gone are the days you will find excuse after excuse, because there isn't anybody to blame but yourself for where you are. I'm not negating the fact that shit happens. I know this, but we have the power to change what we perceive about the shit that happens to us, don't we?! Remember, change doesn't happen without challenge, it's not easy – so we just GOTTA DO IT!

If you don't know how to define your purpose, you need to figure it out. You need to push on in your life and discover it. Once discovered, you need to cultivate your purpose. Through the challenge of cultivating it you will grow, and you will know more about yourself than you ever thought was possible.

My life has certainly not been an easy one. I have gotten where I am today through much trial and error, failure, and adversity.

With that being said, I understand that there are people who have gone through much more adversity than I have ever faced. Regardless of how much adversity a person faces, it is relative. The biggest factor that played a role in my life is when my Dad decided to leave my mom. I was nine years old.

I can still remember very vividly the day my dad came into my room and told me he was leaving my mom. I was sitting on my bedroom floor playing with Legos. The Legos laid scattered across the carpet. I can remember feeling content in what I was doing in that moment. Then I saw my dad walking down the hallway, a somber look on his face. My dad was a giant of a man standing at about 6'2." He had stark black hair, chiseled facial features, and a ton of muscle. Being a police officer, he kept himself in good shape. My dad was my hero growing up. He could do no wrong.

I was devastated, to say the least, when he touched my shoulder and said, "Jay," followed by a long pause, "there is something I need to discuss with you." Another long pause, "me and your mom are breaking up." Immediately my heart began to beat rapidly in my chest, tears streamed down my face. I remember thinking I did something wrong. "But why!" I blurted out. "It just isn't working," he said rather reluctantly. In an instant everything I thought I knew about my dad, everything I adored about my dad, all the admiration I had for him was crushed. "I'm sorry son, I love you," he said, sadly. "But why?" I blurted out again with frustration in my voice. I can remember having a feeling of wanting to save things. "It's not your fault Jason, I want you to know that it has nothing to do with you or your brother." He hugged me once more, said that he loved me, and then turned and walked away. I sat there balling my eyes out as I watched my dad walk away, the silhouette of his back seen through a sea of tears.

Fast forward ahead from that point and I would go on to struggle with alcohol and drug addiction, behavioral issues, suicidal ideation, a codependency on relationships with girls, and ultimately, a complete lack of knowing who God designed me to be. Much of my youth lacked purpose. I was plagued by self-esteem issues; I had no confidence in myself. I was consumed by the FEAR of what other people thought about me. Needless to say, I was miserable.

What I didn't realize at the time is that I had the power to change my life. I had a purpose!

It took me hitting rock-bottom at the age of seventeen to finally make a shift in my life. I got so drunk one night while hanging out with my cousin and friends at a run down, musty, cat-urine-smelling apartment, that I ended up vomiting all over myself. That night is a hazy nightmare. I can vividly remember the quality of the people I was hanging out with and how instead of helping me in my drunk state, they laughed at me and took pictures. I was humiliated and felt completely dejected. All I wanted to do was run, but just like a dream where everything is in slow motion and your feet feel like they are immersed in cement blocks, I couldn't because I was too drunk. I ended up walking the four miles home at 4:00 am, balling my eyes out, still slightly drunk. When I woke up later that day, I vowed to quit drinking and get my life together.

And so, I did. Twenty-one years later here I am about to finish writing this book. Sitting in my own chiropractic office, the diploma for my doctorate sits above my head, a poster of my daughter five minutes after she was born off to my left, with the lyrics from the song *Reckless Love* playing in my headphones.

I am so very thankful that I decided a long time ago to work diligently on my mind, body, and spirit. I hope you do the same.

The reason I share these things is because I believe that no matter how bad life gets, no matter how bad our negative self-image is, we have the power to turn it all around. This is the great news! How well your life is lived is all based on the choices you make? So, the question becomes are you THRIVING in Life or are you just surviving?

What you have just read is something that took approximately 450 days to write. I have laid out my thoughts, opinions, and the research to back it up. I have put my blood, sweat, and tears into writing this thing. I have faith that you are inspired to make the changes you need to make, to live the kind of life you deserve to live.

Remember, you don't have to change everything all at once. You can change things slowly over time, but your changes must be consistent. Over time, you will have made tremendous change. Just as I wrote this book (slowly over time), you can make profound changes in your life. By focusing on your mind, body, and spiritual health, you too can live the life you were designed to live.

BECAUSE YOU ARE DESIGNED TO THRIVE!

Three things in life – your health, your mission, and the people you love. That's it.

-Naval Ravikant

"BE INSPIRED" RESOURCES

Dr. Jay on the Internet and Social Media:

Website
www.thrivespinecenter.com

Facebook
www.facebook.com/groups/Align2Thrive
www.facebook.com/thrivespinecenter

Instagram
Instagram.com/JasonBergerhouse
Instagram.com/ThriveSpineCenter

YouTube
@ Dr. Jason Bergerhouse

Dr. Jay's Affiliate Links:

CBD oil
www.Hempworx.com/SpartanChiro.com

Detoxinated Training Videos
www.ThriveSpineCenter/Blog/affiliate
www.getdetoxinated.teachable.com/p/sauna-detoxification-using-niacin/?coupon_code=DETOX50&affcode=

Smart Meter Guard
www.smartmeterguard.com?afmc=37

EMF Protection
www.emfsol.com/?aff

Suggested Websites

Chiropractic
www.myrcc.com
www.californiajam.org

EMF Protection (microsurge meter to detect dirty electricity)
greenwavefilters.com

EMF Meter
greenwavefilters.com/product/trifield-emf-meter-model-tf2/

EMF Cell phone protection
www.defendershield.com/products/cellphone/

EMF Protective jewelry
www.carpediemnursing.org

Mindset
Dr. Bruce Lipton www.brucelipton.com
Dr. Joe Dispenza www.drjoedispenza.com
Tony Robbins www.tonyrobbins.com

Physical Health
Jason Christoff www.jchristoff.com
Patrick McKeown www.oxygenadvantage.com

Spiritual
www.facebook.com/francisanfuso1/https://crossexamined.org

DR. JAY'S WEEKLY ROUTINE:

Daily habits I perform religiously

EARLY MORNING: *(4:00 – 8:00 am)*

1. 15 minutes of meditation (Mindset)

2. 5 to Thrive Reading (Five pages of a non-fictional book, article, and/or the Bible)

3. Prayer and affirmations

4. 5 to Thrive stretch routine (full body)

5. Emails/Social media post/Blog writing

6. Glass of filtered water with liquid chlorophyll

7. Wheat grass shot 30 minutes after first glass of water

8. Green drink by 8:00 am

> **NOTE:** Healthy snacks throughout the day consisting of things like granny smith apples, nuts, seeds, and healthy all-natural protein bars (usually plant based). I listen to my body when I feel hungry.

MID – MORNING: *(8:00 – 12:00 pm)*

1. 2-4 glasses of highly filtered water

EARLY AFTERNOON: *(12:00 – 2:00 pm)*

1. Light & healthy lunch

2. Glass of highly filtered water with liquid chlorophyll

3. 5 to Thrive stretch routine (full body)

MID – AFTERNOON: (2:00 – 6:00 pm)

1. 2-4 glasses of highly filtered water

EARLY EVENING: (6:00 – 8:00 pm)

1. Light & healthy dinner with family
2. 2 glasses of highly filtered water
3. **STOP EATING BY 7:00 or 7:30 pm**

LATE EVENING: (8:00 – 10:00 pm)

1. 1 glass of highly filtered water
2. Stretch 5-10 minutes before bed
3. Prayer and affirmations
4. Asleep by 9:30 or 10:00 pm

My workout days are Monday, Wednesday, Thursday, and Saturday or Sunday

SAMPLE WORKOUT

11:00-12:00 pm – HIIT full body workout (minimum of 45 minutes)
12:00-1:00 pm – Sauna (minimum of 45 minutes @ 190° F)

Post workout I drink a Cal-Mag recovery drink.

Niacin Protocol

Example:

Weight is 180 lb. = 180 / 2.205 = 81.63 kg

TND = 816.3 mg

The table shows the number of days to reach the TND (or next highest dose) based on a tolerated schedule.

DAY	LIGHT	MODERATE	AGGRESSIVE
1	50	100	100
2	100	300	300
3	200	500	600
4	300	700	**900**
5	400	**900**	1100
6	500	1000	1300
7	600	1100	1500
8	700	1200	1700
9	800	1300	1900
10	**900**	1400	2100
11	1000	1500	2300
12	1100	1600	2500
13	1200	1700	2700
14	1300	1800	2900

"Sauna Detoxification Using Niacin," by Dan L. Root with David E. Root., M.D., M.P.H, Pg. 125

CAL-MAG RECIPE

One batch may last up to three days when covered and properly refrigerated.

Boil one cup of water
1 level tablespoon calcium gluconate powder
½ teaspoon magnesium carbonate powder
1.5 tablespoons of apple cider vinegar
Mix ingredients into a large (1-liter min.) heat resistant, lidded container
Stir/shake well to thoroughly combine all ingredients
Let sit for approximately 3 minutes
Add 1 cup of hot water, stir/shake, and let sit for a few more minutes
Add one cup of cold/ice water and stir
Pour into a glass
Stir in 2 oz. of 100% organic cranberry juice to flavor
Cover and refrigerate remainder for the next session

Sauna Detoxification Using Niacin, by Dan L. Root with David E. Root., M.D., M.P.H, Pg. 126

GREEN SMOOTHIES

- To make a green smoothie add 6-8 ounces of water to your blender. Rinse a handful of greens and remove any thick or fibrous stems. Add greens to the blender. Blend starting on low and then turning your blender up to high. Blend until you can't distinguish any bits of leaf. Add some fruit (bananas, berries, apples, pears, etc.). Add other fruit and berries as you like, removing pits, core scores, and peels if necessary. Blend again until smooth. Serve and drink fresh.

- Greens that go particularly well in green smoothies are kale, spinach, parsley, Swiss chard, romaine lettuce, and young dandelion leaves. Frozen fruits work well in green smoothies, especially in warmer weather. They make a nice cold refreshing drink. You can also substitute some of the water with ice cubes. High powered blenders (at least 800-1000 watts) are best when it comes to making green smoothies.

- If the blender you have isn't that powerful, don't worry. Just chop the ingredients into smaller pieces so you don't put too much strain on your blender. It might also work better if you add half the water and the leafy greens to start, blend them as thoroughly as you can, then add the rest of the water and fruit and blend again.

- Green smoothies are loaded with fiber and therefore are very filling. So, drink about one quart (slowly, do not guzzle it down) which equates to about 32 ounces of fluid. Make sure that you are drinking them on an empty stomach to ensure that you absorb the nutrients at a higher capacity. Also, try drinking the smoothies 2 hours before a meal.

One of the best times to drink a green smoothie is about 30 minutes to an hour after you wake up. Do not eat for about an hour after you drink them as this will affect the quality of absorption as well.

- Rotate your greens. Do not use the same recipe every time, mix it up! For example, instead of spinach use dandelion greens or kale. I have found that rotating the greens you use in your smoothies is crucial to feeling increased energy. You get a variety of different vitamins and minerals when you mix up your greens. Too much of a certain green can build up secondary metabolites in your body. Use only organic greens and don't forget to wash them!

- When designing your green drinks keep it simple. A simple way to do it is think 1:1. One fruit to one green and never go beyond 2 fruits and 2 greens.

Dr. Jay's Green Drink

1/2 organic banana (for flavor and thickens it)

1/2 cup of frozen organic mixed berries (raspberries, blueberries, strawberries etc.)

1 cup of unsweetened almond milk

1 heaping tablespoon of raw almond butter

1-2 cups of raw organic baby spinach

1-2 cups of raw Kale (green, purple, dinosaur)

1/2 - 1 cup of parsley (super green)

1 teaspoon of raw honey (optional)

3/4 cup of crushed ice (optional)

6-8 ounces of filtered water

If needed add Stevia to sweeten

1 scoop vegan protein (optional)

Blend on high for 3-5 minutes to a consistency of your liking. Alternate greens, add Swiss chard, alfalfa, collard greens, dandelion greens, etc.

Medical Doctors and PhD Scientists Speak Out Against Vaccinations

As taken from Jason Christoff's Website: https://jchristoff.com/

Below is a list of videos (*and some articles*) where medical doctors and PhD scientists come forward to discuss the unhealthy effects of vaccines. Each professional presents documented research, facts and statistics to prove, when taken in its' totality, that 1) vaccines aren't safe 2) vaccines aren't effective 3) vaccines haven't been proven to increase immunity or resistance to disease and 4) that vaccines only decrease the health of the people they're injected into. Vaccines are also proven and documented in many cases to kill instantly and cripple for life. The situations of instant child death and permanent injury, due to vaccination, are well documented in the linked information.

Some of the professionals below are straight to the point and some are a little more withdrawn about coming forward to present the exact opposite of what they were taught in medical school and by their society in general. The medical and science professionals listed have nothing to gain and literally everything to lose by speaking up within a system that's designed to punish anyone who moves against the accepted medical standards of care and generally accepted community standards, within our culture. The theme of each presentation is eerily similar, with the common ground always being that this information regarding vaccines being ineffective, unhealthy and dangerous.....is already well documented within the journals of medical science but it's ignored full stop because something else is going on. The weight of the evidence is not only found to be firmly planted against the use of vaccines, due to their unhealthy effects, but the government itself is the very entity spear heading a corrupt and illegal attack upon its' own citizens.....by forcing science, medicine and government policy to keep driving fraudulent vaccine claims and toxic vaccines themselves, deeper into the public at large. This is for parents who want to know more, in order to do the best for their children.

1. Dr. Nancy Banks – http://bit.ly/1Ip0aIm

2. Dr. Russell Blaylock – https://www.youtube.com/watch?v=v5xHV8_Njfc

3. Dr. Shiv Chopra – https://www.youtube.com/watch?v=uDg490zBsmU&t=3s

4. Dr. Sherri Tenpenny – http://bit.ly/2GpCVS4

5. Dr. Suzanne Humphries – http://bit.ly/2Hzn17l

6. Dr. Larry Palevsky – http://bit.ly/1LLEjf6

7. Dr. Toni Bark – http://bit.ly/1CYM9RB

8. Dr. Andrew Wakefield – http://bit.ly/1eXfTTa

9. Dr. Meryl Nass – http://bit.ly/1DGzJsc

10. Dr. Raymond Obomsawin – http://bit.ly/1G9ZXYl

11. Dr. Ghislaine Lanctot – http://bit.ly/1cAIeOt

12. Dr. Robert Rowen – http://bit.ly/1SIELeF

13. Dr. David Ayoub – http://bit.ly/1SIELve

14. Dr. Boyd Haley PhD – http://bit.ly/1KsdVby

15. Dr. Rashid Buttar – http://bit.ly/1gWOkL6

16. Dr. Roby Mitchell – http://bit.ly/1gdgEZU

17. Dr. Ken Stoller – http://bit.ly/1MPVqLl

18. Dr. Mayer Eisenstein – http://bit.ly/2IpHbBC

19. Dr. Frank Engley, PhD – http://bit.ly/1OHbLDI

20. Dr. David Davis – http://bit.ly/1gdgJwo

21. Dr Tetyana Obukhanych – http://bit.ly/16Z7k6J

22. Dr. Harold E Buttram – http://bit.ly/1Kru6Df

23. Dr. Kelly Brogan – http://bit.ly/1D31pfQ

24. Dr. RC Tent – http://bit.ly/1MPVwmu

25. Dr. Rebecca Carley – http://bit.ly/K49F4d

26. Dr. Andrew Moulden – http://bit.ly/1fwzKJu

27. Dr. Jack Wolfson –http://bit.ly/2SDRbjz and http://bit.ly/2tO7luD

28. Dr. Michael Elice – http://bit.ly/1KsdpKA

29. Dr. Terry Wahls – http://bit.ly/1gWOBhd

30. Dr. Stephanie Seneff – http://bit.ly/1OtWxAY

31. Dr. Paul Thomas – http://bit.ly/1DpeXPf

32. Many doctors talking at once – http://bit.ly/1MPVHOv

33. Dr. Richard Moskowitz – http://bit.ly/1OtWG7D

34. Dr. Jane Orient – http://bit.ly/1MXX7pb

35. Dr. Richard Deth – http://bit.ly/1GQDL10

36. Dr. Lucija Tomljenovic – http://bit.ly/1eqiPr5

37. Dr Chris Shaw – http://bit.ly/1IlGiBp

38. Dr. Susan McCreadie – http://bit.ly/1CqqN83

39. Dr. Mary Ann Block – http://bit.ly/1OHcyUX

40. Dr. David Brownstein – http://bit.ly/2pbtD4Z

41. Dr. Jayne Donegan – http://bit.ly/1wOk4Zz

42. Dr. Troy Ross – http://bit.ly/1IlGINH

43. Dr. Philip Incao – http://bit.ly/1ghE7sS

44. Dr. Joseph Mercola – http://bit.ly/18dE38I

45. Dr. Jeff Bradstreet – http://bit.ly/1MaX0cC

46. Dr. Robert Mendelson – http://bit.ly/1JpAEQr

47. Dr. Garth Nicolson – http://bit.ly/2pcGK4R

48. Dr. Marc Girard – http://bit.ly/1iw0smT

49. Dr. Charles Richet – http://bit.ly/2DrLd8Z

50. Dr. Zac Bush – http://bit.ly/1LS19OZ

51. Dr. Lawrence Wilson – http://bit.ly/1kcdirf

52. Dr. James Howenstine – http://bit.ly/1iNyFOy

53. Dr Burton A. Waisbren, Sr., M.D. – http://bit.ly/1Nj8LRe

54. Dr. Sam Eggertsen – http://bit.ly/1Mww9XV

55. Dr. Bonnie Dunbar – http://bit.ly/1N5DXNi

56. Dr. Judy Mikovits – http://bit.ly/1QIzmHU

57. Dr. John Bergan – http://bit.ly/1KYv1yY

58. Dr. Rima E. Laibow – bit.ly/1RmW73C

59. Dr. Lee Hieb – http://bit.ly/1VEIDUv

60. Dr. Daniel Kalb – http://bit.ly/22FPmxv

61. Dr. Rachel Ross – http://bit.ly/1r7Doik

62. Dr. Kathryn H Hale – http://bit.ly/2GsBxym

63. Dr. Gibson – http://bit.ly/2sLINSt

64. Dr. Anthony Phan – http://bit.ly/2squqxN

65. Dr. Daniel Neides – http://bit.ly/2xdg2vz

66. Dr. Christiane Northrup – http://bit.ly/2vWOdqi

67. Dr. James Neuenschwander – http://bit.ly/2gCsl1w

68. Dr. James Meehan – http://bit.ly/2EPLdoU

69. Dr. Christopher Exley – http://bit.ly/2sSVgny

70. Dr. Graham Downing – http://bit.ly/2FUg03G

71. Dr. Judy Wilyman – https://bit.ly/2vUVegp

72. Dr. Jamie Deckoff-Jones – https://bit.ly/1M1DJZm

73. Dr. Ray Andrew – The link no longer works for this. (Look him up on duckduckgo browser

74. Dr Dietrich Klinghardt – https://www.youtube.com/watch?v=sptwNCfC3Ps&feature=youtu.be

Documentaries that Include 100's of Health Professionals WARNING The Public About The Dangers of Vaccination....

1. Vaccination – The Silent Epidemic – http://bit.ly/1vvQJ2W

2. The Greater Good – http://bit.ly/2Cg8PkZ

3. Shots In The Dark – http://bit.ly/1ObtC8h

4. Vaccination The Hidden Truth – http://bit.ly/KEYDUh

5. Vaccine Nation – http://bit.ly/2IrdksA

6. Vaccination – The Truth About Vaccines – http://bit.ly/1vlpwvU

7. Lethal Injection – http://bit.ly/1URN7BJ

8. Bought – https://bit.ly/2NaJ2hK

9. Deadly Immunity – http://bit.ly/1KUg64Z

10. Autism – Made in the USA – http://bit.ly/1J8WQN5

11. Beyond Treason – https://bit.ly/301RuVZ

12. Trace Amounts – http://bit.ly/2ELnUZm

13. Why We Don't Vaccinate – http://bit.ly/1KbXhuf

14. Autism Yesterday – http://bit.ly/1URU2A7

15. Denmark Documentary on HPV Vaccine – Vaccinated Girls – Sick and Portrayed – https://bit.ly/2R4mf8s

16. Vaxxed – http://bit.ly/2pWau9h

17. Man Made Epidemic – http://bit.ly/1XsOi0R

18. 50 Cents A Dose – http://bit.ly/2c0h07P

19. Direct Orders – http://bit.ly/1ivShHg

20. Dtap – Vaccine Roulette http://bit.ly/2dBnc3u

21. Truthstream News: About All Those Vaccines – http://bit.ly/2gCMa4o

22. Hear The Silence – https://bit.ly/35BjMrm

23. Cervical Cancer Vaccine – Is It Safe? – http://bit.ly/2h3Dvsh

24. Vaccines Revealed – https://www.vaccinesrevealed.com/free/

25. The Truth About Vaccines – http://bit.ly/2mX4Tyc

26. Vaccine Syndrome – https://bit.ly/2QBvYnD

27. Injecting Aluminum – http://bit.ly/2qPkFwo

28. Manufactured Crisis: HPV, Hype & Horror – https://bit.ly/2QYzHuG

29. Sacrificial Virgins – http://bit.ly/2xGOfnb

30. Vaxxed II – https://bit.ly/2N6NZYP

31. Shots In The Dark 2020 – https://bit.ly/2T5pwak

Common Sense Vaccine Questions to Ask Your Doctor

If vaccines are safe and effective, why does it state on many vaccines inserts that the vaccine maker will not guarantee that the vaccine will provide immunity to the targeted disease? How does not providing immunity reflect an effective vaccine product?

If vaccines are safe and effective why does it state on all vaccine inserts that each vaccine holds the potential to kill or permanently injure the vaccine recipient? How does the death or permanent crippling of the vaccine recipient reflect a safe vaccine product?

If children encounter viruses via an open orifice in their body (their mouths, eyes, nose, etc.), how is injecting material directly into the blood stream supposed to mimic the body's natural immune reaction?

If vaccines worked for providing immunity, why would the parent of a vaccinated child be afraid of an unvaccinated child?

If we're supposed to be afraid of viruses and avoid them at all costs, why are there live viruses in some vaccines (like the MMR) and why are we asked to inject these live viruses into our children?

If vaccines provide immunity, why do we need booster shots?

The MMR vaccine contains live measles, mumps, and rubella virus. There's the polio vaccine, the flu shot, chicken pox, hep B, diphtheria, tetanus, and pertussis (just to name a few). Some doctors administer several of these vaccines at once to an infant or child. What are the chances my child would be exposed to all those diseases at once in nature and what research do you have that giving all these at once is safe?

(There's no research to prove multiple vaccines are safe so you're asking for research that doesn't exist. That means no child in the world should ever receive more than one vaccine at a time.)

Are you telling me to believe that the only way a child can get sick is by not getting a vaccine and that their lifestyle has nothing to do with the strength of their immune system or their health status? So, you're telling me that we can inject health into sick people, with toxins no less? Please explain?

Why is the third most toxic substance on earth, mercury (also ranked as the most toxic non-radioactive substance on earth), an ingredient in some vaccines.

When mercury is proven to cause adverse neurological damage, why are some of the documented vaccine side effects listed on the vaccine insert exact symptoms of mercury or aluminum poisoning?

Will you personally guarantee on a legal document that this vaccine will not harm my child in any way, now or in the future?

I know you verbally declare vaccines are safe and effective, but will you back that statement with your personal assets to prove to me that you really believe it, as opposed to just saying vaccines are safe because that's what you were taught to say and because your primary source of income is the vaccination of children and infants?

If health authorities wanted to prove to everyone once and for all that vaccines worked at preventing the targeted disease, why aren't you going to track my child after the vaccination to see if he or she gets sick or not?

(Why do you think they don't track the kids after they're vaccinated? It's because they already know what they would find.)

Are you paid extra and compensated in some way (bonus or otherwise) to provide this vaccine to me and my child? How much is that compensation as a percentage of your total income.

(In some cases, family physicians derive 90% of their income from vaccinating the uninformed public.)

If the International Medical Law of Informed Consent applies to any medical procedure that could end the life or permanently injure the patient, why are we not told at every visit that each vaccine can kill or permanently injure my child?

When the vaccine insert declares openly that the vaccine can kill or permanently injure my child, why have I not been given the vaccine insert to read, with enough time to digest it and ask questions when that's the law? By not providing me the vaccine insert which declares the vaccine can kill or cripple my child, are you in contravention of the medical law of informed consent?

If all vaccine inserts document that the vaccine can kill or cripple my child, how is that considered safe?

If you nor the vaccine maker will guarantee this vaccine makes my child immune, how is that considered effective? How did a needle full of documented toxins which have the potential to kill and cripple and doesn't guarantee immunity become sold as something that's safe and effective?

Can you list for me exactly how much neurotoxic aluminum and mercury are in each vaccine you're recommending for my child? And list for me the safe levels of those neurotoxic heavy metals established by the EPA for injection directly into a child's/infant's blood stream?

In the United States our health authorities advise an infant before one year of age receive 26 vaccines. In Canada that number is 24. If vaccines are safe and effective and only provide immunity, would you mind taking shot for shot with my newborn in their first year of life? Would you be willing to take the same 26 or 24 vaccinations you recommend proving to me that you genuinely believe only good and benefit is brought into the body by vaccination?

If we are supposed to listen to doctors who present the science regarding vaccines what are we supposed to do with medical doctors who present the hard science proving vaccines aren't safe or effective? How do we decide between the two sides? One side saying poisons hurt children and the other side saying poison is healthy for children? If science is the unbiased pursuit of truth, why is the science these doctors present not included in the material you provide to patients? Why is the hard science proving vaccines don't provide immunity and that they're dangerous not presented to the public by the mainstream media or the medical profession?

If the media and most medical outlets claim vaccines don't cause autism how do you explain all the sources and citations that confirm vaccines do cause autism?

Can you please explain to me the warning on most vaccines regarding that the vaccine has not been evaluated for its' carcinogenic or mutagenic potentials or impairment of fertility? What exactly does that mean?

If vaccines are safe and effective why did the US government set up the Vaccine Injury Compensation Program in 1987? How safe and effective does this sound to you? If vaccines are safe and effective, why are parents suing vaccine manufactures for causing vaccine induced death or permanent vaccine injury in their children?

Why does the medical industry and government suggest certain vaccines for pregnant mothers when every vaccine (without exception) declares that no vaccine has been tested safe for pregnant mothers or their unborn child?

If vaccines eradicated polio, what's a parent supposed to do with the information proving that vaccines cause polio, yet the paralysis is hidden from the public using a different name?

If hepatitis B is a liver disease caused by someone having unprotected sex with an infected partner or sharing a dirty needle with an infected IV drug user, why is the hepatitis B vaccine recommended in the US on the day of birth? What are the chances my newborn has sex with a hep B infected person or shares a dirty needle with an IV drug addict? I'm confused, please clarify.

Are you willing to take shot for shot with my infant or child based on weight? The average weight of an infant from 0-12 months is 14lbs. The average medical doctor weighs 180 lbs. Adjusted for weight that equates to a medical doctor taking 308 vaccines over one year. Are you willing to take 308 vaccines in the same year you inject 24 vaccines into my infant to prove vaccines are safe and effective? If you won't put your life on the line why do you preach that I should put my children on the line? So you can collect a monetary bonus for a fully vaccinated child? Is this about logic and science or is this about dogma, profit, and sacrifice of the defenseless?

Can you explain to me what you've learned about vaccines in medical school? The medical doctors in this article explain clearly that they didn't learn anything about vaccines in medical school other than the phrase vaccines are safe and effective and when to administer the vaccines, which I've already established as not being tested as safe for any child to receive.

What does injecting me or my baby with the meat of ground up aborted fetuses have to do with making my child or me healthier?

Glycemic Index Chart

LOW GI = 55 or LESS

MEDIUM GI = 56-69

HIGH GI = 70 OR MORE

Glycemic Index
Low GI (<55), Medium GI (56-69) and High GI (70>)

Grains / Starchs		Vegetables		Fruits		Dairy		Proteins	
Rice Bran	27	Asparagus	15	Grapefruit	25	Low-Fat Yogurt	14	Peanuts	21
Bran Cereal	42	Broccoli	15	Apple	38	Plain Yogurt	14	Beans, Dried	40
Spaghetti	42	Celery	15	Peach	42	Whole Milk	27	Lentils	41
Corn, sweet	54	Cucumber	15	Orange	44	Soy Milk	30	Kidney Beans	41
Wild Rice	57	Lettuce	15	Grape	46	Fat-free Milk	32	Split Beans	45
Sweet Potatoes	61	Peppers	15	Banana	54	Skim Milk	32	Lima Beans	46
White Rice	64	Spinach	15	Mango	56	Chocolate Milk	35	Chickpeas	47
Cous Cous	65	Tomatoes	15	Pineapple	66	Fruit Yogurt	36	Pinto Beans	55
Whole wheat Bread	71	Chickpeas	33	Watermelon	72	Ice Cream	61	Black-Eyed Beans	59
Muesli	80	Cooked Carrots	39						
Baked potatoes	85								
Oatmeal	87								
Taco Shells	97								
White Bread	100								
Bagel, White	103								

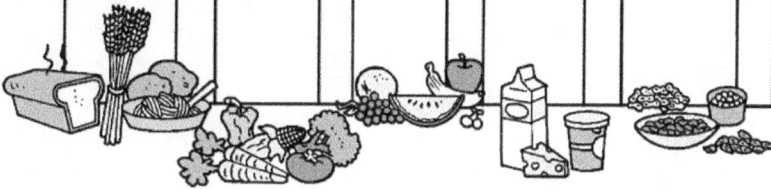

Standing Stretch

STANDNG STRETCH *(Rounded shoulders and FHP)*

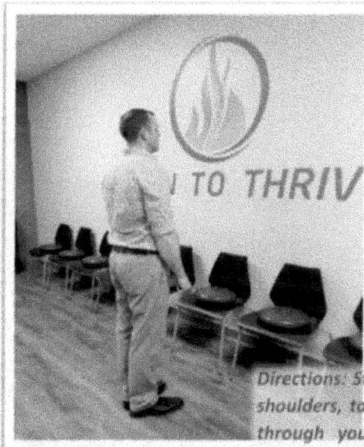

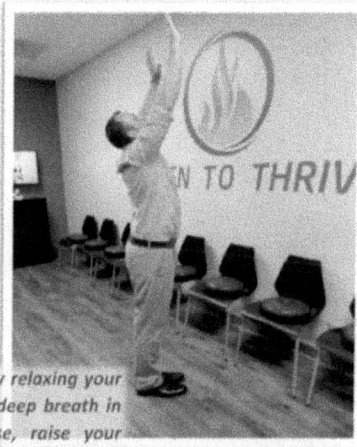

Directions: Start by relaxing your shoulders, take a deep breath in through your nose, raise your arms up and extend your head and neck back (slowly and carefully). Bring your elbows back at a 45 degree angle and exhale through your mouth.

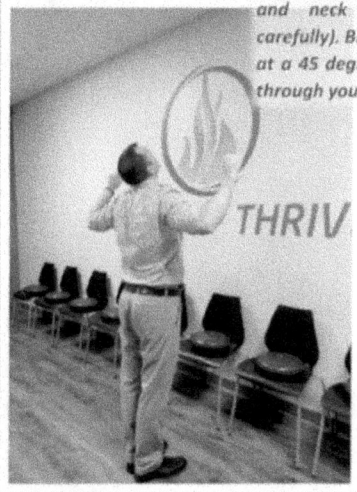

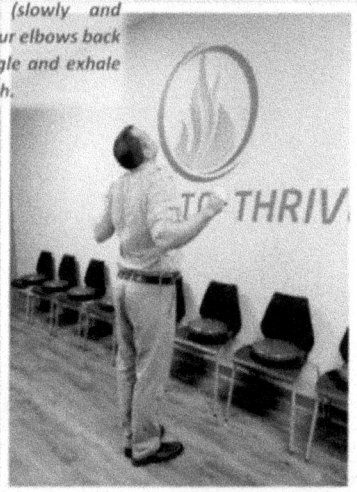

Bibliography

Stephenson, Ralph, "The 33 Chiropractic Principals." Chiropractic Textbook, 1927. Print.

Dispenza, Joe. "You Are the Placebo," 2014, Hay House Inc. Print.

Robbins, A. "Unlimited Power." 1987, Ballantine Books. Print.

Yachter, Dan. "Doctor of the Future," Advantage 2010. Print.

Ruch, William. "Atlas of Common Subluxations of the Human Spine and Pelvis" William J. Ruch. 1995. Print.

Cherniske S. Caffeine Blues: Wake Up to the Hidden Dangers of America's #1 Drug. 1st ed. New York: Warner Books Inc; 1998. Print.

Stevenson, Shawn. "Sleep Smarter." Model House Publishing, 2014. Print.

Richards, Byron. J. Fight for Your Health, Exposing the FDA's Betrayal of America Wellness Resource Books; 2006. Print.

Ingram, Colin. "The Drinking Water Book: How to Eliminate Harmful Toxins from your Water"2nd ed. Berkley: Celestial Arts; 1991, 1995, 2006. Print.

Nora T. Gedgaudas, CNS, CNT. "Primal Body, Primal Mind"

2009, Nora T. Gedgaudas. Print.

Judith Shaw, M.A. "Trans Fats – The Hidden Killer in our Food"

2004, Pocket Books. Print.

Mercola, Joseph, "Fat for Fuel: A Revolutionary Diet to Combat Cancer, Boost Brain Power, and Increase Your Energy." 2018, Hay House Inc. Print.

Bragg, Paul Chappius., and Patricia Bragg. The miracle of fasting: for Agelessness-Physical, Mental & Spiritual Rejuvenation: New Discoveries About an Old Miracle--The "Fast" Fasting Way to Health Science, 1983. Print.

Dr. David E., and Daniel L. Root, "Sauna Detoxification Using Niacin: Following the Recommended Protocol of Dr. Davie E. Root." Dan Root, 2019. Print.

Wigmore, Ann. "The Wheatgrass Book" Wigmore, Ann 1985. Print

McKeown, Patrick, "The Oxygen Advantage." HarperCollins, 2015, Print.

Greenfield, Ben. "Beyond Training." Ben Greenfield, 2014. Print.

Humphries, Suzanne, and Bystrianyk, Roman. Dissolving Illusions: Disease, Vaccines, and the Forgotten History." 2013, Print.

Stevenson, Shawn. "Sleep Smarter." Model House Publishing, 2014. Print.

Cherniske S. Caffeine Blues: Wake Up to the Hidden Dangers of America's #1 Drug. 1st ed. New York: Warner Books Inc; 1998. Print.

Halpern, Jonathan. "Electromagnetic Radiation Survival Guide: Step by Step Solutions." Halpern, Jonathan; 2013. Print.

Gittleman, Ann. "ZAPPED: Why Your Cell Phone Shouldn't be your Alarm Clock and 1,268 Ways to Outsmart the Hazards of Electronic Pollution" New York, HarperCollins, 2011. Print.

Body by God: The Owner's Manual for Maximized Living, Ben Lerner, Thomas Nelson 2007. Print.

Dr. Lisa Dunne, Multigenerational Marketplace. Print.

End Notes

Introduction

1. "15 Powerful Les Brown Quotes that Will Inspire You." https://motivationgrid.com/15-powerful-les-brown-quotes-will-inspire/

Chapter 1

2. Thornton, Alex – World Economic Forum, "These are the World's Healthiest Nations." 2019, Feb. 25th https://www.weforum.org/agenda/2019/02/these-are-the-world-s-healthiest-nations

3. Carr, T., "Too Many Meds? America's Love Affair with Prescription Medication." Aug. 3, 2017 https://www.consumerreports.org/prescription-drugs/too-many-meds-americas-love-affair-with-prescription-medication/

4. Mayo Clinic, "Nearly 7 in 10 Americans are on prescription drugs." ScienceDaily, 19 June 2013, www.sciencedaily.com/releases/2013/06/130619132352.htm.

5. Lutz, Rachel, "Pharmacists Underreport Adverse Drug Reactions Due to Inadequate Training." 2014, Nov. 6, https://www.pharmacytimes.com

6. Lazarou, J. "Incidence of Adverse Drug Reactions in Hospitalized Patients: A Meta-analysis of Prospective Studies." 2000 et all. JAMA 1998 Apr 15th; 279(15): 1200-1205

7. FDA, "Preventable Adverse Drug Reactions: A Focus on Drug Interactions," https://www.fda.gov

8. Wikipedia, "Years of Potential Life Lost." https://en.wikipedia. org/wiki/Years_of_potential_life_lost

9. Wikipedia, "List of the Verified Oldest People," https:// en.m.wikipedia.org

9. Sidrah, "The Health Secrets of the Hunza People who Live Over 100 Years and are Cancer-Free." 2017, Apr 18, 2017, https:// www.shughal.com

10. World Affairs, 2017, "How Rockefeller Founded Modern Medicine and Killed Natural Cures." worldaffairs. blog

11. Null, G., Dean, C. Feldman, M. Rasio, Debora. "Death by Medicine," 2010

12. Berenson, A. Gardiner, H. Meier, B. Pollack, A., "Despite Warnings, Drug Giant Took Long Path to Vioxx Recall." 2004, Nov. 14th, https://www.nytimes.com

13. Sukkar, Elizabeth, "Still Feeling the Vioxx Pain." 2014, Sep. 19th https://www.pharmaceutical-journal.com

14. Groningen, Nicole, "Big Pharma Gives Your Doctor Gift. Then Your Doctor Gives You Big Pharma's Drugs." 2017, June 13, https://www.washingtonpost.com.

15. Gyles, C., "Skeptical of Medical Science." Can Vet J. 2015, OCT; 56(10): 1011-1012 https://www.ncbi.nlm.nih.gov/pmc/articles/PMC4572812/#_ffn_sectitle.com

Chapter 2

16. Medline Plus, "How Wounds Heal," https://medlineplus.gov

17. Wikipedia, "Health," https://en.m.wikipedia.org/wiki/health. com

18. Stephenson, Ralph, "The 33 Chiropractic Principals." Chiropractic Textbook 1927

19. Lynne, Planet Chiropractic. "What is Chiropractic Retracing." 2004, May 5th, https://planetc1.com

CHAPTER 3

20. Bible Gateway, Ephesians 5:11-16, https://www.biblegateway.com

21. Lipton, Bruce, "The Wisdom of your Cells." 2012, June 7th, https://www.brucelipton.com

22. Bible Gateway, Proverbs 23:7, https://www.biblegateway.com

23. Inglis-Arkell, E., "How the 'Nocebo Effect' can trick us into actually dying." 2015, Jan. 26th, https://www.Io9.gizmodo.com

24. Rankin, Lissa. "The Nocebo Effect: Negative Thoughts can Harm your Health." 2013, Aug. 6th, https://www.psychologytoday.com

25. Wikipedia, "Autosuggestion," https://www.en.m.wikipedia.org/wiki/autosuggestion

26. "Understanding the Conscious & Subconscious Mind with Bruce Lipton"

27. Neuroscience, "Prefrontal Cortex." 2017, Jan. 4th, https://www.thescienceofpsychotherapy.com/prefrontal-cortex/

28. Brian Tracy International, "Subconscious Mind Power Explained." Retrieved on 03/20/2019, https://www.briantracy.com

29. Dispenza, Joe. "You Are the Placebo," 2014, Hay House Inc.

30. Robbins, A., "Unlimited Power," 1987, Ballantine Books

31. Chalupa, Andrew, "How to Win the Lottery – Yes you Read that Correctly – by Visualizing it." 2009, May 22, https://www.aol.com

32. Cochrane Database System Review, "Exercise for Depression," 2013, SEPT 12th, https://www.ncbi.nlm.nih.gov/pubmed/24026850.com

CHAPTER 4

33. Yachter, Dan. "Doctor of the Future" Advantage 2010

34. Franklin, Cory. "When are you Officially Dead?" Chicago Tribune, 2014, January 10th https://www.chicagotribune.com/opinion/ct-xpm-2014-01-10-ct-death-jahi-brain-legal-perspec-0110-20140110-story.html

35. Staughton, John. "The Human Brain Vs. Supercomputers... Which One Wins?" https://www.scienceabc.com/humans/the-human-brain-vs-supercomputers-which-one-wins.html

36. CSU, Chico, McCaffrey, Patrick, PHD. "Chapter 3. The Meninges and Cerebrospinal Fluid," https://www.csuchico.edu/~pmccaffrey//syllabi/CMSD%20320/362unit3.html

37. Burnier, Arno, "A Marvel of Design." Care of Life, 2015, April 7th, http://cafeoflife.com/articles/amarvel-of-design/

38. Romano, Luis, "Riding Accident Paralyzes Actor Christopher Reeves," 1995, JUNE 1st, http://www.washingtonpost.com/wp-dyn/articles/A99660-1995Jun1.html?noredirect=on

39. Stuart, Courtney, "100% Preventable: Reeves Didn't Have to Die."2004, OCT 24th, http://www.readthehook.com/95937/news-100-preventable-reeve-didnt-have-die

40. Ruch, William, "Atlas of Common Subluxations of the Human Spine and Pelvis," 1995 William J. Ruch.

41. Chirotrust, "Chiropractic and Hypertension." 2018, AUG 6th, https://chiro-trust.org/whole-body-health/chiropractic-and-hypertension/

42. Rickards, "Dr. Henry Winsor: Chiropractic Research" https://rickardschiropractic.com/dr-henry-winsor-chiropractic-research/

43. Des Toups, "How Many Times will you Crash Your Car?" https://www.forbes.com/sites/moneybuilder/2011/07/27/how-many-times-will-you-crash-your-car/

44. WHO "Fact sheet 344: Falls" World Health Organization. 2018. JAN 16th, https://www.who.int/news-room/fact-sheets/detail/falls

45. "10 Facts & Statistics About Slip and Fall Accidents." https://www.askadamskutner.com/slip-and-fall/10-facts-statistics-slip-fall-accidents/

46. Lephart, Kim, "Toddlers Weeble, Wobble, and Fall Down. When is it Cause for Concern?" 9th, January 2014. https://veipd.org/earlyintervention/2014/01/09/toddlers-weeble-wobble-and-fall-down-when-is-it-cause-for-concern/

47. HistoryExtra "Call the Roman Midwife." 2019, MARCH 2019. https://www.historyextra.com

48. "Sylvester Stallone's Slurred Conversation Is Actually Caused by an Accident in the Beginning that Brought on Semi-paralysis in Parts of His Face." https://www.mindblowing-facts.org

49. Gustitus, David. "Thoughts, Traumas and Toxins: Three Causes of Subluxation." Blog, Issue #38, https://www.pathwaystofamilywellness.org

50. Stephenson, R.W. "Chiropractic Textbook," 1927, The Palmer School of Chiropractic.

51. In Touch Chiropractic, "The Truth by BJ Palmer." (Blog) https://www.sandiegonucca.com

CHAPTER 5

52. Helmenstine, Anne. "How Much of Your Body Is Water?" 2019, MAY 13th https://www.thoughtco.com

53. Cooper, M. Geoffrey. "The Cell: A Molecular Approach. 2nd Edition." Sunderland (MA): Sinauer Associates; 2000, https://www.ncbi.nlm.nih.gov/books/NBK9879/

54. Medi Resource Inc. "Dehydration (Low Body Fluids)," https://medbroadcast.com/condition/getcondition/dehydration

55. Biller A, Reuter M, Patenaude B, Homola GA, Breuer F, Bendszus M, Bartsch AJ. Responses of the Human Brain to Mild Dehydration and Rehydration Explored In Vivo by 1H-MR Imaging and Spectroscopy. AJNR Am J Neuroradiology. 2015 Dec;36(12):2277-84 https://www.ncbi.nlm.nih.gov/pubmed/26381562

56. Cherniske S., Caffeine Blues: Wake Up to the Hidden Dangers of America's #1 Drug. 1st ed. New York: Warner Books Inc; 1998. Print.

57. E-Imports "How Many Cups of Coffee are Consumed Daily in the US?" Retrieved 3/01/2019, https://www.e-importz.com/coffee-statistics.php

58. Stevenson, Shawn. "Sleep Smarter." Model House Publishing, 2014. Print.

59. Gerben B. Keijzers, "Caffeine Can Decrease Insulin Sensitivity in Humans." Diabetes Care 2002 Feb; 25(2): 364-369, https://doi.org/10.2337/diacare.25.2.364

60. Chan, Casey "The Average American Drinks 45 Gallons of Soda a Year." 2011, JUNE 27th, https://www.gizmodo.com

61. Mercola, Joseph. "Give up Soda" Mercola. Jan. 10, 2018 https://articles.mercola.com/sites/articles/archive/2018/01/10/drinking-soda-health-risks.aspx

62. Briffa, John. "Aspartame and its effects on health Independently funded studies have found potential for adverse effects" BMJ. 2005 Feb 5; 330(7486): 309–310. https://www.ncbi.nlm.nih.gov/pmc/articles/PMC548217/

63. Food and Nutrition Board, "Dietary Reference Intakes: Water, Potassium, Sodium, Chloride, and Sulfate." 2004, FEB 11th https://www.nationalacademies.org

64. Mercola, Joseph. "Hydration is about More than Just Drinking Water – How to Hydrate at the Cellular Level to Improve Health and Longevity." 2018, MAY 6th https://www.articles.mercola.com

65. Axe, Josh. "7 Fulvic Acid Benefits & Uses: Improve Gut, Skin & Brain Health." 2017, OCT 12th https://www.draxe.com

66. Berkeley Wellness, "CDC: The Top 10 Public Health Achievements in the 20th Century." Retrieved on 8/13/2019, https://www.berkeleywellness.com

67. Neurath, C. (2005). "Tooth Decay Trends for 12-Year-Old in Non-fluoridated and fluoridated countries." Fluoride 38:324-325.

68. Pochelli, Marianna. "15 Facts Most People Don't Know About Fluoride." 2019, JULY 19th https://www.wakingtimes.com/2019/07/17/15-facts-most-people-dont-know-about-fluoride/

69. Richards, Byron. J. "Fight for Your Health, Exposing the FDA's Betrayal of America." Wellness Resource Books; 2006. Print.

70. Whitford GM. (1987a). Fluoride in dental products: safety considerations. Journal of Dental Research 66: 1056-60.

71. Fluoride Alert "Fluoride Content of Bottled Water." 2012 AUG. https://fluoridealert.org/content/bottled-water/

72. Michaels, Ann. "Top 5 Sources of Fluoride (It's Not your Toothpaste)" 2018, SEPT 19th https://www.cheeseslave.com/top-5-sources-of-fluoride-its-not-your-toothpaste-or-drinking-water/

73. DianeDi. "Water Fluoridation is a Crime. Dr. David Kennedy, D.D.S." YouTube, June 20, 2013. Web 10 December 2018.

74. "Chlorine." Wikipedia: The Free Encyclopedia. Wikimedia Foundation, Inc. 22 July 2004. Web. 12 December 2018, https://en.wikipedia.org/wiki/Chlorine

75. Ingram, Colin. "The Drinking Water Book: How to Eliminate Harmful Toxins from your Water"2nd ed. Berkley: Celestial Arts; 1991, 1995, 2006. Print.

76. Kogevinas, Manolis. "Genotoxic Effects in Swimmers Exposed to Disinfection By-Products in Indoor Swimming Pools" 12 September 2010, https://ehp.niehs.nih.gov/doi/10.1289/ehp.1001959

77. Mercola, Joseph. "Is Your Water Safe: How Modern Water Sanitation Can Damage Your Health" https://www.mercola.com/downloads/bonus/chlorine/default.htm

78. CDC. "Water Fluoridation Basics" 17 June 2016. https://www.cdc.gov/fluoridation/basics/index.htm

79. Group, Edward. "12 Toxins in Your Drinking Water" 3 May 2016. https://www.globalhealingcenter.com/natural-health/12-toxins-in-your-drinking-water/

80. Heil, DP "Acid-base balance and hydration status following consumption of mineral-based alkaline bottled water." J Int Soc Sports Nutr. 2010 Sep 13; 7:29. https://www.ncbi.nlm.nih.gov/pubmed/20836884

81. Link, Rachael, MS RD "Alkaline Water: Beneficial or All Hype?" 2018, OCT 4th, https://draxe.com/nutrition/article/alkaline-water/

82. Dr. Surat P, Ph.D. "pH in the Human Body." Retrieved on 8/17/2019 https://www.news-medical.net/health/pH-in-the-Human-Body.aspx

83. Aniys, Aqiyl "Drink Spring Water to Support the Health of Your Organs." 2016, JUNE 14th, https://www.naturallifeenergy.com/alkaline-water-benefits/

84. Wikipedia, "Electrolysis of Water" Retrieved on 8/18/2019 https://en.wikipedia.org/wiki/Electrolysis_of_water

85. Vivo Pathophysiology "Free Radicals and Reactive Oxygen." Retrieved on 8/18/2019 https://www/vivo.colostate.edu

86. Bestwater, "Ionized Water, also Known as "Microclustered" water." 2016, JULY 25th https://waterionizer.org

87. Canadian Wildlife Federation, "Eight Quotes That Illustrate Why Water is Life." https://www.blogcwf-fcf.org

CHAPTER 6

88. Stephenson, R.W. "Chiropractic Textbook," 1927, The Palmer School of Chiropractic. Print.

89. Harding, K. "Drank too much Water, Woman Dies." 2007, January 15th. https://www.theglobeandmail.com

90. JH Bloomberg School of Public Health, "Industrialization of Agriculture." http://www.foodsystemprimer.org

91. Peta, "The Chicken Industry." https://www.peta.org/issues/animals-used-for-food/factory-farming/chickens/chicken-industry/

92. Organic Consumers Association, "What's Wrong with Food Irradiation." 2002, February.

93. Mateljan, George, "The World's Healthiest Foods." https://www.whfoods.org

94. Wikipedia, "Max Gerson." https://www.wikipedia.org

95. Dr. Carney, "Big Industries Influence USDA Food Guidelines." https://www.drcarney.com

96. AnimalPlace (Website) "Life of a Dairy Cow." https://animalplace.org/life-dairy-cow/

97. Wikipedia, "Somatic Cell Count." 2019, March. 13th https://en.wikipedia.org/wiki/Somatic_cell_count

98. Healthy Holistic Living, "How Pasteurized Dairy Destroys Your Bones from the Inside." 2016, Jan. 16th, https://www.healthy-holistic-living.com

99. Harkinson, Josh. "Turns Out Your Hormone-Free Milk is Full of Sex Hormones." 2014, April, http://www.motherjones.com

100. Maruyama K1, Oshima T, Ohyama K. "Exposure to exogenous estrogen through intake of commercial milk produced from pregnant cows." https://www.ncbi.nlm.nih.gov/pubmed/19496976

101. Hormone Clinic (Website) "Bone Loss and 5 Other Symptoms of Low Testosterone in Men." 2017, FEB 15th, https://www.hormoneclinics.com

102. Info Clinic (Website); Julian Whitaker, MD "Cow Milk, Milk: A Deadly Poison." https://www.infoclinic.co.za

103. Organic Authority (Website) "61 Names for Sugar Used to Sweeten Your Food." 2018, OCT. 22nd, https://www.organicauthority.com

104. Sugar Science, "How much is Too Much? The Growing Concern Over Too Much Added Sugar in our Diets." https://www.sugarscience.ucsf.ed

105. Cherney, K. "Simple Carbohydrates Vs. Complex Carbohydrates." https://www.healthline.com

106. Wikipedia, "Glycemic Index," https://en.wikipedia.org/wiki/Glycemic_index

107. IDM, "Understanding Digestion: Why You Should Eat Carbohydrates with Fat, Fibre, and Vinegar." https://www.idmprogram.com

108. Diabetes.co.uk (website) "Insulin." https://www.diabetes.co.uk/body/insulin.html

109. Stanford Health Care (Website), "How PET Scans Work." https://www.stanfordhealthcare.org

110. Hewing-Martin, Y, "Sugar and Cancer: A Surprise Connection or a 50-Year-Cover-Up." 2017, Nov. 24th, https://www.medicalnewstoday.com

111. Gershenson, G. "A Brief and Bizarre History of Artificial Sweeteners." 2017, Feb. 23rd https://www.saveur.com

112. Healthline Editorial Team, "The Truth About Aspartame Side Effects." https://www.healthline.com

113. Mohamed, Benyagoub & EL-Masry, Eman & Abdel-Rahman, Ali & Mclendon, Roger & Schiffman, Susan. (2008). Splenda Alters Gut Microflora and Increases Intestinal P-Glycoprotein and Cytochrome P-450 in Male Rats. Journal of toxicology and environmental health. Part A. 71. 1415-29. 10.1080/15287390802328630.

114. Hardick, BJ. "Does Stevia Make You Sterile," 2016, June. 15th https://www.drhardick.com

115. Healthline (website), "Xylitol: Everything You Need to Know." https://www.healthline.com

116. Nora T. Gedgaudas, CNS, CNT. "Primal Body, Primal Mind" 2009, Nora T. Gedgaudas. Print.

117. Judith Shaw, M.A. "Trans Fats – The Hidden Killer in our Food," 2004, Pocket Books. Print.

118. Carnivore Aurelius, "How Ancel Keys Brainwashed the Masses into Fearing Meat (He's Wrong)." https://www.carnivoreaurelius.com/ancel-keys/

119. Fell, James, "10 Things We Learned from Jack Lalanne." 2011, Jan. 31st https://www.chatelaine.com

120. Mercola, Joseph, "Fat for Fuel: A Revolutionary Diet to Combat Cancer, Boost Brain Power, and Increase Your Energy." 2018, Hay House Inc. Print.

121. Salynn Boyle, "Trans Fat May Increase Infertility." 2007, JAN. 12th https://www.webmd.com

122. Cherney, Kristine, "5 Ways to Avoid Hydrogenated Oil." 2018, JULY 31st, https://www.healthline.com

123. Center for Science in The Public Interest, (CSPI) "Trans Fat." https://www.cspinet.org

124. Mercola, Joseph "What are Coconuts Good For?" 2016, OCT 13th. https://www.foodfacts.mercola.com

125. Pasquale, Neka, "What are Fats? The Real Skinny on Healthy Fats and Harmful Fats." 2017, JULY 18th, https://www.urbanremedy.com

126. Freydis Hjalmarsdottir, "17-Science-Based Benefits of Omega-3 Fatty Acids." 2018, Oct. 15th, https://www.Healthline.com

127. Zimmerman, Edith "What is Autophagy?" 2019, APRIL 25th. https://www.thecut.com

128. Bragg, Paul Chappius., and Patricia Bragg. The miracle of fasting: for Agelessness-Physical, Mental & Spiritual Rejuvenation: New Discoveries About an Old Miracle--The "Fast" Fasting Way to Health Science, 1983. Print.

129. Mercola, Joseph, "The Beginners Guide to Intermittent Fasting." 2013, NOV. 8th, https://www.fitness.mercola.com

130. Dr. David E., and Daniel L. Root, "Sauna Detoxification Using Niacin: Following the Recommended Protocol of Dr. Davie E. Root." Dan Root, 2019

131. Tello, Monique MD, MPH, "Eat More Plants, Fewer Animals." 2018, November 29th https://www.health.harvard.edu

132. J. Agric. Food Chem., 1998, 46, 1, 206-210

133. Quan R, et al. Pediatrics, 1992 Apr;89 (4 Pt 1): 667-9

134. Harvard Health, "Microwave Cooking and Nutrition." 2019, FEB. 6th. https://www/health.harvard.edu

135. Ducharme, Jamie, "Eating too Quickly May be Bad for Your Health." 2017, NOV. 14th, https://www.time.com

136. Price, Annie. "Pink Himalayan Salt Benefits: Better Than Regular Salt?" 2019, AUG. 19th, https://www.draxe.com

CHAPTER 7

137. "Western Pattern Diet" https://en.wikipedia.org/wiki/Western_pattern_diet

138. Wigmore, Ann. "The Wheatgrass Book" Wigmore, Ann 1985

139. "Why Wheatgrass is a Super-Powerful Health Food" http://www.healthymuslim.com/articles/izogj-why-wheatgrass-is-a-super-powerful-health-food.cfm

140. Link, Rachel, MS, RD, "7 Evidence-Based Benefits of Wheatgrass." 21, Feb. 2018 www.healthline.com

141. Villines, Zawn. "What are the Benefits of Wheatgrass?" 2017, 3. Dec. www.medicalnewstoday.com

142. NCBI, "How Does the Liver Work?" www.ncbi.nlm.nih.gov/books/nbk279393/

143. ACG, "Non-Alcoholic Fatty Liver Disease." http://patients.gi.org/topics/fatty-liver-disease-nafld/

144. NIH, "Definition & Facts of NAFLD & NASH." https://www.niddk.nih.gov/health-information/liver-disease/nafld-nash/definition-facts

145. Durairaj V, et al. "Effect of Wheatgrass on Membrane Fatty Acid Composition During Hepatotoxicity Induced by Alcohol and Heated PUFA" Journal of Membrane Biology, Jun;247(6):515-21, https//www.ncbi.nlm.nih.gov/m/pubmed/24706101/

146. Daya, Shabir. "Go Super Green with Chlorophyll." https://www.victoriahealth.com/editorial/go-super-green-with-chlorophyll

CHAPTER 8

147. Ergotron, "Almost 70% of Full Time American Workers Hate Sitting, but They Do it all Day Every Day." 2013, JULY 17th, https://www.prnewswire.com

148. "Prolonged Sitting Responsible for More Than 430,000 Deaths." 2016, MARCH 24th https://www.medicalnewstoday.com

149. University of Illinois, "Brief Diversions Vastly Improve Focus, Researchers Find." 2011, FEB 8th, https://www.sciencedaily.com/releases/2011/02/110208131529.htm

150. Kilpatrick, M., Sanderson, K., Blizzard, L., Teale, B., Venn, A. (2013), Cross-sectional associations between sitting at work and psychological distress: Reducing sitting time may benefit mental health. Mental Health and Physical Activity, 6(2), 103–109.

151. University of Cambridge, "Lack of Exercise Responsible for Twice as Many Deaths as Obesity." American Journal of Clinical Nutrition; 14 Jan 2015, https://www.cam.ac.uk

152. Firger, Jessica, "When Moms Exercise, So Do Kids." 2014, MARCH 24th https://www.cbsnews.com/news/when-moms-exercise-so-do-kids/

153. Slordahl, S.A., Madslien, V.O., Støylen, A., Kjos, A., Helgerud, J., and Wisloff, U. (2004). Atrioventricular plane displacement in untrained and trained females. Medicine and Science in Sports and Exercise, 36(11), 1871-1875.

154. Anderson, Charlotte, "Eight Benefits of High Intensity Interval Training (HIIT)." https://www.shape.com/fitness/workouts/8-benefits-high-intensity-interval-training-hiit

155. Quinn, Elizabeth "Interval training Workouts Build Speed and Endurance." 2019, MARCH 12th, https://www.verywellfit.com

156. Perry CG, Heigenhauser GJ, Bonen A, Spriet LL, "High-intensity Aerobic Interval Training Increases Fat and Carbohydrate Metabolic Capacities in Human Skeletal Muscle." Appl Physio Nutr Metab. 2008 Dec;33(6):1112-23. https://www.ncbi.nlm.nih.gov/pubmed/19088769/

157. ACSM, "High Intensity Interval Training." https://www.acsm.org/docs/default-source/files-for-resource-library/high-intensity-interval-training.pdf?sfvrsn=b0f72be6_2

158. "Testosterone Responses to Intensive Interval Versus Steady-State Endurance Exercise." Retrieved on 8/19/2019, J Endocrinol Invest. 2012 Dec;35(11) https://www.ncbi.nlm.nih.gov/pubmed/23310924

159. Hayes LD, Herbert P, Grace FM, "HIIT Produces Increases in Muscle Power and Free Testosterone in Male Masters Athletes." Endocrine Connections 2017 Oct; 6(7): 430-436 https://www.ncbi.nlm.nih.gov

160. L. Jonathan, E. Monique, "Effectiveness and Safety of High-Intensity Interval Training in Patients with Type 2 Diabetes." Diabetes Spectrum. 2015 Jan; 28(1): 39-44 https://www.ncbi.nlm.gov

161. Brain, Marshal, "Is it Harmful to Breathe 100- Percent Oxygen?" https://science.howstuffworks.com/question493.htm

162. National Heart, Lung, and Blood Institute, "How the Lungs Work." https://www.nhlbi.nih.gov/health-topics/how-lungs-work

163. Rakhimov, Artour. "Breath Control (Regulation of Respiration): O2 vs. CO2" 2018, AUG 9th, https://www.normalbreathing.com/CO2-breath-control.php

164. Brown, Ann, "How Many Breaths Do You Take Each Day?" 2014, APRIL. 28th Blog Blog.epa.gov

165. Rakhimov, Artour "Exercise Effects on the Respiratory System: Short – and Long-Term CO2 Changes." 2018, AUG 9th https://www.normalbreathing.com/c-effects-of-exercise-on-the-respiratory-system.php

166. Sloan, Jim "How to Improve Heart and Lung Strength." https://www.livestrong.com/article/429497-how-to-improve-heart-lung-strength/

167. Wikipedia, "Buteyko Method." https://en.wikipedia.org/wiki/Buteyko_method

168. McKeown, Patrick, "The Oxygen Advantage." HarperCollins, 2015, Print.

169. Rifkin, Rachael, "How Shallow Breathing Affects Your Whole Body." https://www.headspace.com/blog

170. Faceology, posted by Sarah, "Mouth Breathing Article by Patrick McKeown." 2015, APRIL 5th, https://www.myfaceology.com

171. Tanner, Claudia "Struggling to Lose Weight? The Way you BREATHE May Be to Blame..." 2017, AUG 30th, https://www.Dailymail.co.uk/health

172. Healthline, "5 Ways to Increase Nitric Oxide Naturally." https://www.healthline.com

173. Rakhimov, Artour, "Running Benefits: Higher Body O2 Only with Nose Breathing" 2018, AUG 9th https://www.normalbreathing.com

174. Pollock, Anastasia, "The Power of Breath in Calming the Nervous System." 2016, NOV. 30th, https://www.goodtherapy.org

175. Cohen, Andrew, "Breathing is Crucial; I Like Tony Robbin's Approach to Breathing" 2011, SEPT. 3rd, https://www.proactivesf.com/2011/09/breathing-is-crucial-i-like-tony-robbins-approach-to-breathing/

176. Ruggeri, Christine, "Hyperbaric Oxygen Therapy Benefits for Specific Healing." 2019, JUNE 7th, https://www.draxe.com (Blog)

177. Krishnamurti, Chandrasekhar, "Historical Aspects of Hyperbaric Physiology and Medicine." 2019, APRIL 18th. https://www.intechopen.com/online-first/historical-aspects-of-hyperbaric-physiology-and-medicine

178. McCabe, Ed, "Flood Your Body with Oxygen." Ed McCabe, 2003. – 6th edition. Print.

179. Howell, Taras, "Why do Athletes Use Hyperbaric Oxygen Therapy." https://www.progressivemedicalcenter.com

180. Vadas, Dor & Kalichman, Leonid & Hadanny, Amir & Efrati, Shai. (2017). Hyperbaric Oxygen Environment Can Enhance Brain Activity and Multitasking Performance. Frontiers in Integrative Neuroscience. 11.25.

181. Veronique Desaulniers, "Can Hyperbaric Oxygen Therapy Help Heal Cancer?" 2017, JAN. 24th https://beatcancer.org/blog-posts/can-hyperbaric-oxygen-therapy-help-heal-cancer

182. Poff AM, Ari C, Seyfried TN, D'Agostino DP. The ketogenic diet and hyperbaric oxygen therapy prolong survival in mice with systemic metastatic cancer. PLoS One. 2013;8(6): e): e65522.

Published 2013 Jun 5. doi: 10.1371/journal.ponedoi: 10.1371/journal.pone.0065522

183. Greenfield, Ben, "A Surgeon's Little-Known Secret to Biohacking Your Body with Oxygen Therapy." https://www.Bengreenfieldfitness.com

184. Science Meets Nature (website) "LiveO2 is Exercise with Oxygen Therapy (EWOT): Oxygen Multistep Therapy." https://www.sciencemeetsnature.org

185. Ruggeri, Christine, "What is Exercise with Oxygen Therapy." 2019, MAY 17th https://draxe.com/health/treatments/ewot-exercise-with-oxygen-therapy/

186. Harvard Medical School, "Strength Training Builds More Than Muscles." https://www.Health.harvard.edu

187. Chris Iliades, MD "7 Ways Strength Training Boosts Your Health and Fitness." 2019, MAY 5th, https://www.everydayhealth.com

188. Harvard, School of Public Health, "Weight Training Associated with Reduced Risk of Type 2 Diabetes." 2012, AUG. 6th, https://www.hsph.harvard.edu.com

189. Airborne Academy, "The Importance of Stretching." 2019, JAN 15th https://www.airborneomaha.com

190. Greenfield, Ben. "Beyond Training." Ben Greenfield, 2014. Print.

190. Dolen, Michelle, "How to Stretch." 2019, June 21st https://www.wikihow/stretch.com

191. Athletico, "What is a Muscle Knot and How to Treat it." 2014, MAY 1st https://www.athletico.com/2014/05/01/what-is-a-muscle-knot/

192. Santa Barbara Deep Tissue "Fascia Massage, and Fuzz." 2019, JULY 18th https://www.Santabarbaradeeptissue.com

193. Wikipedia, "Fascia." Retrieved on 9/9/2019 https://en.wikipedia.org/wiki/Fascia#cite_note-15

194. Notable Quotes, "Jack Lalanne Quotes." Retrieved on 9/10/2019 https://www.notable-quotes.com

CHAPTER 9

195. Environmental Working Group, Body Burden: The Pollution in Newborns, 2005, JULY 14th, https://www.ewg.org/research/body-burden-pollution-newborns

196. Dr. David E., and Daniel L. Root, "Sauna Detoxification Using Niacin: Following the Recommended Protocol of Dr. Davie E. Root." Dan Root, 2019. Print.

197. The people's Chemist (blog). "How the AMA Hooks You on Drugs, Harms Your Health and Hurts the Earth." May 11th, 2011, 2011, https://thepeopleschemist.com

198. Dr. Baillie-Hamillton, Paula "The Detox Diet: Eliminate Chemical Calories and Restore Your Body's Natural Slimming System." Hamilton, 2012

199. "What in the World Are They Spraying." G. Edward Griffin, Michael Murphy, Paul Wittenberger

200. https://www.geoengineeringwatch.org/

201. Mitchel, Jamie. "On This Day in 1961: JFK Reveals 'Weather Control' Plans." https://www.bluegreentomorrow.com

202. https://www.raytheon.com

203. FPO, "Creation of Artificial Ionization Clouds Above the Earth." http://www.freepatentsonline.com/4999637.html

204. Watts, Jonathan, "Geoengineering May Be Used to Combat Global Warming Experts Say." 2018, OCT. 8th, https://www.theguardian.com

205. Walia, Arjun. "If You Think That These are Just Contrails, Think Again: Here's What They Really Are." 2013, 29th April, https://www.collective-evolution.com

206. Chemtrail Research, "Dr. Russel Blaylock Talks About Chemtrails." YouTube, Oct. 14th, 2016. Web July 2019

207. Alzheimer's Association, "Facts and Figures." https://www/alz.org

208. Ultra Cleanse Guide. "Bentonite Detox" July 10th https://www.ultracleanseguide.com

209. West, Jim, "Pesticides and Polio: A Critique of Scientific Literature." 2003, FEB. 8th https://www.westonaprice.org

210. Peter Miller "Suzanne Humphreys, MD, Speaking on Polio and DDT." Published on June 10th, 2013, 2013, https://www.youtube.com/watch?v=rZMn7oapJD4&t=146s

211. Merriam Webster (online) definition of polio, https://www.merriam-webster.com/dictionary/polio

212. Brogan, Kelly MD "What We Can Learn From DDT." https://kellybroganmd.com/can-learn-ddt/

213. CDC, "National Biomonitoring Program, DDT," https://www.cdc.gov

214. Find Law, "Monsanto PCB Lawsuits." www.https://injury.findlaw.com

215. Seattle Organic Restaurants, "The 10 Poisons That are the Legacy of Monsanto." https://www.seattleorganicrestaurants. com

216. Woodruff, Tracey, "UCSF Study Identifies Chemicals in Pregnant Women." 2011, JAN. 14th, https://www.ucsf.edu

217. Fandom, "Agent Orange," https://www.vietnamwar.fandom. com/wiki/agen_orange

218. Ruggeri, Christine, "Monsanto Lawsuit: Agricultural Giant Ordered to Pay $289 Million in Cancer Case." 2018, AUG 23rd, https://draxe.com

219. Honeycutt, Zen, "Glyphosate Found in Childhood Vaccines." 2016, SEPT 10th https://www.ecowatch.com

220. Kaja, "Have GMOs Been Around for Centuries." 2016, July 24th https://ichooseorganic.wordpress.com/2016/07/24/have-gmos-been-around-for-centuries/

221. Hilbeck, Angelika, "No Scientific Consensus on GMO Safety." 2015, JAN 24th Journal of Environmental Sciences Europe https://enveurope.springeropen.com/articles/10.1186/s12302-014-0034-1

222. "10 Reasons to Avoid GMOs." Retrieved on 07/17/2019 https://responsibletechnology.org/10-reasons-to-avoid-gmos/

223. Wikipedia, "TAPPED (Film)" https://en.wikipedia.org/wiki/Tapped_(film)

224. Made Safe, "How to Avoid Toxic Chemicals in Plastics." 2016, DEC 13th https://www.madesafe.org

225. Pawlowski, A. "Left Your Bottled Water in a Hot Car? Drink it with Caution, Some Experts Say." 2018, JULY 6th https://

www.today.com/health/bottled-water-hot-plastic-may-leech-chemicals-some-experts-say-t132687

226. NaturallySavvy.com "How to Avoid BPA Exposure from Cash Receipts." Retrieved on 07/18/2019, https://health.howstuffworks.com

227. Sholl, Jessie. Experience Life (Blog) "8 Hidden Toxins: What's Lurking in Your Cleaning Products." Oct. 2011, https://experiencelife.com

228. Grace, Emily. "Cleaning without Chemicals: Thieves Household Cleaner" https://www.graceandgoodeats.com

229. Moram, Stephanie. "Homemade Cleaners Using Vinegar" https://goodgirlgonegreen.com

230. Michael, Dawn. "Toxic Carpet: Dangerous Chemicals that Live in Your Carpeting." http://www.greenandhealthy.info/toxiccarpeting.html

231. Schrock, Monica. "Is My Makeup Toxic" May 9th, 2018, 2018 https://www.nontoxicrevolution.com

232. Congletan, Johanna. "Exposing the Cosmetics Cover up: Is Cancer-Causing Formaldehyde in Your Cosmetics." https://www.ewg.org

233. PD Darbe, "Aluminum, Antiperspirants and Breast Cancer." J Inorg Biochem. 2005 Sep;99(9):1912-9, https://www.ncbi.nlm.nih.gov

234. Skincare Ox, "20 Best Organic Shampoos That are Actually Non-Toxic." https://www.skincareox.com/20-best-organic-shampoos-that-are-actually-non-toxic/

235. Ingram, Colin. "The Drinking Water Book: How to Eliminate Harmful Toxins from your Water" 2nd ed. Berkley: Celestial Arts; 1991, 1995, 2006. Print.

236. Scranton, Alex. "Toxic Tampons." 2014, June 30th https://www.womensvoices.org/2014/06/30/toxic-tampons/

237. Nelson, Marilee, "Dangerous Detergent: Is My Laundry Soap Toxic?" 2018, MAY 2nd, https://www.branchbasics.com

238. Laforge, John. "Mammograms Still Doing More Harm than Good." 2012, SEPT 20th https://duluthreader.com

239. Kresser, Chris. "The Downside of Mammograms." 2017, APRIL 6th https://kresserinstitute.com/the-downside-of-mammograms/

240. Mercola, Joseph. "Your Greatest Weapon Against Breast Cancer (Not Mammograms)." https://www.articles.mercola.com

241. Chun, Christina. "Comparing Mammography and Thermography." 2019, JUL 22nd https://www.medicalnewstoday.com

242. Fischer, Mary, "When Medicine Makes You Sick." Retrieved online 07/23/1019 AARP The Magazine, Sept/Oct. 2010 Issue. https://www.aarp.com

243. Bishop, Vic. CNN and NBC Caught Faking Photo of Baby with Measles." 2019, APRIL 25th https://www.wakingtimes.com

244. California Legislative Information, SB-276 Immunizations: Medical Exemptions. (2019-1000) Author Senator Richard Pan. https://leginfo.legislature.ca.gov/faces/billTextClient.xhtml?bill_id=201920200SB276

245. O'Shea, Tim. "Vaccination Is Not Immunization." 14th Edition Immunization ltd 14 Edition. Print.

246. Pappas, Stephanie. "How Do Vaccines Work?" 2010, JUNE 1st https://livescience.com

247. "Measles Outbreak in a Highly Vaccinated Population – Israel, July – August 2017." 2018, OCT. 26th, https://www.cdc.gov

248. Karlamangla, Soumya. "30 Harvard-Westlake Students Diagnosed with Whooping Cough Amid Wider Outbreak." 2019, FEB 27th, https://www.latimes.com

249. Seck, Hope. "Navy Ship Changes Schedule After Outbreak of Mumps-Like Disease Aboard." 2019, MAR 15th, https://www.military.com

250. My Health Alberta, "Parotitis: Care Instructions." https://www.myhealth.alberta.ca

251. Dorey, S. "Louis Pasteur Recants His Germ Theory." http://www.susandoreydesigns.com/insights/pasteur-recant.html

252. Humphries, Suzanne, and Bystrianyk, Roman. Dissolving Illusions: Disease, Vaccines, and the Forgotten History." 2013, Print.

253. Arthur Charles Cole, "The Irrepressible Conflict 1850-1865: A History of American Life Volume VII, Macmillan, New York," 1934, p. 181. Taken from Dissolving Illusions

254. Merriam Webster, definition of cesspool https://www.merriam-webster.com/dictionary/cesspool

255. Bernard Guyer, MD, Mary Anne Freeman, MA, Donna M. Strobino, PhD, Edward J. Sondik, PhD., Pediatrics, Dec 2000, Vol. 106, No. 6.

256. "Antione Bechamp" Retrieved on 8/07/2019 https://www.Arizonaenergy.org/bodyenergy/antione_bechamp.htm

257. JB Handley, "The Impact of vaccines on Mortality Decline Since 1900 – According to Published Science." 2019, MARCH 12th https://childrenshealthdefense.org/news/the-impact-of-vaccines-on-mortality-decline-since-1900-according-to-pub-lished-science/

258. Walter, Edward. Scott, Mike. "The Life and Work of Rudolf Virchow 1821-1902: "Cell Theory, Thrombosis and the Sausage Duel." J Intensive Care Soc. 2017 Aug; 18(3): 234-235

259. Szalay, Jessie. "Black Mamba Facts," 2014, DEC 22nd https://www.livescience.com/43559-black-mamba.html

260. Gherardi RK, Aouizerate J, Cadusseau J, Yara S, Authier FJ. "Aluminum Adjuvants of Vaccines Injected into the Muscle: Normal Fate, Pathology and Associated Disease. Morphologie. 2016 Jun;100(329):85-94. doi: 10.1016/j.morpho.2016.01.002. Epub 2016 Apr 6., https://www.ncbi.nlm.nih.gov/pubmed/26948677 https://www.learntherisk.org/injection/

261. Shaw CA, Tomljenovic L. "Aluminum in the Central Nervous System (CNS): Toxicity in Humans and Animals, Vaccine Adjuvants, and Auto-Immunity. Journal of Immunology Research 2013 July; 56(2-3): 304-16 https://www.ncbi.nlm.nih.gov/pubmed/23609067

262. Focus for Health, "Vaccine Adverse Events Reporting System (VAERS) https://www.focusforhealth.org

263. Lyon-Weiler, J. Rickerson, R. "Reconsideration of the Immunotherapeutic Pediatric Safe Dose Levels of Aluminum." Journal of Trace Elements in Medicine and Biology Vo. 48, 2018, JULY, pages 67-73 https://www.sciencedirect.com/science/article/pii/S0946672X17300950

264. "Babies are Getting More than 1,000 Micrograms of Aluminum in Vaccines." 2017, AUG. 12th https://vaccinesbytheoutliers.

wordpress.com/2017/08/12/babies-are-getting-more-than-1000-micrograms-of-aluminum-in-vaccines/

265. Redshaw, Megan. "God Does Not Support Vaccines." 2014, JULY 7th https://www.livingwhole.org. Referenced source: https://www.cdc.gov/vaccines/pubs/pinkbook/downloads/appendices/b/excipient-table-2.pdf

266. Deisher TA, Doan NV, et al. "Impact of Environmental Factors on the Prevalence of Autistic Disorder after 1979." J Public Health Epidemiology 2014 Sep; 6(9): 271-86.

267. Deisher, Theresa. "Open Letter to Legislators Regarding Fetal Cell DNA in Vaccines." https://healthimpactnews.com/2019/fetal-dna-contaminants-found-in-mercks-measles-vaccines/

268. Mostafa et al. 2014, J Neuroimmunol, Vol. 272, pp. 94–98;98. Mostafa et al. 2015, J Neuroimmunol, Vol. 280, pp. 16–20

269. Group, Edward. "The Hidden Formaldehyde in Everday Products." 2015, OCT 21st https://www.globalhealingcenter.com/natural-health/formaldehyde/

270. Reference, "What Foods Contain Formaldehyde?" https://www.reference.com/food/foods-contain-formaldehyde-704cb5d19fe0e730

271. CDC, "What's in Vaccines?" https://www.cdc.gov/vaccines/vac-gen/additives.htm

272. Tenpenny, Sherry "Formaldehyde in Vaccines" 2013, JAN 29th http://tenpennyimc.com/2013/01/29/formaldehyde-in-vaccines/

273. Vaxopedia, "Polysorbate in Vaccines." https://vaxopedia.org/2016/09/07/polysorbate-80-in-vaccines/

274. Pardridge, William. "The Blood-Brain Barrier: Bottleneck in Brain Drug Development" NeuroRx. 2005 Jan; 2(1): 3–14. https://www.ncbi.nlm.nih.gov/pmc/articles/PMC539316/

275. Parpia, Rishma "Polysorbate 80: A Risky Vaccine Ingredient." 2019, AUG 9th https://healthimpactnews.com/2016/polysorbate-80-a-risky-vaccine-ingredient/

276. Truth Wiki "Mercury in Vaccines." https://www.truthwiki.org

277. Kennedy, Robert. "Mercury in Vaccines." Retrieved on 8/10/2019 https://www.childrenshealthdefense.org

278. Piper-Terry, Marcella. "Dr. Oz Warns About Mercury in Flu Shots." Retrieved on 8/10/2019, https://www.healthimpactnews.com, https://www.vaxtruth.org

279. World Truth "List of Vaccine Ingredients and Their Known Side Effects" Retrieved on 8/10/2019, https://www.worldtruth.tv

280. Neustaedter, Randall "The Vaccine Guide, Making an Informed Choice." 1996 North Atlantic Books

281. HRSA "National Vaccine Injury Compensation Program." https://www.hrsa.gov

282. Kids Health "Immunization Schedule." https://www.kidshealth.org

283. Skeptical Raptor "Argument by Vaccine Package Inserts – They're not Infallible." https://www.skepticalraptor.com

284. Parpia, Rishma "Is There a Link Between Vaccines and the Rise in Pediatric Cancer." 2018, MAY 28th https://thevaccinereaction.org

285. Freed, David MLS, "The Vaccine Controversy, Does the Benefit Outweigh the Risk? 2011, DEC 1st, https://www.ponderingconfusion.com

286. Christoff, Jason, "Common Sense Vaccine Questions to Ask Your Doctor." Blog, https://www.Jchristoff.com

287. Adventures in Autism "We Finally Get a Vaxxed v. Unvaxxed Study, Vaccinated Primates Have Brain Changes Seen in Autism" 2010, JULY 15th https://adventuresinautism.blogspot.com/2010/07/we-finally-get-vaxxed-v-unvaxxed-study.html

288. Passingham, Richard "How Good is the Macaque Monkey Model of the Human Brain?" Current Opinion in Neurobiology Volume 19, Issue 1, February 2009, Pages 6-11 https://www.sciencedirect.com

289. Law Firms "CDC Members Own More than 50 Patents Connected to Vaccinations." https://www.lawfirms.com

290. FDA "The FDA's Drug Review Process: Ensuring Drugs are Safe and Effective." https://www.fda.gov

291. McGovern, Celeste. "Vaccinated vs. Unvaccinated: Mawson Homeschooled Study Reveals Who is Sicker." 2019, MARCH 14th. https://www.Prepareforchange.net

292. Handley, J.B. "How to End the Autism Epidemic." Chelsea Green Publishing, [2018]

293. http://www.vacinfo.org/educate.html

294. Fisher, Loe Barbara "Is the Childhood Vaccine Schedule Safe?" 2017, OCT. 1 https://www.nvic.org/nvic-vaccine-news/october-2017/is-the-childhood-vaccine-schedule-safe.aspx

295. Dr. Levine, B Jonathan, "Toxic Teeth: Are Amalgam Fillings Safe?" Retrieved on 9/11/2019 https://www.doctoroz.com/article/toxic-teeth-are-our-amalgam-fillings-safe

296. Kroschel, Steve, "The Beautiful Truth" Film, 2008

297. Weintraub, Karen, "Can You Sweat Out Toxins?" 2017, AUG. 18th https://www.nytimes.com

CHAPTER 10

298. National Institutes of Health, "How Sleep Clears the Brain." https://www.nih.gov/news-events/nih-research-matters/how-sleep-clears-brain

299. CDC, "Perceived Insufficient Rest or Sleep." https://www.cdc.gov/mmwr/preview/mmwrhtml/mm5708a2.htm

300. Mark R. Rosekind, PhD, Kevin B. Gregory, BS, Melissa M. Mallis, PhD, Summer L. Brandt, MA, Brian Seal, PhD, and Debra Lerner, PhD "The Cost of Poor Sleep: Workplace Productivity Loss and Associated Costs." JOEM • Volume 52, Number 1, January 2010 http://www.norcalbaa.org/uploads/NCBAA_ARTICLES_20110825_Alertness_Solutions_Cost_of_Poor_Sleep.pdf

301. www.tuck.com "Stages of Sleep and Sleep Cycles." https://www.tuck.com/stages/

302. www.tuck.com "Sleep and Human Growth Hormone." https://www.tuck.com/sleep-hgh/

303. J R Davidson, H Moldofsky, and F. A. Lue "Growth Hormone and Cortisol Secretion in Relation to Sleep and Wakefulness." J Psychiatry Neurosci. 1991 Jul; 16(2): 96–102. https://www.ncbi.nlm.nih.gov/pmc/articles/PMC1188300/

304. Millard Elizabeth. "The Cortisol Curve." March 2016 https://experiencelife.com/article/the-cortisol-curve/

305. Brazier, Yvette, "Sleep Well to Avoid Insulin Resistance." 2015, NOV. 4th https://www.medicalnewstoday.com

306. Taheri S, Lin L, Austin D, Young T, Mignot E (2004) "Short Sleep Duration is Associated with Reduced Leptin, Elevated Ghrelin, and Increased Body Mass Index." PLoS Med 1(3): e62

307. Gittleman, Ann. "ZAPPED: Why Your Cell Phone Shouldn't be your Alarm Clock and 1,268 Ways to Outsmart the Hazards of Electronic Pollution," New York, HarperCollins, 2011. Print.

308. Dun-Xian Tan, "Melatonin and Brain." Current Neuropharmacology. 2010 Sep; 8(3): 161. https://www.ncbi.nlm.nih.gov/pmc/articles/PMC3001209/

309. Stevenson, Shawn. "Sleep Smarter." Model House Publishing, 2014. Print.

310. Wikipedia, "Suprachiasmatic Nucleus." https://www.en.m.wikipedia.org

311. Wooten Virgil, "How to Fall Asleep." Howstuffworks.com https://health.howstuffworks.com/mental-health/sleep/basics/how-to-fall-asleep2.htm

312. Lewis, Tanya. "How the Brain Resets its Biological Clock." 5, June. 2013 LiveScience https://www.livescience.com/37179-how-brain-sets-its-clock.html

313. Tan DX, Xu B, Zhou X, "Pineal Calcification, Melatonin Production, Aging, Associated Health Consequences and Rejuvenation of the Pineal Gland." Reiter RJ2.Molecules. 2018 Jan 31;23(2). https://www.ncbi.nlm.nih.gov/pubmed/29385085

314. Cherniske S. Caffeine Blues: Wake Up to the Hidden Dangers of America's #1 Drug. 1st ed. New York: Warner Books Inc; 1998. Print.

315. Mann, Denise. "Alcohol and a Good Night's Sleep Don't Mix." 2013, January, 13 https://www.webmd.com/sleep-disorders/news/20130118/alcohol-sleep#1

316. Sleep Doctor "The Truth About Alcohol and Sleep." https://www.thesleepdoctor.com/2017/11/15/truth-alcohol-sleep/

317. Merriam Webster, definition of white noise. https://www.merriam-webster.com

318. Sleep Doctor "Understanding CBD: The Calming and Sleep Promoting Benefits of Cannabidiol." https://thesleepdoctor.com

319. Jamison, Jr. "Insomnia: Does Chiropractic Help?" JMPT. 2005 Mar-Apr; 28(3):179-86. https://www.ncbi.nlm.nih.gov/m/pubmed/15855906/

320. NIH "Brain Basics: Understanding Sleep." https://www.ninds.nih.gov/Disorders/Patient-Caregiver-Education/Understanding-Sleep

321. Upper Cervical Awareness, "How Upper Cervical Chiropractic Helps Fight Insomnia." https://uppercervicalawareness.com/how-upper-cervical-chiropractic-helps-fight-insomnia/

322. Chevalier G, Sinatra S, Sokal P, "Earthing: Health Implications off Reconnecting the Human Body to the Earth's Surface Electrons." Journal of Environmental Public Health. 2012; Published online 2012 Jan 12th Ncbi.nlm.nih.gov

CHAPTER 11

323. Bellis, Mary. "Who Created Wi-Fi? Everything you Need to Know about Wireless Internet." 29 Sept. 2018. https://www.thoughtco.com/who-invented-wifi-1992663

324. Physics Wiki. "Electromagnetic Radiation" http://physics.wikia.com/wiki/Electromagnetic_radiation

325. Halpern, Jonathan. "Electromagnetic Radiation Survival Guide: Step by Step Solutions." Halpern, Jonathan; 2013. Print.

326. Statista. Number of Smartphone Users in the United States from 2010 to 2022 (in millions). https://www.statista.com/statistics/201182/forecast-of-smartphone-users-in-the-us/

327. Daws, Ryan. "Research: 90% of US Consumers Own a Smart Home Device." IoT News, 15 May 2008. https://www.iottechnews.com/news/2018/may/15/research-us-consumers-smart-home-device/

328. Plante, Amber. "How the Human Body Uses Electricity." University of Maryland Graduate School. https://www.graduate.umaryland.edu/gsa/gazette/February-2016/How-the-human-body-uses-electricity/

329. Gittleman, Ann. "ZAPPED: Why Your Cell Phone Shouldn't be your Alarm Clock and 1,268 Ways to Outsmart the Hazards of Electronic Pollution" New York, HarperCollins, 2011. Print.

330. Bioinitiative 2012, https://www.bioinitiative.org/

331. Dellorto, Danielle, CNN, "Cell Phone Use Can Increase Possible Cancer Risk." 31 May 2011 http://www.cnn.com

332. McGlade, Jacqueline, European Environment Agency. "Statement on Mobile Phones for Conference on Cell Phones and Health: Science and Public Policy Questions." Washington 15 Sept. 2009. www.emrpolicy.org

333. Marjanovic Cermak AM, Pavicic I, Trosic I, "Oxidative Stress Response in SH-SY5Y Cells Exposed to Short-Term 1800 MHz Radiofrequency Radiation. J Environ Sci Health A Tox Hazard Subst Environ Eng. 2018 Jan 28;53(2):132-138 https://www.ncbi.nlm.nih.gov/pubmed/29148897

334. Moustafa YM, Moustafa RM, Belacy A, Abou-el-ela SH, Ali FM. Effects of acute exposure to the radiofrequency fields of cellular phones on plasma lipid peroxide and antioxidase activities in human erythrocytes. J Pharm Biomed Anal. 2001;26(4):605-8. https://www.ncbi.nlm.nih.gov/pubmed/11516912

335. The University of Melbourne. "The Truth About Mobile Phone and Wireless Radiation" – Dr. Devra Davis. YouTube, 2, Dec. 2015. https://youtu.be/bwydchf5Icy

336. Perez, Sarah. "U.S. Consumers Now Spend 5 Hours per Day on Mobile Devices." Techcrunch.com

337. Alster, Norm. Captured agency: How the Federal Communications Commission is dominated by the industries it presumably regulates. Cambridge, MA: Edmund J. Safra Center for Ethics, Harvard University. 2015. https://www.saferemr.com

338. Reuters. "AT&T Plans 5G Network Trial for DirecTV Customers." 4, Jan 2017. http://fortune.com/2017/01/04/att-5g-directv/

339. Burrell, Lloyd. "5G Radiation Dangers - 11 Reasons to Be Concerned" 12. May 2017. https://www.electricsense.com/12399/5g-radiation-dangers/

340. safespaceprotection.com

341. https://smartmeterguard.com/pages/faq

342. "Dirty Electricity," Green Wave. Retrieved on 11/22/2019 https://greenwavefilters.com/dirty-electricity/

CHAPTER 12

343. Body by God: The Owner's Manual for Maximized Living, Ben Lerner, Thomas Nelson 2007. Print.

344. Tony Robbins

345. Merriam-Webster Dictionary Online, definition of stress https://www.merriam-webster.com

346. Merriam-Webster Dictionary Online, definition of eustress https: www.merriam-webster.com

347. Merriam-Webster Dictionary Online, definition of distress, https: www.merriam-webster.com

348. TIME, "The Science of Stress: Manage It. Avoid It. Put It to Use." 2019 Meredith Corporation.

349. Harvard Health Publishing, "Understanding the Stress Response." 2011, MARCH. https://www.health.harvard.edu

350. McKeown, Patrick, "The Oxygen Advantage." HarperCollins, 2015.

351. Healthline, "Emotional Signs of Too Much Stress." Retrieved on 9/18/2019. https://www.healthline.com

352. Hamilton, Lisa Dawn, and Cindy M Meston. "Chronic stress and sexual function in women." The journal of sexual medicine vol. 10,10 (2013): 2443-54. doi:10.1111/jsm.12249

353. Giles, Grace E et al. "Stress effects on mood, HPA axis, and autonomic response: comparison of three psychosocial stress paradigms." PloS one vol. 9,12 e113618. 12 Dec. 2014, doi: 10.1371/journal.ponedoi: 10.1371/journal.pone.0113618

354. Gesch, Bernard. "Adolescence: Does good nutrition = good behaviour?" Nutrition and health vol. 22,1 (2013): 55-65. doi:10.1177/0260106013519552

355. Sheahan, William T et al. "Testosterone Replacement Therapy: Playing Catch-up with Patients." Federal practitioner: for the health care professionals of the VA, DoD, and PHS vol. 32,6 (2015): 26-31.

356. Power Thoughts Meditation Club, "Info on 432Hz Music." https://www.powerthoughtsmeditationclub.com

357. Leeds, Marty, "The Numerology of the Holy Name of Jesus." 2013, FEB. 13th https://blog.world-mysteries.com/uncategorized/the-numerology-of-the-holy-name-of-jesus-christ/

358. Insight Timer (Website) "Positive Affirmation Meditation: Empower Yourself." https://www.insighttimer.com

359. Mercola, Joseph "How LED Lighting May Compromise Your Health." 2016, OCT 23rd, https://www.articles.mercola.com

360. Stevenson, Shawn. "Sleep Smarter." Model House Publishing, 2014. Print

361. Wooten Virgil, "How to Fall Asleep." Howstuffworks.com https://health.howstuffworks.com/mental-health/sleep/basics/how-to-fall-asleep2.htm

362. Fox, Maggie, "One in 6 Americans Take Antidepressants, Other Psychiatric Drugs: Study." 2016, DEC. 12th. https://www-nbcnews.com

363. Harvard Medical School, "What are the Real Risks of Antidepressants." 2014, MARCH. https://www.health.harvard.edu

364. Jacobs, Sam, "Prescription for Violence: The Corresponding Rise of Antidepressants, SSRIs & Mass Shootings." 2019, MAY 20th https://www.libertarianinstitute.org

365. Citizens Commission on Human Rights of Colorado, "The Real Lesson of Columbine: Psychiatric Drugs Induce Violence." https://www.psychiatricfraud.org

366. Third Eye Blind, "Semi-Charmed Life." Songwriter, Stephan Jenkins. https://www.lyricfind.com

367. NBC News, Better, (Website) "What the Beach Does to Your Brain." https://nbc.com/better/health

368. Color Wheel Pro, (Website) "Color Meaning." https://www.color-wheel-pro.com

369. McCabe, Ed, "Flood Your Body with Oxygen." Ed McCabe, 2003. – 6th edition.

370. Muhammad Ahmad Ali, "Nick Vujicic's Success Story." https://www.awakenthegreatnesswithin.com

371. TED Talks, "Overcoming Hopelessness | Nick Vujicic | TEDxNoviSad." YouTube, Oct. 17, 2012. Web Oct. 2, 2019.

372. Joy Christians, "Nick Vujicic's Testimony, Christian Testimonies." 2018, JUNE 4th, https://www.joychristians.com

373. Hyat, Kamila, "Hunza an Oasis of Peace and Order in Crime – Infested State." 2010, APRIL 24th, https://gulfnews.com

374. Sandoiu, Ana, "Religious Belief May Extend Life By 4 Years." 2018, JUNE 18th, https://www.medicalnewstoday.com/articles/322175.php

375. Dr. Lisa Dunne, Multigenerational Marketplace, print.

376. The Journal of Popular Culture, Vol. 38, No. 2, 2004r 2004
Blackwell Publishing, 350 Main Street, Malden, MA 02148, USA,
and PO Box 1354, 9600 Garsington Road, Oxford OX4 2DQ, UK

CHAPTER 13

377. Definition of purpose, https://www.dictionary.com

378. Tony Robbin's quote, "Life Deserves for More of You to Show
Up." Unknown Origin

379. https//www.warrioronfire.com

380. Habits for Wellbeing, "6 Core Human Needs by Anthony
Robbins." https://www.habitsforwellbeing.com

381. Google, Zig Ziglar quotes

382. Wikiquote, Patch Adams, https://www.en.m.wikiquote.org

383. Psalms 139:13-14, https://www.biblehub.com

Index

Cholesterol 122, 123, 126, 130, 131, 132, 149, 199, 204, 228, 321

Chromium 93, 94, 208

Concentric 183, 184

Conscious 41, 42, 141, 169, 276, 341, 389

CoQ10 131

Cortisol 82, 130, 132, 168, 264, 265, 267, 268, 269, 307, 316, 416, 417

CSF 58, 59, 261

D

DDT 94, 136, 212, 213, 214, 407

Degeneration 64, 68, 197, 213, 321

Dehydration 79, 80, 81, 83, 87, 88, 99, 141, 187, 189, 392

Dental 90, 92, 255, 394

Depression 37, 39, 40, 48, 50, 51, 119, 163, 310, 313, 315, 327, 331, 390

Detox 136, 150, 151, 156, 196, 197, 198, 199, 200, 201, 203, 204, 205, 211, 257, 261, 406, 407

Diabetes 10, 13, 24, 25, 114, 118, 124, 149, 168, 183, 190, 203, 255, 265, 393, 397, 402, 405

Diet 3, 11, 25, 28, 83, 85, 99, 105, 108, 109, 110, 115, 116, 117, 118, 119, 120, 122, 123, 129, 130, 131, 134, 135, 136, 137, 139, 143, 147, 148, 149, 150, 164, 178, 210, 217, 235, 266, 316, 384, 398, 400, 404, 406

Dioxins 94, 211, 214, 217, 224

Discs 38, 60, 64

Disease viii, xi, 10, 13, 16, 23, 24, 25, 26, 31, 33, 36, 40, 47, 62, 64, 68, 85, 104, 106, 114, 119, 120, 122, 123, 124, 125, 130, 131, 148, 150, 156, 162, 179, 195, 196, 197, 203, 208, 209, 210, 212, 213, 215, 217, 222, 227, 232, 233, 234, 235, 236, 237, 238, 239, 243, 247, 254, 255, 265, 285, 304, 305, 310,

Minerals 83, 94, 95, 96, 97, 105, 129, 130, 137, 142, 148, 201, 202, 364

Mitochondria 88, 97, 115, 166, 321

Molecule 148, 166

Monoculture 105

Monsanto 94, 119, 214, 215, 216, 407, 408

Movie 36, 43, 44, 93, 215, 216, 256, 313, 340, 346

N

Nature xiv, 18, 52, 83, 96, 105, 122, 148, 234, 248, 256, 279, 317, 374, 405

Neck 60, 62, 65, 66, 67, 68, 69, 70, 71, 72, 74, 169, 185, 256, 276, 292, 322, 328

Nerve system 3, 28, 57, 58, 59, 60, 61, 62, 64, 69, 72, 73, 74, 81, 142, 151, 171, 174, 202, 244, 265, 267, 272, 276, 285, 305, 306

Niacin xv, 197, 199 , 200, 203, 257, 355, 359, 361, 384, 399, 406

Nitric Oxide 172, 173, 403

Nutrition vii, 3, 16, 28, 103, 104, 125, 138, 143, 165, 187, 210, 235, 316, 393, 399, 401, 422

O

Occiput 60, 61

Omega 87, 122, 127, 128, 129, 130, 138, 142, 399

Omnivore 108

Organic 13, 92, 103, 109, 110, 113, 121, 130, 136, 138, 139, 142, 153, 154, 157, 201, 202, 205, 207, 216, 219, 220, 221, 222, 223, 297, 361, 364, 365, 396, 397, 408, 409

Orgone 297

Osteoporosis 112, 183

Oxidation Reduction Potential 98

Oxidative Stress 88, 97, 211, 267, 286, 321, 420

www.ingramcontent.com/pod-product-compliance
Lightning Source LLC
Chambersburg PA
CBHW080555030426
42336CB00019B/3198